Cultural Studies
Interdisciplinarity
and Translation

Critical Studies

Vol. 20

General Editor
Myriam Díaz-Diocaretz

Assistant Editor
Esther von der Osten-Sacken

Rodopi

Amsterdam - New York, NY 2002

Cultural Studies Interdisciplinarity and Translation

Edited by

Stefan Herbrechter

The paper on which this book is printed meets the requirements of "ISO 9706:1994, Information and documentation - Paper for documents - Requirements for permanence".

ISBN: 90-420-0893-8 (bound)

Printed in The Netherlands

To my colleagues at Trinity and All Saints who helped and encouraged me with this project, especially Derek McKiernan and Amy Kenyon.

CONTENTS

INTRODUCTION: CULTURAL STUDIES – INTERDISCIPLINARITY AND TRANSLATION

STEFAN HERBRECHTER

The history of cultural studies is a contested issue. The extreme self-reflexivity which has always been characteristic of cultural studies – whether understood as a specific methodology, a particular set of questions, an (anti- or interdisciplinary) discipline (or 'interdiscipline'), as a specific (academic or non-academic) analytical practice, or simply as a subject area of studies – prevents the establishment of traditional forms of (disciplinary) consensus. It is in fact this 'foundation' on productive dissensus that has made the rise of cultural studies such an impressive success story. The challenge – the future of cultural studies – will be to find a working compromise between tendencies of increasing self-centeredness, a detachment of theory from practice and the development of a specialised vocabulary (jargon), on the one hand; and the demand for disciplinarity (teachability, marketability, quality assessment, and all the requirements connected with the ongoing process of cultural studies' institutionalisation within higher and possibly even secondary education), on the other.

The practitioners of cultural studies – including the contributors to this volume – are drawing their strength from crossing, even ignoring, disciplinary boundaries and combining methodologies, without really being too concerned with the question of what 'properly' constitutes the 'baggy monster' called 'cultural studies'. They either deliberately transgress boundaries and disown what is 'proper' (to) cultural studies, or problematise the notions of 'propriety' and 'belonging' as such (see for example Bowman and O'Sullivan). While the question: 'What is cultural studies?' – a question which has been asked all too often – might not reveal too many 'useful' answers, the discussion of interdisciplinarity promises to be more productive. In fact, it is the main concept – together with translation – that allows people working in and with cultural studies to think through issues like the relation between theory and practice. This is a concern which is voiced throughout the essays in this volume – sometimes in more theoretical discussions about the project of cultural studies (see Section A); sometimes in relation to cultural studies as an educational enterprise; sometimes in the form of a critique and a redirecting of cultural studies as a reading practice; or, indeed, all of these together. The strength of the essays in the first part of this volume – which from one angle may appear quite eclectic – is that they all already constitute practical (or one might say 'performative') interdisciplinarity while remaining self-aware of the 'praxical' problematic. What they combine are theory, critical practice and praxis.

From the start cultural studies as a more or less openly political movement was inspired by a desire for inter-, trans-, anti- and sometimes post-disciplinarity (see Grossberg, Nelson and Treichler 1992: 1ff). The fact of its institutionalisation within the academy – especially in the English-speaking countries, but also increasingly outside (which raises all sorts of issues related to its translation, some of which are addressed in Sections C, D, E and the Afterword) – poses the question of its inter- and antidisciplinarity anew. The problem is often that of the discrepancy between the current 'sexiness' of interdisciplinary programmes and a *de facto* lack of funding and expertise in institutions. For marketing purposes, cultural studies very often is represented as *the* interdisciplinary field, or even as being founded on interdisciplinarity, or as interdisciplinarity *itself*. But if cultural studies claims interdisciplinarity as its *own*, while in practice it continues to be hostile to disciplinary boundaries as such, it seems quite inevitable that its situation within the academy will remain precarious and its relation to the traditional disciplines rather superficial. The resulting 'lack' of identity might also explain why cultural studies has been so obsessed with problems of identity and its construction(s) – a theme that, in the present volume, quite deliberately, plays a less prominent part.

The prefix 'inter-' (e.g. in interdisciplinarity) is, of course, polysemous. Its meaning is not fixed, which is precisely, what makes a conceptual discussion possible and necessary. The contributions reveal the great variety of meanings the word 'interdisciplinarity' can acquire. 'Inter-' is one of many possible notions signifying 'inbetweenness'. These fuzzy, deconstructive conceptual areas carry the potential for change (for better or for worse), affirmation, consolidation, but also destruction, dissolution, dissemination, etc.; but 'inbetweenness' cannot be prescribed, captured, declared. It 'happens' – which is why it seems extremely difficult, if not undesirable, to develop a didactic, prescriptive methodology for cultural studies that is founded on interdisciplinarity. Interdisciplinarity rather seems to *ex-sist*, in scholarly events and projects of radical singularity, as the result of something radically different each and every time. The kind of phenomena cultural studies sets out to describe and analyse usually demand specific adaptation rather than prefabricated conceptual frameworks. This is also due to the 'anti-disciplinary' objects of study and 'non-disciplinary' practices to which cultural studies applies itself: texts, images, discourses, phenomena, the notion of culture and its production. What unites – without agreement – the contributions in this volume is a certain interdisciplinary eventfulness. Interdisciplinarity and cultural studies 'happen' in these pages.

Acknowledging the problematic nature of the 'inter-' seems to be the only way of respecting the political project of cultural studies and its undeniable past achievements, safeguarding its radicality and its dynamic involvement in the politics of cultural change. The essays therefore also aim to regenerate the discussion on interdisciplinarity as the motor of the cultural studies project. What seems political about cultural studies, which loses, finds and reinvents itself through interdisciplinary transgressive acts, differently every time, is this singularity of the transfer (or translation – between disciplines, but also between languages, cultures, methodologies, mentalities) and the possibility and the specificity of a dialogic knowledge this process may encourage. What is political is the difference that is also the driving force for any act of translation and transgression, and for 'dissent' (see Nelson and Gaonkar 1996). Interdisciplinarity is therefore always connected with a certain economy of desire and anxiety (see Coles and Defert 1998), an economy which reveals itself within the history of its concept (Klein 1990). It is these anxieties and desires of interdisciplinarity which constitute not only the common thread of the essays to follow, but they also are what demands the continual self-questioning and thus the (im)possible identity of cultural studies.

As Andrew Carlin in his contribution points out, it is the 'editor's work' to provide coherence to an essay collection. The price for this identity work is that it is achieved *via* the (implicit or explicit) appeal to (disciplinary) boundaries. What this volume does is, of course, to legitimate 'performatively' (i.e. by speaking about it) *and* to (re)create/rewrite cultural studies as a discipline, merely by providing a framework. So in creating coherence where there may be none, a selection process is already underway – e.g. 'good' interdisciplinarity *versus* 'bad' interdisciplinarity. While this process seems inevitable it is also culturally, historically and contextually specific. It is not only the editor who merely constructs or 'invents' the coherence but also the context. It is for example no coincidence that certain themes recur in several contributions. There is frequent reference to Bill Readings' *The University in Ruins* (1996). It seems that the anxiety about 'the university of excellence' and the role attributed to cultural studies by Readings seems to have caught on (see e.g. Maton, Bowman, and Quinn). There is a certain (however critical) hope for cultural studies and its interdisciplinary character to play a major role in the change towards a 'postmodern' and 'postdisciplinary' university.

The other event that has inscribed itself into several contributions is the 'Sokal affair'. Cultural studies, of course, could not remain indifferent towards the accusations Alan Sokal (and Jean Bricmont) put forward in their *Intellectual Impostures* (1997; see Quinn below). From a certain perspective the Sokal hoax may be seen as an attack not only on institutionalised programmes of cultural studies, on cultural studies as an intellectual enterprise, as a field of knowledge, a discourse, but also on the practice and the idea of interdisciplinary work as such. It remains to be seen whether any productive discussion can be generated from this latest of a long series of 'wars' (Culture Wars, Science Wars, etc.) or contests between faculties (Derrida 1992), or between human, social, natural etc. sciences.

Section A ('Redirections') groups essays by scholars from a variety of backgrounds who start their analysis of cultural studies and interdisciplinarity from a theoretical point of view and then go on to argue for changes in cultural studies' practices. Michael Hayes argues for a "marriage between Saussure's structuralism and Bakhtin's dialogics". While structuralism can be said to reveal the relative positioning of all the cultural events that go to make a culture, dialogics analyses the dynamic human processes that inform the cultural scheme of things. Hayes believes that, in this way, cultural studies becomes the systematic regulated search for, rather than assertion of, the myriad preconceptions that inform, maintain and evolve our cultural life.

Karl Maton's analysis of the 'current state of cultural studies' focuses on the contradictory nature of an 'antidisciplinary discipline' that has been institutionalised 'against itself'. Vibrant and in disarray, the two faces of cultural studies are intermingled in accounts. Maton asks how cultural studies has come to be in such a curious position and why, and whether there is something intrinsic to cultural studies, something internal to the way it is structured as a knowledge formation, which enables its strange position in higher education. While the central theme of legitimation in cultural studies is non-disciplinarity, the emphasis lies on people rather than procedures to guarantee its identity. What Maton's analysis shows is that: "any account of cultural studies – past, present or future – needs to address not only issues of agency or social structure but also the internal features of cultural studies as a knowledge formation".

Paul Bowman's contribution provides a rereading of some central Derridean texts to elaborate on the question of the 'proper' of cultural studies. He is interested in the avoidance of the question of cultural studies' identity. He argues that:

> all disciplines impose enabling limits; that is, a set of conditions within which one can work, in a well policed, 'legitimate', 'correct', or 'proper', way. To transgress, ignore or refute these conditions is to question the validity of everything done within and in the name of that discipline. It is to move 'outside' of that space, to call it into question, and also to incur the wrath of its judgement, a judgement that will inevitably come from a position that agrees with the premises, hypotheses, and proper procedures, that have been transgressed.

This 'wrath' that cultural studies continues to attract seems endemic to interdisciplinarity itself. The inevitable paradox (or aporia) of interdisciplinarity, following Derrida, is thus that:

> *On the one hand*, the claim of interdisciplinarity signals an eminently pure academic activity, consisting, as it would seem, of a redoubling of academic effort, in order to *master* more than one discipline, to be hyper-academic, to *be* more and *do* more than 'single' disciplines themselves. But, *on the other hand*, the 'interdiscipline' will be less, or at least other than, *improper in terms of*, each discipline it travels between.

The 'interdiscipline', according to Bowman, therefore, cannot help but both reassure and upset the academy. It at once promises to add a new dimension in its overall aim of omniscience; yet it threatens to rattle the order of things, to reorder and potentially disorder; it is both promise and threat. A (properly?) deconstructive move therefore consist in focusing on the risks of the opening towards, and the resulting strategies of containment, of interdisciplinarity.

Malcolm Quinn's essay starts off from a reading of the Sokal affair as a sign of academia losing the form of its translation from 'academic' to 'nonacademic'. In a bold, almost Baudrillardian, move Quinn claims that the institutionalised versions of cultural studies are merely there to promote the double meaning that academic work is both itself and cultural, in order to retain a fantasy of distinction through a discourse on transgression. He asserts that:

> "Transgressing the Boundaries" was simply another reminder that the multivocal, multidisciplinary cultural debate that academia wants to see itself as engaging in with is a fiction, and that what seems to guarantee the 'conversation' is a mute, unreadable and meaningless object no longer attached to the 'enculturation' of disciplinary orthodoxy but instead solely to a process of modernisation which is ultimately driven by extra-academic forces; new objects discovered by constantly updated modes of production for new markets such as 'science studies', as exemplified in the 'Science Wars' edition of *Social Text* in which [Sokal's hoax] article appeared.

The quasi-disciplinary, quasi-intellectual project of institutionalised cultural studies may, thus, be one of the few remaining means of securing a difference between the University sector and the free market in knowledge goods, of retaining the connection between the institution and its historical devotion to ideals of knowledge for knowledge's sake.

Simon O'Sullivan follows a somewhat different trajectory. Equally critical of institutionalised forms of cultural studies, he turns towards Deleuze's and Guattari's work and calls for a 're-invention' of cultural studies as a project that does not rely on disciplinary notions of knowledge; instead he understands: "cultural studies as an affirmative and strategic mapping of the possibilities of life". For O'Sullivan the project of cultural studies as 'rhizomatics' might provide an access to the (virtual) potentialities of culture, a pragmatics that would go beyond traditional disciplinary analysis and instead would take into account the work of (cultural) imagination.

Necdet Teymur's essay is a witty and original deliberation on the first of a series of non- or anti-disciplinary concepts that have migrated across disciplines and have also traversed cultural studies: space. To be more precise, the space of the 'inbetween', e.g. of interdisciplinarity. With its focus on cultural studies' 'anti-disciplinary objects' (see Mowitt 1992) and practices, the contributions in Section B deal with 'conceptual' objects/practices like space, music, art, bibliography, and the ways in which they have been appropriated or translated by traditional disciplines but also by cultural studies. The questions these essays ask are whether cultural studies' interdisciplinary or anti-disciplinary practices allow for a different form of appropriation, one that could do more justice to the complexity of these objects/practices.

Teymur, for example, argues that all practices, arts, institutions and disciplines have some concern with space. Space is not entirely culturally specific but to a large extent intercultural. His ambition is to demonstrate the "incredible combination of the mysterious undefinability of space on the one hand, and its concrete materiality on the other".

Andrew Carlin, in his essay, focuses upon bibliographies *as* disciplinary boundaries. He understands textual artefacts (bibliographies, footnotes, textbooks) as loci of disciplinary boundaries and, therefore, of interdisciplinary bases. Bibliographies, in this context, are "texts in which are embodied the interpretive practices whereby [scholars] realise their disciplinary boundaries". Bibliographies are 'sites of interdisciplinarity' and, as such "they define a field of study". Although Carlin's case study focuses on sociology textbooks, he is, of course, right in claiming that:

> Whether Cultural Studies constitutes the attempt to reinvent wheels, or invent different kinds of wheels with different kinds of spokes, its bibliographic bases and boundaries are not exempt from scrutiny in terms of disciplinary provenance and the history of ideas.

In conclusion, Carlin reiterates one of the most fundamental points to remember for 'good' interdisciplinary practice: the realisation of cognate forms of inquiry. When doing interdisciplinary work, Carlin argues, we must avoid the creation of "category-mistakes", which result from analysts making moves between incompatible "language games". The translation of concepts within and between disciplines, should not undermine their logical coherence. Thus, appreciating the endogenous 'rules' of disciplines is crucial to the realisation of any meaningful programme of interdisciplinarity.

Duncan Campbell focuses on the ways in which music (and popular music in particular) has been appropriated as an object of study and submitted to, and changed by, traditional ways of reading. His key target in this context is inscription which "as an operator opens the way to reconceptualization of the relationship between the sensible and the intelligible, between the two senses of sense, that is, as the meaning of the body and the body of meaning." The result is that despite the vast proliferation of readings of popular music that treat it seriously, either as another branch of cultural studies or as a discipline in its own right, the gesture of phonographic inscription, with which Campbell is concerned, is still reduced, placed as secondary to other disciplines which determine its form and function:

> Popular music is thought of as a sociological phenomenon, a debased classical music, a literary-critical narrative (personal, political, and so on), always determined from the outside by a *disciplinarity* that pays no attention to the status of the musical

> inscription; the multiple disciplinary codes of reading popular music – whether they are sociological, musicological, poetical, phenomenological, psychological, political – mirror the classical subordination of aesthetics to logic (or, in a more general sense, to philosophy). The sensuous particularity of music disappears in the face of external determination.

Instead, it should be recognised that popular music is neither simply a debased form of high culture, nor a pacifier produced by the military-industrial-entertainment complex; neither, though, is it necessarily a source of anti-hegemonic resistance as some cultural studies readings seem to suggest.

In a similar vein, Jen Webb's article criticises the fact that cultural studies' interest in art seems to lie not so much in considering its part in 'the existence of the world' but in problematising art and, at least implicitly, questioning its 'right to exist'. It thus seems that, ironically, cultural studies tends not to take into account the identity of art objects and artists *qua* art, or as aesthetic experience, thus denying its own roots in aesthetics; she claims that:

> In short, while cultural studies writings contribute many valuable and interesting perspectives on the field, they typically fail to address what for me is the central point about art: that it is committed to the production of works which 'demand to be experienced aesthetically'.

But, as Webb argues, if we ignore aesthetics, or engage with it only critically, we risk alienating and rejecting the private and the affective spheres in favour of the public and the rational. The potentially liberating perspectives that aesthetic questions offer – investigating the 'outside' of reason, the sensual, visual etc. – should be at the centre of cultural studies' interests.

Webb's contribution is a good conclusion to Part I because it also provides a very neat summary of the gains and losses in interdisciplinary work. It can thus also serve as a kind of reflection on interdisciplinarity in general and as discussed in the previous essays. It is worth quoting Webb's essay at length here:

> Interdisciplinarity… has a number of practical benefits in the research community: working and publishing across disciplines means we have to write for extra-peer audiences, and hence minimise that opacity of style which is a feature of much aesthetic/philosophical and cultural studies writing in the interests of achieving a greater transparency and accessibility. Further, interdisciplinarity in the academy parallels contemporary practice in the workplace and professions, where it's no longer sufficient (in many cases) to have expertise, however sophisticated, in just one area. Developing an interdisciplinary approach makes it easier to structure courses which will train students for the sorts of environments in which they will be working. And there are other advantages; working across the disciplines offers a point of entry to the liminal which in turn provides access to synergetic energies and transgressive possibilities, and demonstrates the permeability of the arbitrary boundaries of conventional disciplines. Working across disciplines can also be a way of breaking down particularised interest, and hence extending knowledge and thought in a field.

Of course, interdisciplinarity can also be viewed in more negative terms, as Webb continues: "with the increasing fragmentation of knowledge that is a result of this perspective and structure come the loss of coherent research or knowledge communities and, potentially, of specialised knowledge".

Altogether, however, I think it is no exaggeration to say that the gains of working 'at the intersections of disciplines and professions' by far outweigh the (institutional, personal, etc.) costs.

It is the claim of this volume that interdisciplinarity and translation constitute the two main challenges for cultural studies at present. Each of these conceptual issues is related to specific historical and cultural contexts. Interdisciplinarity is interlinked with the ongoing process of institutionalisation of cultural studies within the academy – mainly in the English-speaking world, but also, increasingly, as a result of its exportation elsewhere, outside it, internationally and even globally. The second half of this volume deals specifically with the issues that arise out of this translation of cultural studies.

Cultural studies translates and cultural studies is (being) translated; this is what the phrase 'the translation *of* cultural studies' in both its subjective and objective aspects, implies. There is a normative-political, an ethical and a historical-geographical dimension to this phrase. Some urgent questions that arise out of this problematic are: what should cultural studies translate? Or is there, apart from a politics of translation (i.e. translation as strategic appropriation), an ethics of translation (e.g. what demands translation?)? What has cultural studies been translating (which involves a critique of cultural studies' translation choices and practices; a historical and geographical analysis of cultural studies as both the product and the producer of translations)? Which processes of translation are responsible for cultural studies (for its history, its evolution and institutionalisation and, maybe, today, for its dissemination)? It would be important to write the history of cultural studies as an interdisciplinary movement with its own 'teleology' of academic institutionalization. However, at a time when cultural studies is being exported as a model into a variety of academic contexts worldwide (a process which shadows but maybe also constitutes a certain 'global(ized) culture'; see Bauman's "Postscript") it would be even more necessary to write a geography of cultural studies, tracing its origins (which, of course, already lie in translation) and mapping its trajectories, its effects.

Cultural theory in general, throughout the Twentieth Century, has become increasingly aware of a certain paradox of translation. More recently, it was deconstruction, in particular, which has been engaging with and even, in a sense, defined itself according to a certain 'aporetic' understanding of translation (Derrida 1985; see also Gentzler 1993; and Niranjana 1992). The emphasis has been on the 'supplementarity' of translation (the necessity for translation and its denial), on the politics of translation (translation as a cultural strategy of dissemination and appropriation); and on the '(in)visibility' of the translator or mediator (Venuti 1992, 1995, and 1998). The complex relation between translation or mediation and the construction and protection of identity can be traced on levels as various as the individual, cultural, social, national, etc. Neither the history of the modern university and its disciplines, nor that of transnational movements like Marxism, structuralism, postmodernism, nor, as argued in this volume, that of cultural studies, can be thought without the disseminative structure of translation processes that, although strategic and appropriative, never leave the translator, or the translated unchanged.

The history of cultural studies – as a movement, an institution, a discourse etc. – cannot be thought without considering the transfer of ideas, i.e. without a set of concepts starting with 'trans-': transnationalism, transdisciplinarity, translation. One reason why cultural studies suffers from but also continues to indulge in the sometimes obsessive problematisation of identity, orthodoxy and canonicity, is that its origins lie in translation, or in the 'inbetween'. The founding gestures of the cultural studies movement in Britain, in the 1960s (and even before), already lay in the 'inbetween': between (institutional) politics and adult education (see Steele 1997), between the academic and the non-academic, between disciplines, subject areas and centres, etc.). The development of cultural studies, first in Britain, later in America and the rest of the English-speaking world, would have to remain inexplicable were it not for certain strategic translations: e.g. of a certain adaptation of continental Marxism, of the structuralists (Lévi-Strauss, Barthes, Lacan, Althusser), of so-called 'postmodernists' (Lyotard, Derrida, Baudrillard), of 'German' philosophy (from Nietzsche and Heidegger to Adorno and The Frankfurt School) – already in their translation, or translation of a translation (see for example the 'French' Nietzsches and Heideggers, but also Kojève's Hegel and Kant, who have fulfilled their own specific purposes in the French context). On closer inspection, it would be impossible to find a single modern discipline whose development did not rely on some kind of translation (linguistic, cultural, disciplinary, etc.) as the norm rather than the exception.

In addition to this, cultural studies seems to be having more than its fair share of mediators and translators. A large number of cultural studies practitioners are themselves hybrids – they would find it very difficult to commit themselves to one discipline, one nation, one language, one culture, etc. This is also true for the present volume, which is full of these curious 'go-betweens'. This is certainly a sign of the internationalism of cultural studies, its foundation in translation. However, this situation is not without dangers.

What is particularly interesting – in a time when (international) cultural studies' main interest is shifting towards the global (global culture, or the globalisation of culture) – is cultural studies' own implication in effects of cultural imperialism, hegemony and political economy. This becomes particularly evident when one asks the question: what language does cultural studies speak? Here, institutionalisation plays a major role. Since the process of institutionalisation is far more advanced in the English-speaking world, and given the rise of 'Global English' in general, cultural studies enters the academy, and also national popular cultures in strange ways. Cultural studies often remains uncritically associated with Anglo-American (global) cultural hegemony through its very Anglo-centric perspective on hegemony and processes of globalisation. Speaking about culture in the way cultural studies does is – despite its origins in translation – perceived and translated in a culturally specific way. It would be ironic for cultural studies to forget its own implication in processes of translation (subjective and objective).

For example, in most European countries cultural studies is translated and practised in English departments under the name 'British (Cultural) Studies' or 'American Studies' – the perspective is that of cultural studies as 'the kind of thing they do in the British or the US academy'. This takes away the national-hegemonic aggressiveness that often remains unreflected in even the most circumspect of cultural theorists, writing, teaching and thinking in the Anglo-American context. The hyphen in Anglo-American, here, of course silences a whole area of misperception in and of Britain, Australia, New Zealand, Canada, etc. who are dealing with their own Anglo-English problematics of translation and their own specific threats of globalisation and 'Americanisation'.

The essays in the second half of this volume, more or less explicitly, express this unease and this awareness of cultural studies' growing internationalisation. More or less openly they ask: can cultural studies become truly transnational, or is there – in the very process of its dissemination and implantation within institutional contexts – an unthought or unthinkable nationalism it cannot, of its own, address? A horizon of a national culture, an Anglocentrism which affects even the most critical analyses of the global? I take this to be the underlying and unexpressed question that echoes in Zygmunt Bauman's afterword.

It remains to be seen how cultural studies will deal with its others – other disciplines, cultures, languages – that it keeps invoking, mostly quite egoistically, in order to keep its translation processes at work. The essays in this volume set out to revisit some highly controversial questions within and around cultural studies: questions about cultural studies' legitimation as an academic discipline; its identity as 'non-discipline' and interdisciplinary practices; and its role in the various translation processes that constitute its dynamics, its success and also its international expansion.

The contributors to this volume are from a great variety of disciplinary and national backgrounds. Many also are submitting their ideas to translation, i.e. they have adopted a language which is not their 'own'. One could even follow Derrida and describe cultural studies' current situation as that of an 'unhappy' monolingual: '[cultural studies] speaks only one language, yet, it is not [its] own' (Derrida 1996). What the contributors have in common is the desire to resist simplistic definitions of culture and unproblematic translations of cultural studies. What they share is a certain anxiety about the process of institutionalisation and internationalisation in which they themselves are taking part, but also a confidence that good interdisciplinary and transnational practice is more in demand than ever. They agree that cultural studies at its best produces self-reflexive and critical interdisciplinary work and translations which constitute a genuine contribution to the production of knowledge and create advances in the development of methodologies that benefit more than one discipline, more than one culture, more than one language. As a result, cultural studies must accept anew that the price for this 'more than' is a 'no longer one' (i.e. Derrida's aporia of the *plus d'un*; see e.g. Derrida 1996).

What separates these contributions from each other are questions of focus, priority and location. It seems quite clear that there cannot, and indeed should not, be a consensus about the political agenda and the future of cultural studies. It is precisely these differences that constitute cultural studies' success and dynamism. The best way of understanding the elusive identity of cultural studies (its (self)questionings, its methodologies, its practices) seems to be through the notion of translation. Cultural studies would be unthinkable without the ongoing strategic translation of texts, concepts and intellectual currents from and into different cultural, linguistic, disciplinary and institutional contexts. The volume unites practitioners of cultural studies from very diverse cultural and institutional backgrounds who all have submitted their specific cultural experiences and identities to questions they have come to associate with cultural studies. It is therefore fascinating to compare the various adaptations cultural studies undergoes in these essays and the ways in which they perform translations of cultural studies.

These processes of translation – cultural studies as a product of both importation and exportation – today co-occur with fundamental changes in the ways in which economic, social, juridical and political aspects of culture are structured. Cultural studies cannot remain indifferent to these changes – rightly or wrongly referred to as globalisation and 'global(ized) culture'. Indeed, it is probably the most urgent question for cultural studies to determine its own implication within such processes of cultural translation, hybridisation and globalisation that could constitute forms of intellectual and cultural hegemony.

The question of inevitable exclusion and repression that takes place in the process of forming an identity is something that comes back to haunt cultural studies today, during its process of institutionalisation. But this process of establishing itself as an academic discipline in its own right is not taking place in an academic, social and cultural void. It is co-occurring with 'global(ized) cultural', political and economic developments. In his "Postscript", Zygmunt Bauman differentiates between 'global culture(s)' and the 'globalisation of (a) culture'. Today, it seems to be cultural studies' task – given its reliance on acts of (disciplinary, theoretical and cultural) translation – to ask itself what its alliance with the process of globalisation is. Will cultural studies be an agent of (a) global culture or will it attend to the singularity of cultural translations of globalized culture(s)? The role of translation – and of disciplinary and cultural transgression – can hardly be overestimated, as Bauman explained (in *Culture as Praxis*):

> Translation is an ongoing, unfinished and inconclusive *dialogue* which is bound to remain such. The meeting of two contingencies is itself a contingency, and no effort

> will ever stop it from being such. The act of translation is not a one-off event which will put paid to the need of further translating effort. The meeting ground, the frontierland, of cultures [and disciplines, *SH*] is the territory in which boundaries are constantly obsessively drawn only to be continually violated and re-drawn again and again – not the least for the fact that both partners emerge changed from every successive attempt at translation.
> Cross-cultural [and cross-disciplinary, *SH*] translation is a continuous process which *serves* as much as *constitutes* the cohabitation of people who can afford neither occupying the same space nor mapping that common space in their own, separate ways. No act of translation leaves either of the partners intact. Both emerge from their encounter changed, different at the end of the act from what they were at its beginning – and so with the translation left behind the moment it has been completed, in need of 'another go' – and that reciprocal change is the work of translation. (Bauman 1999: xlviii)

The question that cultural studies, as both the subject and the object of translation today (i.e. as a translator of ideas and as an academic discipline or a methodology translated into various national institutional contexts) has to address is to what extent (cultural and disciplinary) translation can be 'dialogic' (in Bauman's 'Bakhtinian' terms). The contributions to this volume should be seen as a first step towards answering this question.

In many ways, Russell West's 'critique of translation' is an ideal opening for Section C (The Translation of Cultural Studies – Translation Studies). As he claims, translation has been at the heart of some of the most momentous interdisciplinary innovations in the social sciences in the twentieth century. Lacan's 'translation' of Freud using the instruments of structuralist linguistics produced a novel theory of subjectivity; Lévi-Strauss, similarly wielding Saussurean linguistics, resulted in a translation of traditional ethnography; and Marx found himself translated by Althusser in a further application of the notion of 'structure'. West's idea that translation is an operation which establishes continuity across a space of discontinuity, making heterogeneity productive for intellectual pursuit, is particularly true for cultural studies with its 'translative' interdisciplinary operations. West follows Bhabha, who points out that translation is primarily "a process by which, in order to objectify cultural meaning, there always has to be a process of alienation and of secondariness in relation to itself. In that sense there is no 'in itself' and 'for itself' within cultures because they are always subject to intrinsic forms of translation" (Bhabha 1990: 209-210). West then goes on to confront Anglo-American cultural studies with a double translation – on the one hand its translation into the specific pedagogic context of teaching translation studies, and on the other, beyond its own national sphere into the European context. West concludes that, in accordance with Paul Gilroy, in *The Black Atlantic* (1993), "cultural studies has been dogged in its emergence as a radically critical interdisciplinary pursuit by its clinging to a national (English) paradigm". This maintenance of national boundaries as the defining framework for cultural studies constitutes a blind spot which elides the inherently syncretic and hybrid influences not only of British society but of cultural studies as well.

Cultural studies should not ignore that, in a postmodern era national cultures and cultural identities in general "increasingly constitute each other in processes of reciprocal if not symmetrical translation".

The practitioner of (international and intercultural) cultural studies therefore must rely on an awareness of identity-as-translation. Or as Rosi Braidotti, quoted by West, suggests about the polyglott, who "also knows intimately what de Saussure teaches explicitly: that the connection between linguistic signs is arbitrary. [...] Thus the polyglot becomes the prototype of the postmodernist speaking subject; struck by the maddening, fulminating insight about the arbitrariness of linguistic meanings and yet resisting the free fall into cynicism" (Braidotti 1994: 14). West goes on to demonstrate, through a close reading of Robert Dessaix's novel *Night Letters* (1996), the relevance of Appadurai's concept of "cultural studies conceived [as] the basis for a cosmopolitan (global? macro? translocal?) ethnography" (Appadurai 1996).

David Katan points out that cultural studies and translation studies have traditionally trodden separate paths, even though both have been fundamentally concerned with the processes of communication and meaning. To a large extent the former has viewed translation as a necessary but unimportant vehicle (and necessary only because many cultural studies scholars are 'foreign'), while those involved in translation have tended to assume that culture, and the study of it, has little to do with the art of translating a text. Katan sets out to address this problem by focusing on the addressee of the translation process: the reader, who, in interpreting a succession of words as coherent discourse (locutions or signifiers) will give the words meaning, and experience a certain effect, known in speech act theory as the perlocutionary effect. Katan's point is that the interpretation of the reader will, to a large extent, be determined by decisions made by the translator, both as critical reader and as (re)writer. Cultural studies and translation studies thus share a common interest in these 'perlocutionary effects' and their mediation.

The section on translation studies is completed by Eduardo Vior's (com)passionate analysis of the imperialist translation politics that has been taking place between 'the two Americas'. Vior's is a detailed historical analysis of international political relations and political economy, based on the translation of technical texts, mainly from American into (South-American) Spanish.

In Section D (Translating Cultural Studies) a series of essays looks at the processes of cultural studies' institutionalisation in various national contexts. Stephen Chan, starting from Bill Readings' analysis, in *The University in Ruins* (1996), provides an attempt at "translating the significance of (post)culture in pragmatic pedagogic terms through a 'strategic border re-alignment' of some institutional realities". In particular, he focuses on present Hong Kong as "a case of critical cultural studies". He does this by writing about his experience in creating a cultural studies programme for students in Hong Kong.

Sebastian Berg, and Lawrence Raw, in their contributions also focus on the nationally specific reception of cultural studies. While Berg looks at 'British

(Cultural) Studies' in Germany, Raw focuses on his experience in teaching and developing cultural studies in Turkey. In both cases, it becomes clear that the translation of cultural studies is closely associated with national cultural and institutional politics.

Mandy Oakham provides another, highly entertaining episode within the history of cultural studies' translations. Her perspective is that of the Australian academy where cultural studies (similar to Britain) has found entrance to departments of media and journalism. The inter and intra-institutional battles and their international and intercontinental dimensions are interwoven with images of the imperialism of other 'wars' – culture wars, science wars and *Star Wars*.

Finally, Karima Laachir returns the message of cultural studies to the national context from which many of its foundational texts were translated: postcolonial France. Laachir focuses on recent issues of racism and republicanism in the French context which sees itself threatened from all sides: in the face of global (in particular Anglo-centric) cultural imperialism France has been unwilling or unable to address, or work through its own colonial past and remains blind to its own cultural imperialist aftermath. Laachir argues for a careful translation of cultural studies into the specifically French republican context, i.e. for an opening up of republican ideals in terms of cultural studies. On the other hand, it may be argued that the predominantly Anglo-American critical discourse on race, ethnicity, identity and multiculturalism could benefit from other, e.g. European models, focusing on citizenship and integration (developed for example by thinkers like Habermas, Balibar, Taguieff, Wieviorka etc.).

Section E (Cultural Studies: Translation and Globalisation) contains an essay by Holger Rossow, who looks at the most recent stage of the dialogue between America and Europe in an age of rapid processes of globalisation and growing interconnectedness. Rossow argues for a longterm historical view in which recent fears of Americanisation should rather be seen as part of a longer process of Europeanisation. He reminds us that cultural studies – especially in its international translated form – should not overlook a close analysis of international politics and international relations.

In the "Postscript" to this volume Zygmunt Bauman summarises many of the questions raised in the essays and in this introduction within the problematic of the opposition between 'cultural variety' and 'cultural specificity'. These questions cannot only be objects of analysis for a culturally neutral cultural studies but also have to be applied to cultural studies itself, as a historically and culturally specific practice. Bauman concludes, despite claims to the contrary by many cultural studies theorists and practitioners, that "there is nothing remotely reminiscent of a 'global culture' in the sense of a cultural choice shared by the whole of the human species; neither is it certain that such world-wide 'cultural sameness', were it to become reality, would be necessarily a good thing". Global culture instead often means "the world-wide spread of various 'globalized localisms' like the 'basic English' of the internet addicts, car sellers and car park attendants, McDonald burgers, Coca-Cola bottles, Pizza parlours, explosive births and instant deaths of a Pokemon/Digimon craze, Princess Diana's mourning or American soap-operas and the Sydney Olympics beamed by television channels throughout the world". The question is, whether cultural studies – while working towards transnationalism and global culture has merely become one more globalized localism, spread thanks to what Bauman calls a certain 'globality of culture' (as opposed to a truly 'global culture') – namely "world-wide 'virtual travel' and world-wide display of locally born forms of life".

Cultural studies needs to look behind the current scene of this globality in order to critically analyse what its own role within that scene is or should be. Cultural studies would do good to follow Bauman's distinction between 'cultural variety' and a 'variety of cultures' (i.e. between cultural pluralism and the plurality of cultures). Highlighting issues of cultural specificity, relativism and universalism through processes of translation should be cultural studies' foremost aim, without forgetting, however, that as a mediator of processes of globalisation it may be implicated in the very logic it was hoping to unhinge.

Bibliography:

Appadurai, Arjun (1996) *Modernity at Large: Cultural Dimensions of Globalization,* Minneapolis: University of Minnesota Press.

Bauman, Zygmunt (1999) *Culture as Praxis*, 2nd edition, London: Sage.

Benjamin, Andrew (1989) *Translation and the Nature of Philosophy: a New Theory of Words*, London: Routledge.

Bhabha, Homi (1990) "The Third Space", Interview by Jonathan Rutherford, in Jonathan Rutherford, ed. (1990) *Identity: Community, Culture, Difference*, London: Lawrence and Wishart, 207-21.

Braidotti, Rosi (1994) *Nomadic Subjects: Embodiment and Sexual Difference in Contemporary Feminist Theory,* New York: Columbia University Press.

Coles, Alex; and Bentley, Richard, eds. (1996) *Interdisciplinarity: Art/ Architecture/Theory - de-, dis-, ex-,* Vol. I. (Excavating Modernism), London: Backless Books/Black Dog.

Coles, Alex; and Defert, Alexia (1998) *The Anxiety of Interdisciplinarity – de-, dis-, ex-,* Vol. II., London: Backless Books/Black Dog.

Derrida, Jacques (1996) *Monolingualism of the Other, Or, The Prosthesis of Origin*, trans. D. Wills, Stanford, Ca: Stanford University Press.

Derrida, Jacques (1992) "Mochlos, or, The Conflict of the Faculties", trans. R. Rand and A. Wygant, in: Rand, Richard, ed. *Logomachia*, Lincoln and London: University of Nebraska Press, 1-34.

Gilroy, Paul (1993) *The Black Atlantic,* London: Verso.

Grossberg, Larry; Nelson, Cary; and Treichler, Paula; eds. (1992) *Cultural Studies*, New York: Routledge.

Klein, Julie Thompson (1990) *Interdisciplinarity: History, Theory, and Practice*, Detroit: Wayne State University Press.

Morley, David; and Chen, Kuan-Hsing (1996) *Stuart Hall: Critical Dialogues in Cultural Studies*, London: Routledge.

Mowitt, John (1992) *Text: The Genealogy of an Antidisciplinary Object*, Durham and London: Duke University Press.

Nelson, Cary; and Gaonkar, Dilip Parameshwar, eds. (1996) *Disciplinarity and Dissent in Cultural Studies*, New York: Routledge.

Peters, Michael, ed. (1999) *After the Disciplines: The Emergence of Cultural Studies*, Westport and London: Bergin & Garvey.

Readings, Bill (1996) *The University in Ruins*, Cambridge, Ma: Harvard University Press.

Said, Edward W. (1991) *The World, the Text and the Critic*, London: Vintage.

Sokal, Alan; and Bricmont, Jean (1997) *Impostures intellectuelles*, Paris: Odile Jacob.

Spivak, Gayatri Chakravorty (1992) "The Politics of Translation", in: Barrett, Michele; and Phillips, Anne; eds. *Destabilizing Theory: Contemporary Feminist Debates*, Cambridge: Polity Press, 177-200.

Steele, Tom (1997) *The Emergence of Cultural Studies 1945-65*, London: Lawrence and Wishart.

Steiner, George (1992) *After Babel*, 2nd edition, Oxford: OUP.

Section A:

Cultural Studies and Interdisciplinarity – Redirections

CULTURAL STUDIES AT THE CROSSROADS

MICHAEL HAYES

As the need to take account of context has grown so the place of culture in the human sciences has become more insistent. In disciplines that study culture, such as anthropology, sociology and cultural studies, and as a result of the recent focus on inter-textuality, the nature of change versus purpose in human evolution has become more problematic. Saussure's contribution was to foreground relationships between elements, whether words or behaviour, as the key to their definition. Structuralism opened up the discussion, but ignored the capacity of human individuality and eccentricity to kill off or re-invent meaning by re-mapping structural relationships. This essay suggests that the 'discipline' of cultural studies might investigate the ground between stability and evolution whose dynamic contains the roots of growth and decline. The suggestion for a methodology draws essentially on linguistics – for 'stability': Saussurean structuralism, for change: Bakhtinian dialogics. In other words the essay proposes a strategy for projecting the diachronic onto the synchronic, in whose nexus lie those preconceptions which account for the enigmas of human re-mapping of meaning.

'The past is not dead. It is not even past.' William Faulkner

Introduction

When Oedipus got to the crossroads he could carry on the way he was going or he could confront the King. He chose confrontation and was eventually lost in darkness, but his contribution to the Western imagination was inestimable.

So too with Cultural Studies (CS), it can go on as a conglomeration of disciplines such as sociology, psychoanalysis, anthropology all investigating the matter of culture or it can lay claim to a kind of knowledge proper to itself with procedures specifically its own. The latter course is the more grandiose venture but there are already intimations of the emergence of such a discipline.

In chapter eight of John Storey's *Cultural Theory and Popular Culture* (1993: 193) he has a sub-section entitled "A paradigm crisis in cultural studies". The section not only identifies disjunctions in CS but the use of the word "paradigm" places the discussion within the conceptual framework of Thomas Kuhn's *Structure of Scientific Revolutions*. In this book Kuhn argues that major shifts in scientific theories are accompanied by paradigm shifts – the geometric regularities of Newton's universe give way to Einstein's relativity.

Of course the inclusion of the popular within "Kulchur" is by no means concluded, but the argument for separation between high and low culture seems to me no more rational than saying chemistry should not include my lead soldiers. It comes down to a question of what explanations do and what they do not do.

What Storey emphasises in the chapter is that the emergence of the popular has led to a breakdown of the old hierarchical determination of Cultural Value. Consequent on this change, as with changes in scientific theories, a new approach or paradigm for culture is trying to emerge. Various factions of intellectuals are stating their positions, from resurrectionists who want to restore the old certainties of judgement by values imposed, to those who see popular culture as a form of resistance movement. In order to move beyond this "impasse of intellectuals… debating with other intellectuals about theories about popular culture" what is needed is an "ethnographically informed cultural analysis" (Storey 1993: 193).

CS will not "explain" anything. Nothing can explain the awful event of Oedipus blinding himself but what we can have are "classes of explanations". The totality of the event, albeit fictional, is open to a variety of explanations "attempt[s] to cover with explanatory devices – and thereby to obscure – the vast darkness of the subject".[1]

- Psychiatry explains psychopathology;
- Sociology explains taboo;
- Theology explains divine ordinances of transgression and retribution,

and so on. What darkness might CS seek distinctively "to cover with explanatory devices"?

Intimations of Cultural Studies

The word 'culture' in both its human and biological senses suggests organism, purpose and process. Penicillin in a Petri dish is an organism with the purpose of replicating itself in order to grow. Fifty people breathing in a large room consists of an organism undergoing the process of staying alive, but we would not consider that process as constituting a purpose except at a very basic level. To accept that our fifty people had 'a purpose' they would need to be intentionally breathing, for example, in unison. The more sophisticated the organism the stricter become our definitions of purpose – in human beings that notion is associated with meaningfulness. Fifty people intentionally breathing in unison entails some kind of meaning directed behaviour that could be the object of study

---

[1] This section is deeply indebted to Gregory Bateson (1958) "Epilogue 1958", *Naven*, Second Edition, Stanford University Press, 280-303.

of sociology, anthropology, even religion or drama. But what kind of distinctive explanation might arise from the proposed CS?

The emergence of CS as a discipline in its own right has already been variously adumbrated. Analysts of the popular have predominantly deployed theoretical approaches such as M.D.F. Their failure has been in applying theories which have inevitably revealed what they seek when so profligately applied. Steve Dixon in an adroit and ironic intervention reads the film 'The Wizard of Oz' through a variety of theoretical perspectives all of which fit admirably, but without a relevance or appropriateness test, so what! (Dixon 1997). As Charles S. Peirce wrote, "if all the world was red then red wouldn't exist".

But there have been a large number of studies from a variety of disciplines which I am suggesting foreshadow CS. They intimate, to borrow from Ferdinand de Saussure writing about semiology, that CS "has a right to existence, a place staked out in advance." Bateson as anthropologist in *Naven* sets out to describe "culture as a whole in such a manner that each detail shall appear as the natural consequence of the remainder of the culture" (Bateson 1958: 1). This is quite clearly in part a structuralist undertaking as he himself writes in the "Epilogue 1936". In the "Epilogue 1958" he moves on to discuss the causal inter-relations of what he calls "each detail", or what from the present point of view would be considered "cultural events". In broader terms it is the working of purpose in process.

Mary Douglas, the sociologist, in *Thought Styles* considers occasions of disagreement with a view to understanding:

> a point at which private thought, after it has come into being, either vanishes or slots into a ready frame of stock connections, and then stays on as part of the local ambience that catches future thoughts and holds them steady. The process of culture in action. (Douglas 1996: xi)

From a CS point of view thought is being demonstrated as purpose within process and the stability/instability problem being explored.

Janet Mueller in 'Complications of Intertextuality' ends her philosophical discussion of Katherine Parr's 'The Book of the Crucifix' with:

> some reflections on what for me remains a conjoint dilemma of methodology and interpretation; how to describe which factor to treat as determinative when more than one option seems to be available and what interpretative difference it makes to decide one way or the other. (Mueller 1997: 16)

Clearly there are a multiplicity of connections between one cultural event and another; the problem as Mueller states is deciding what the implications are for interpretation. How, in other words, do our "classes of explanation" interact and how do we select among different possible determinants?

These three examples, coming from very different disciplines can, like many more, be linked through a common interest in cultural events. Moreover all three tacitly agree that there is an inner landscape of connection between cultural events which I have chosen to designate as *purpose within process*. Within the complex landscape of culture individuals are in a state of becoming, orientating themselves to the system of rules that supports the network. Finally and crucially for CS what determines participants' choices?

The Subject Matter of Cultural Studies

When Oedipus arrives at the crossroads and confronts Laius there are already a number of cultural systems or determinants in play. Among them is the kingship of Laius, his Theban kingdom terrorised by the Sphinx, and Oedipus himself in flight believing he is thus avoiding killing his father. When Oedipus is jostled by the King's herald and attacked by the King he responds by killing the King and the accompanying servants, all but one, who escapes. The event and its outcomes as presented by Sophocles have led to various interpretations – if Oedipus is culpable then his punishment by the Gods is just retribution; it is also arguable that if he is guilty his sufferings might be disproportionate, mere teasings of unjust Gods. Yet another interpretation is that the piece is an ironic comment, that guilt and suffering are not connected, their relatedness an invention of man.

These interpretations of course do not relate to a real Oedipus, they are the speculations of Sophocles – that is what fiction is all about. If Oedipus did exist, as a distant historical figure, and the events of his life had actuality we would have to have a methodology to scrutinize the real events and try to disentangle the cultural meaning. Fictions are a speculative play of possible or likely patterns of process and purpose for entertainment and instruction.

In a highly accomplished article A. L. Becker argues for a development in philosophy of "a specialist in contextual relations" that would bring together humanities (literary scholarship) and science (linguistics):

> Any meaningful activity is a conjunction of *pre-existing* constraints (or rules, or structures, or laws, or myths) with the present, the unpredictable, the particular *now*. (Becker 1995: 27)

The foregoing discussion first with its presentation of examples and then of interpretations is not merely to justify CS, but suggest that there is a current of enquiry running through a diversity of disciplines all concerned with identifying a similar kind of explanation. What participant purposes sustain the processes of cultural events? In other words what preconceptions mental, emotional and behavioural do participants form, related to cultural contexts, to sustain, renew or even end entry into new cultural phenomena? How does our existing cultural knowledge equip us for the ongoing life of culture?

Suggesting a Methodology

To get beyond the anecdotal account of individual cultural events we need a system that has its own internal logic. We might draw, for example an analogy with topography in Euclidean geometry. If the measurements of a field and wood combined are longer than the individual measurements of the field and wood added together then either the measurements are wrong or Euclidean geometry needs revising (Bateson 1973: 27).

Arising out of the papers quoted as well as my own predilection the methodological exploration begins with structuralism. Its formalisation may be seen to start with Ferdinand de Saussure, its major developments were by Nicolai Trubetzkoi and Claude Lévi-Strauss, since which time it has been deployed and criticised variously. As a linguist Saussure was confronted with the problem of trying to make general statements about spoken language while being aware that every speaker of the language had his own unique variation, so much so that now many courts accept voice prints as readily as finger-prints. In order to make statements about language knowledge as a whole (*langue*) the unique variant of each individual (*parole*) had somehow to be subsumed within a system.

Continuing with his characteristic device of creating dichotomies he next divides language study into the diachronic and synchronic. Diachronic study is language through time, the sort of historical linguistics that for him, as an Indo-European expert, had been the foundation of his nineteenth century training and was the subject of his early papers. Synchronic, in opposition to this, is a cross-section of language at any given time, or as Saussure calls it a study of the language state.

Taken as a defining series we have a progression of dichotomies which although not representing Saussure faithfully does give some idea of the systemic relationships he proposed as the foundation of linguistics:

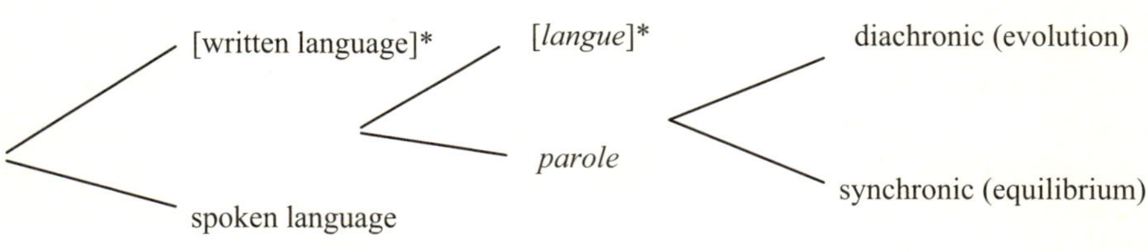

diagram I

* Square brackets indicate a branch of the system irrelevant to the present purpose.

The synchronic gives rise to structuralism, whose key notion is that meaning is defined by the system, not by reference to the real world. We avoid the individuality of language by allowing words to define words rather than individual people, put simply 'work' gets its meaning from opposition to 'leisure', 'good' from opposition to 'bad' and 'religious' from opposition to 'secular'. "It is good, we feel, to know the exact antonym of a word, for not only will it give us a firmer grasp of the meaning of the word to which it is opposed, but inversely, to itself."[2]

The advantage of structuralism was that it brought order and control not only to the study of language but to Saussure's envisaged science of semiology (hereafter semiotics). In structuralism we have a means of studying subjects as diverse and apparently individual as Lévi-Strauss on eating habits and Roland Barthes on fashion. Saussure's achievement was to define a class whose membership depended on the necessary and sufficient condition of being mutually defining. The relationship between language and the real world is ignored in favour of the relationship with other words all of which help to define its "meaning".

I have no wish to enter here discussions about the relationship between language and semiotics, or semiotics and cultural events. My point is simply that the Saussurean or structuralist class is a feasible and invigorating way of bringing into discussion disparate events and objects. But however productive this separation of the relational, mutually defining element, might be the elision of the human aspect has been the source of much criticism. What many critics fail to acknowledge, however, is that Saussure was there before them: "Speech always implies both an established system and an evolution: at every moment it is an existing institution and a product of the past" (Saussure 1966: 8). The division, like all intellectual divisions, is to further discussion, when that discussion is no longer relevant then the division or classification is no longer useful.

To this point my argument has been that so many disciplines seem to be pre-figuring a place for Cultural Studies that we should be trying to delineate its characteristics. Those characteristics are that cultural contexts or events are connected to all other cultural contexts or events and that they are sustained, renewed, transformed or obliterated by their human participants. In Mueller's apt phrase I see CS as "surmount[ing] disjunctions between world and word." (Mueller 1997: 15). Or as Lévi-Strauss put it "the systems with which we are concerned are not easily 'mythologizable' as systems because their virtually synchronic nature is engaged in a never-ending struggle with diachrony" (1972: 231).

---

[2] I am indebted to my colleague Steve Jones for this quotation (Egan, cited in Muehleisen 1997: 4) and for directing me, through his forthcoming work on antonyms (Routledge), to the notion that dichotomies may well be a predisposition of mind (Jones, forthcoming, 2002: Chap. 2 pp. 9-24).

To re-introduce the human into our structuralist identification of cultural events to include process within and between cultural systems we need an account of the inheritance that humans bring to their initiation into specific cultural systems. Taking as an analogy Roman Jakobson's work on metaphor we could say the diachronic has to be projected onto the synchronic in an orderly way. This orderliness will consist in realisation procedures for the history of cultural events within the synchronic state, specifying how the human past is actualised in the present. To return to diagram I, CS can be placed as the interplay between evolution and equilibrium:

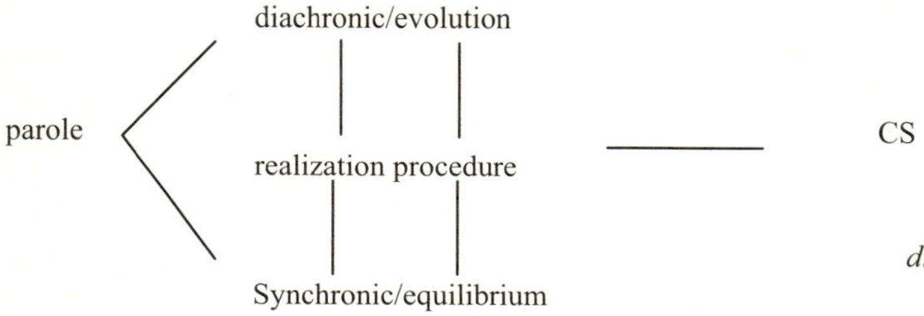

diagram II

The result is a new look at the semiotic systems of the individual within culture. In this way the meanings of cultural events take definition from their place in culture as a whole as well as being grounded in the variable human processes that constitute their meanings. If structuralism delimits the cultural event and places it within the overall state of culture how do we tackle the problem, crucial to our proposed CS, of projecting the historical onto the synchronic state, so getting a description which accounts for breaks and disruptions in culture?

The determinant of either cultural continuity or cultural change resides in a balance between the preconceptions of the participants and the structural positioning of the specific event. If we return to Oedipus we find him caught unwittingly between two cultural states. Having saved the kingdom from the Sphinx he married Laus' widow, Queen Jocasta, in the properly ordained manner. But on learning that she is also his mother he is caught up in the transgressive position of having broken a solemn taboo – mothers and sons never have sexual relations, not even when ordained by marriage. Without the preconception of that taboo in the kinship system there would be no tragedy.

I have come across no discussion of the play suggesting that the original cultural state of his marrying the Queen was wrong, thus inevitably causing the tragedy. Criticism concentrates, following Freud, on the interdiction. Any play which approved of Jocasta marrying her son Oedipus would be the sort of wicked comedy that might have come from the pen of the mischievious Joe Orton – so ingrained is the preconception of the taboo. Of course it is not nearly as universal a taboo as we like to think – there is good anthropological evidence that even in the recent past among isolated peasant communities in Europe some mothers and sons had sexual relations in order to keep the young males as part of the working unit.[3]

That part of the determining preconceptions that comes from the overall cultural state remains a force for stability and will only change if there is a major shift in the culture. In Oedipus the hierarchical state validates his marrying Jocasta, it is of interest to modern observers of the play only in so far as it is seen as a plot device to create the transgressive situation we recognise. The more interesting preconceptions are those which bring about system change. We need strategies to identify them and assess their impact on the cultural state.

Initiation into cultural events or situations, ranging from sheltering refugees to taking someone to an art gallery, all involve communication. There is entry into the cultural system, interaction within the system, and choices about maintenance, change or abolition of the system. This complex of communicative exchanges includes linguistic and non-linguistic modes all of which have a sophisticated and specialised methodology. It is not intended that CS will simply become a branch of any one of these methodological approaches but rather that students of CS will deploy what is most appropriate to their expertise in understanding the system and the preconceptions which provide its evolutionary character.

Taking the language part of communication, linguistic expertise may range from grammar to discourse. Someone interested in grammar might well choose to investigate the transitivity system which is detailed in the work of M.A.K. Halliday. But this would not preclude a non-linguist deploying a less technical work-a-day version provided they were consistent and replicable in their analysis. The transitivity system seeks to identify the nature of intensity of the relationship that exists in clauses, the type of relationship expressed by subject–verb–object.

If we compare:

(a) Oedipus hit the herald,
(b) The herald was jostled by Oedipus,

it does not need a syntactic analysis to reveal manifest differences. (a) has a great deal more 'force' than (b). Partly it is the choice of 'hit' as against 'jostle' and we also note that the subject is different in each case. Combined with other factors such an observation might contribute to the identification of a preconception about Oedipus.

At first sight discourse studies rather than grammatical studies might seem to be the only realistic choice for investigating preconceptions. Even transitivity has one foot in the discourse camp, its investigation by M.A.K. Halliday placing

---

[3] Several accounts of the serial murderer Fred West suggest that he had sexual relations with his mother. The resultant psychopathology could in part arise from a residue of traditional behaviour coming into conflict with presently held taboos.

it firmly in the functional grammar camp while the work on systematizing the parameters of transitivity by Paul Hooper and Sandra A. Thompson is overtly discoursal. However even as strictly abstract a grammar as Noam Chomsky's Transformational Generative Grammar has been used by Leonard Bernstein to generate music; so it surely has the potential as an investigative tool for revealing aspects of preconceptions.

My favoured choice for investigating preconceptions, the companion piece for structuralism, is Mikhail Bakhtin's Dialogics which in essence is the closest approach to both culture and discourse. Central to Bakhtin's thinking about language is the proposition that it is fashioned in dialogue:

> The word is born in dialogue as a living rejoinder within it; the word is shaped by dialogic interaction with an alien word that is already in the object. A word forms a concept of its own object in a dialogic way. (Bakhtin 1981: 279)

Indeed we do not have a language *of our own* but are always using other voices, voices which come out of their own contexts and concepts:

> the word does not exist in a neutral and impersonal language… but rather it exists in other people's mouths, in other people's contexts, serving other people's intentions: it is from there that one must take the word, and make it one's own. (ibid: 294)

So far as CS is concerned "other people's mouths" are speaking in a variety of culturally positioned contexts, their mutual contentiousness a contribution to the evolution of the synchronic cultural state.

Central to Bakhtin's discussion of the word is the notion of intertextuality. Not only are our words borrowed from former speakers but on occasion whole chunks of discourse. The borrowings may take different forms, from outright quotation to a much looser borrowing of the intention but they are all manifestations of past dialogues. Also we must consider not only the borrowing but also the context of the borrowing. My earlier examination of Storey's use of "paradigm" made use of the *context* within which his usage takes its colouration – I might also have gone on to discuss the *situation* within which Kuhn's text established its dialogic place.

A marriage between Saussure's structuralism and Bakhtin's dialogics then, in general, is what I am proposing. Structuralism reveals the relative positioning of all the cultural events that go to make a culture. Dialogics reveals the dynamic human processes that inform the cultural scheme of things. In this way cultural studies becomes the systematic regulated search for, rather than assertion of, the myriad preconceptions that inform, maintain and evolve our cultural life.

Case Study

The following case study is an experimental attempt at a working analysis to illustrate the methodology suggested, with all its gaps and weaknesses. The event chosen has been identified retrospectively; certain anomalies struck me at the time and so I have elected to scrutinise them through the proposed analysis. This analysis will be effected with a broad pencil, but the possibility should always be open to others to collaborate by performing technically rigorous operations within their own field of expertise and comparing results. The superordinate cultural event chosen is a university conference. It is the sort of activity very familiar to both staff and graduate students and has an honourable history in academic life. Certain conferences like the Macy conferences and the first Major Semiotics Conference have proved landmarks in the development of their subjects.

Our point of departure is identifying structurally the distinctiveness of this particular conference. It was organised by ISSEI, the International Society for the Study of European Ideas, whose goal is a multidisciplinary interest in European intellectual and cultural history. Participants came from USA, Canada, Israel, most from Europe with a few from as far as Ghana, Japan, Cameroon and Australia as well as the host nation, Norway. If we consider the fundamental structural division as between the universities' obligations to the state, as against their obligation to learning, then such an idealistic mix representing different political accommodations has to seek a resolution elsewhere, typically in the subject matter. But the subject of the conference 'Approaching a New Millenium' could be considered equally contentious in its idealism or, more cynically, its vagueness.

If we construct oppositional pairs we have from the broadest constituency to the most particular:

a) national versus *international*
b) state versus *academia*
c) *general subject* versus specific subject
d) group versus *individual*

We find an international academic group of individuals dealing with a general subject matter. The compromise point, as so often, was to have plenary sessions bringing the community together for a bravura academic performance counter-pointed by workshops. The workshop I joined was 'The Future of Beauty' convened by Daniel Meyer-Dinkgraffe, a member of the Drama Department at the University of Wales, Aberystwyth.

Structurally we have another problem: were the eleven speakers at this topic-specific workshop there as individuals, or as members of an academic group? There was one group of three with a very clear subject agenda – the trouble was they were put into the group at short notice because their workshop had not formed: an idealistic solution but running counter to the academic ambitions of the workshop. The topic itself has exciting possibilities, very obviously wishing to engage with changing notions of art and beauty, but with no class of explanations to inform the discussion where it could go?

In the failure of the subject as an organising force institutional constraints took over. Not having group identity within the subject, parameters of academic behaviour took over – evidenced by most of the papers being 'read' when the conference expressly asked for papers to be 'presented and not read'. With a subject more emotive than rational it is not surprising that norms of academic behaviour predominated – one does not desire to be thought an idiot by colleagues who are strangers.

Structuralism has helped us to understand the idealism in a new and uncertain world as well as the positioning of participants in that world. The new dynamics of education, where states now want higher education for all rather than an elite academic community, has not been accompanied by new practices. It has simply provided the academic system with more initiates and the old practices congeal around them.

At this point the diachronic is demanding its voice be heard so I will briefly apply a dialogic consideration to the topic of the workshop consisting of two parts, 'future' and 'beauty'. Only one paper addressed the future, two addressed the problematic present and the others reiterated the past. Exemplification consisted of one original poem read to a video compilation by an academic who is also an artist, some photocopies of photographic reproductions of paintings and of photographs of Gorden Craig's Moscow 'Hamlet', one reading of an Elizabeth Bishop poem and one tape of Ravi Shankar/Philip Glass 'Passengers'.

Since the discussion of future 'beauty' was virtually absent what prevailed were the disembodied shadows of past dialogic encounters. In this way there was a deliberate acquiescence in a concept whose dialogic credentials and vitality have largely been lost. Whatever of interest is revealed in the institutional setting the failure of the dialogue hinged on the absence of a dialogically accessible concept of beauty.

What I feel the analysis reveals is that in the absence of a secure framework of academic dialogue, purposes are adjusted. The topic of the workshop becomes less secure in its futurity – institutional norms are no longer fully comprehended so there is a retreat into an imagined past. Individuals seek a role they can fulfil in the group, and the topic of 'beauty' has recourse to its previous sanctions. At the moment such adventurous departures are viewed with some trepidation as uncertain paths.

Bibliography

Bakhtin, Mikhail (1981) "Discourse in the Novel", in: *The Dialogic Imagination*, Austin: University of Texas Press.

Bateson, Gregory (1958) *Naven*, 2nd Edition, Stanford: Stanford University Press.

Bateson, Gregory (1973) *Steps to an Ecology of Mind*, London: Paladin.

Becker, A. L. (1995) "Text-building, Epistemology and Aesthetics in Javanese Shadow Theatre", in: *Beyond Translation*, Ann Arbor: University of Michigan Press.

Dixon, Steven (1997) "Hermeneutics and The Wizard of Oz", in: Costa de Beauregard, R., et Menegaldo, G., eds. *Le Cinéma et ses objets*, Paris: La Licorne.

Douglas, Mary (1996) *Thought Styles*, London: Sage.

Duranti, Alessandro and Goodwin, Charles, eds. (1992) *Rethinking Context*, Cambridge: CUP.

Jones, Steven (2002) *Antonyms: a corpus based perspective*, London: Routledge.

Levi-Strauss, Claude (1972) *The Savage Mind*, New York: Weidenfeld and Nicolson.

Mueller, Janet (1997) "Complications of Intertextuality: John Fisher, Katherine Parr and 'The Book of the Crucifix'", in: Brown, C.C. and Marotti, A.F., eds, *Texts and Cultural Change in Early Modern England*, London: Macmillan.

Saussure, Ferdinand de (1966) *Course in General Linguistics*, New York: Mcgraw-Hill.

Storey, John (1993) *Cultural Theory and Popular Culture,* London: Harvester Wheatsheaf.

POPES, KINGS & CULTURAL STUDIES: PLACING THE COMMITMENT TO NON-DISCIPLINARITY IN HISTORICAL CONTEXT

KARL MATON

Cultural studies is janus-faced, describable as intellectually blooming and in disarray, institutionally booming and in decline. This essay examines how cultural studies reached this paradoxical position, investigating the role played by a factor hitherto ignored: the structuring of cultural studies as a knowledge formation. The analysis begins by historically outlining how knowledge has been legitimated within Western thought, including the *Ancien Régime* of popes and kings, the Enlightenment, Romanticism and cultural studies. Two principal forms of legitimation are defined, emphasising either *knowledge* or *knower*. A thought experiment then shows how the 'knower mode' (of cultural studies) generates processes of proliferation which fragment subject areas and tend towards narcissistic autobiography, methodological individualism, historical amnesia and institutional vulnerability. Showing this to represent an inverted form of the *Ancien Régime*, I argue it is inimical to the proclaimed ends of cultural studies and that a culture of consequence is required to augment its level of commitment if real change is to be effected.

...the first time as tragedy, the second as farce...
Karl Marx *The Eighteenth Brumaire of Louis Bonaparte*

Farce is but tragedy turned upside-down.

Introduction

This essay is prompted by apparent paradoxes in the intellectual and institutional positions of British cultural studies in higher education.[1] Ask a number of academics or consult examples of the voluminous literature on cultural studies and you'll soon find two basic pictures emerging of its current position. One is a story of institutional and intellectual success. Cultural studies is, educationally speaking, big business, with journals, professional associations, conferences and

[1] I am grateful to Basil Bernstein, Rob Moore, Gemma Moss and Parlo Singh for encouragement and discussion of earlier versions of ideas which underpin this article.

textbooks proliferating.[2] There is now, for example, an *International Journal of Cultural Studies*, a *European Journal of Cultural Studies*, as well as *Cultural Studies*. The British-based Media, Communication and Cultural Studies Association had its first annual conference in January 2000; five months later a proposal to establish an International Association for Cultural Studies was accepted at a biannual conference ('Crossroads in Cultural Studies') of nearly one thousand delegates. Where a decade ago one struggled to find cultural studies texts amid Literary Criticism, Sociology, Criminology and other sections of bookshops, cultural studies now has large sections of its own, often dwarfing its past classificatory homes. Courses in cultural studies are often viewed as a formula for guaranteeing student numbers – every higher education institution has to have one. Even the British Government appears to have caught on to its chic: what was a Department of National Heritage is now rebranded the Department of Culture, Media and Sport. Institutionally, the signs seem to indicate, to some at least, that cultural studies is in bloom.

Intellectually, such adjectives as 'energetic', 'vibrant', 'fresh' and 'original' abound; cultural studies appears to be an exciting area of intellectual activity, generating new substantive foci and theories at astonishing speed. Everyone seems to want a piece of the action; geographers, historians, sociologists, psychologists, amongst others, have adopted 'cultural' as a prefix to describe their work. Further, cultural studies is often described as cutting-edge, radical and progressive, a site for critical theory and practice, at the forefront of movements for cultural, social and political change. Regular attacks by the media and self-styled guardians of the cultural heritage are held up as badges of honour, testament to its crackling political energy. From one angle, then, the stock of cultural studies is riding high.

The second picture, however, is somewhat less triumphant. Institutionally, cultural studies has a marginal and limited presence within British higher education (Maton 1996, 2000a). For all its apparent popularity, the actual number of courses, departments, students and staff *named* as 'cultural studies' remains relatively small. If it has found a place in the sun, this has largely been as an adjunct or adjective to other disciplines (e.g. 'English and cultural studies', 'cultural geography'), rather than as a distinct entity. Even where cultural studies has managed to carve out an institutional home of its own, this has consistently been in lower status institutional positions: adult education, schools, technical colleges, art colleges, polytechnics and distance learning.[3] Further, this existence

---

[2] I should emphasise that this brief sketch is of *British cultural studies* within *British* higher education. Subject areas typically regarded as related to cultural studies, such as media and communication studies, have divergent emphases, and the development of cultural studies in other national contexts have differed (see, for example, Blundell *et al* 1993).

[3] See Maton (2000a) for more detail of this institutional trajectory. In the course of ongoing research into the institutionalisation of cultural studies within higher education, I have constructed a database of every course, option and module in cultural, media and

is typically precarious: the famous Centre for Contemporary Cultural Studies at Birmingham University had very limited resources and staffing, minimal institutional support, and was threatened with closure at least twice; the first full degree course in 'cultural studies' (Portsmouth Polytechnic, 1975) was closed down in the late 1990s despite healthy student numbers; and until recently professional subject associations have been *ad hoc* and short-lived. The institutional position of cultural studies has, it appears, been marginal and insecure.

Intellectually, one may find the field characterised as in disarray, in decline, inchoate, fragmented, exhausted, beset by internecine strife and otherwise on the wane. If the first picture was of letting a hundred flowers bloom, this picture is less rosy – an unkempt and overgrown garden. Cultural studies has been depicted as frivolous and undermining academic standards, more an indulgence of whimsy or hobby-horse of political grievance than rigorous intellectual activity. The huge size and kaleidoscopic nature of the *Crossroads* conference signals from this perspective not health but unmanaged and unmanageable gargantuanism, the outward expression of an amorphous and directionless collection of interests, easily swayed by fads and fashions. If the subject had a founding project, it has, such characterisations maintain, fallen into parody, a spent force politically, its purpose little more than providing a punchbag for media and intellectual élites in search of signs of cultural decline:

> It would seem we are forging a gullible generation of media-soaked teenagers, narcotically duped into fashionable but vacuous quasi-disciplines, by careerist culture junkies high on their own incestuous theorising. (Golding 2000)

From this angle, the stock of cultural studies is in terminal decline.

Cultural studies it would seem is everywhere but nowhere, vibrant and in disarray. Moreover, these two faces of cultural studies are often intermingled in accounts. It is not unusual to find cultural studies described as both intellectually blossoming and institutionally marginal, or intellectually exhausted but institutionally booming. (Indeed, these are the typical accounts by its most vociferous protagonists and opponents, respectively). Moreover, this janus-faced character is not simply another example of academics always having two hands ('But on the other hand...') – both have a basis in reality (Maton 1996, 2000a). This raises the questions I address in this article: how has cultural studies come to be in such a curious position and why?

---

communication studies (and variants thereof) offered in British institutions of higher education since the early 1960s. Analysis of this database, as well as unpublished archival course materials and student data, will be made available in future publications.

Conventional Accounts

The development of cultural studies is a dangerous and confused topic in which authors have often lost their sense of direction. One can, however, identify at least two broad approaches to these questions. The first focuses on intention and commitment, typically either making a virtue of necessity, claiming that the position of cultural studies is just as intended, or calling for more vigilance and effort in the face of threats to its original project(s). Debate over institutionalisation is often couched in these terms, perceived as a 'moment of profound danger', in Hall's oft-quoted phrase, or a moment of profound opportunity.[4] Both positions, however, focus on commitment and agency. A second approach looks beyond cultural studies, focusing on the impact of social relations of power, such as the relations of class, race and gender to curricula and pedagogy or the role of social change in shaping the disciplinary map. What both approaches have in common is that whilst they highlight the couplet power/knowledge, they tend to reduce knowledge to power, whether located in subjective agency or external social structures. In other words, they highlight relations *to* cultural studies but neglect relations *within* cultural studies – an (albeit tacit) externalist and reductive sociology of knowledge which lacks an analysis of knowledge itself (Bernstein 1990: 165-180, Maton 2000a, Moore 2000). In contrast to this, I here address a relatively neglected dimension of academic subjects, namely the question of whether there is something *intrinsic* to cultural studies, something internal to the way it is structured as a knowledge formation, which enables this curious position in higher education.[5] Specifically, I focus on how cultural studies has been legitimated by its proponents.

It is tempting to view claims made by actors on behalf of their academic subjects, practices and thus themselves as little more than bombast to be dismissed or ideological camouflage whose social basis in power relations needs to be revealed. The dominance of a sociologically reductive approach to knowledge – which one can summarise as 'You would say that, wouldn't you?' – encourages an attitude of uncompromising scepticism towards the claims of actors. Although we often make such proclamations about our own practices in good faith, to take seriously those of others, even as an object of study, is to be 'taken in'. Approaches such as Pierre Bourdieu's 'field theory' (e.g. 1988, 1991, 1993) highlight that such claims are based in struggles over status and resources, they are *interested* and thus to conceive them as anything but reflecting power

[4] Compare, for example, Johnson (1983), Hall (1992), Miller (1994) and Bennett (1996) with various articles in Nelson & Gaonkar (1996) and Striphas (1998).

[5] It cannot be overemphasised that I am not suggesting that externalist issues are unimportant in the development of intellectual fields; as I argue elsewhere, *both* are essential to a non-reductive account of knowledge (see Maton 2000a). My focus here is to highlight the significance of the neglected dimension of knowledge itself.

struggles represents a failure to rise above the doxic 'bad faith' of the intellectual field. The aim is to reveal the situated character of knowledge claims and any mismatch between rhetoric and reality. There is, of course, much of value in such an approach (Maton 1999, Swartz 1997), but when taken alone it tends to result in knowledge becoming little more than an epiphenomenon of power. I have elsewhere detailed how conceiving knowledge in terms of *legitimation* enables the synthesis of the insights of such sociological approaches with philosophical accounts which highlight the potentially legitimate nature of knowledge claims (Maton 2000a). Suffice to say here that the ways in which actors legitimate their knowledge claims represent, first, a proclaimed ruler of participation within the subject area and criteria by which achievement should be measured, and, secondly, the basis of claims to status and material resources and so are crucial in carving out intellectual and institutional spaces within higher education. In other words, how actors portray themselves, however distanced from empirical reality, has effects.

Specifically, I will suggest that the way cultural studies is legitimated shapes its intellectual and institutional development and so sheds light on its paradoxical position in higher education. Cultural studies is often discussed without historical perspective (Moore & Maton 2001). So, I begin by embarking on a whistle-stop tour of the history of legitimation in Western thought, to both bring its present condition into sharper relief and open up for analysis such oft-stated but little analysed claims as a radical break with disciplinarity. My aim, above all, is to provide food for thought by raising questions and suggesting possible answers.

The Legitimation of Knowledge: A Very Brief Historical Account

Any review of the ways in which knowledge has been legitimated in Western thought must of necessity be selective and partial. Moreover, my aim here is to illustrate a suggestive (rather than historically comprehensive) account of two fundamental ways of conceiving the legitimate basis of legitimate knowledge. These, which I have termed knowledge and knower modes of legitimation (Maton 2000a), have dominated thinking at different times, though they are ever-present and competing (I return to this in due course).

The Ancien Régime*: Popes and Kings*

Prior to roughly the seventeenth century, official knowledge in the West was much more circumscribed in quantity compared to today and much slower to change, but also much more certain (Gellner 1974b, 1978). As contemporary debate over the nature of society illustrates, the enormous growth of knowledge characterising modernity has also raised more uncertainty; every answer, as

Popper (1972) points out, leads in turn to more questions. In contrast, prior to this explosion of understanding and uncertainty, the relative stability and certainty of knowledge was ostensibly based primarily on the authority of the Crown and the Papacy. Official knowledge, that is to say, was held to be legitimated by the personal authority of the King / Queen or Pope and, ultimately, via notions of the divine right of kings and the Petrine primacy, on the authority of the ultimate knower, God (Bloch 1962, Critchley 1978, Shapin 1994). Like Platonic notions (see below), this held a monist conception of knowledge – the truths proclaimed by monarchs or Popes were immutable and universal – but one based on the characteristics of a single knower rather than a specific method.

Taking England as an example, the King's authority was legitimated according to divine right, delegation from the King of Kings (e.g. Morton 1643, Burrell 1683). What the King decreed as the truth was right because he was the King.[6] Thus, James I, King of England, told Parliament in 1614:

> Monarchy is the greatest thing on earth. Kings are rightly called gods since just like God they have power of life and death over all their subjects in all things. They are accountable to God only... so it is a crime for anyone to argue about what a king can do.

Similarly, King Charles I was called 'the little God' and, after losing the English Civil War of 1642-9, many argued that he could not be tried by his peers as he had none (Norbrook 1999). At his trial in January 1649, Charles refused to answer the court, claiming they had no lawful, God-given authority:

> I demand to know by what authority, I mean lawful authority I am called here. Remember, I am your King, your lawful King. And what sins you bring upon your heads, and the judgement of God upon this land, think well upon it, before you go from one sin to a greater one. I have a trust committed to me by God, by lawful inheritance. I will not betray it to answer to a new and unlawful authority.

The feudal arrangements underlying this legitimation of knowledge represented a pyramidal structure of authority descending from God, via lawful descent, to the King and then down through Barons, Knights, Yeoman to the peasant majority (see Figure 1).[7]

The other principal source for legitimacy of knowledge was the Church, with a similar structure of divine delegation. According to the Roman Catholic

---

[6] I use 'King' here only to avoid any confusion with the present.

[7] Feudal relations in England varied over time, but the overall pyramid shape remained relatively constant. Thus, for example, the structure in England under William after 1066 was: God - King - approximately 200-300 Barons and Bishops (or Tenants-in-Chief) - 100-2,000 Knights / Lords (or Under-Tenants) – 1-1.5 million Peasants. Similarly, England in 1500 was: God - King - Nobles (about 50 families) - Knights or gentry and gentlemen (10,000 families) - Yeoman (100,000 families) - Tenant farmers and the poor (400,000 families).

Church, Jesus Christ, God's representative on Earth, conferred primacy of jurisdiction upon Saint Peter as prince of the apostles and visible head of the Church. His authority to pronounce infallibly was to pass down in perpetuity to his papal successors. This Petrine primacy, a monopoly of legitimacy, was affirmed by the Council of Florence in 1439, but evident even earlier.[8] Cyprian of Carthage, writing about 256, asked 'Would the heretics dare to come to the very seat of Peter whence apostolic faith is derived and whither no errors can come?'; and Pope Sixtus III, for example, declared in 433 that 'all know that to assent to [the Pope's] decision is to assent to St. Peter, who lives in his successors and whose faith fails not.' Underneath the Pope was a hierarchy of positions, from Cardinals, Archbishops, Bishops, down to Parish Priests. Both bases for legitimate knowledge thus represented a hierarchical system of divine delegation, from one at the top to many at the bottom, where the higher up the hierarchy one was, the nearer to God, the supreme and all-knowing knower, and the more legitimacy one could draw upon in making knowledge claims.

Figure 1:
Simplified Schematic of Feudal & Papal Hierarchies

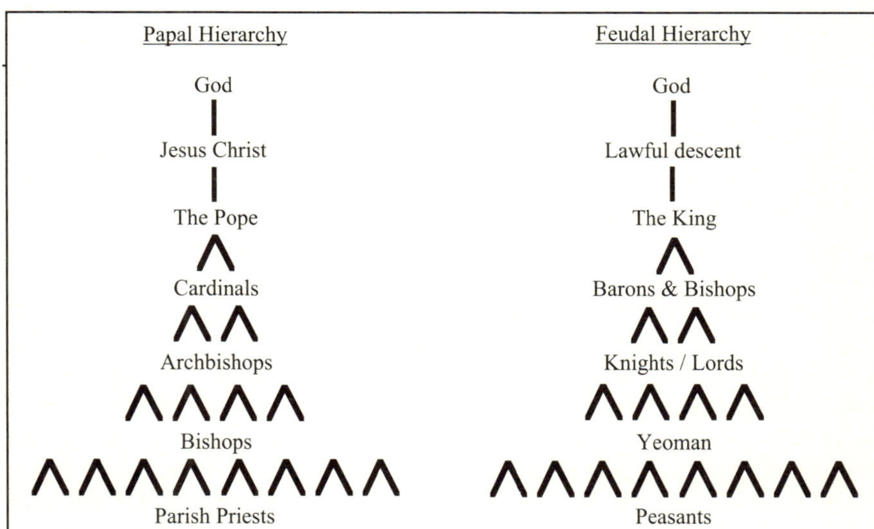

[8] Papal Infallibility was more famously defined as a matter of faith by the First Vatican Council in 1870, but (as illustrated) the legitimacy of knowledge based on the Pope as a privileged knower was already well established. That the Pope may claim infallibility only when speaking on specific issues and in a particular way was only declared in 1870, prior to which it was far less restricted. (Thus the Vatican's explanation for why the behaviour of so-called 'bad popes' does not undermine papal infallibility: they had overstepped their remit).

The central point here is not their proclaimed basis in religion but the *form* taken by claims to legitimate knowledge, namely that the King or Pope was right because of *who* they were. Although specific popes had been chosen by election since 1179 by the Sacred College of Cardinals, once elected they assumed this status as the privileged knower and repository of legitimacy. Similarly, once established on the throne, the basis of monarchs' claims to legitimacy regarding knowledge focused on their status as a divinely privileged knower, regardless of how they reached the throne. Thus the basis of legitimacy resided in attributes of the claimant, the privileged knower; there were strong boundaries around and strong control over *who* can make truth claims, and attempts to do so could meet extreme and violent censure. (A famous example of this clash between knowers saw the Pope's representative in England, Thomas Becket, Archbishop of Canterbury, murdered in 1170 on the orders of King Henry II). In contrast, *what* the privileged knower could claim knowledge about and *how* they arrived at it were much less restricted – *weak* boundaries and control regarding subject matter and procedures. Thus knowledge itself also resembled a pyramid, with all phenomena brought under the infallible gaze of a single knower.

The Reign of Reason: Science

Moving forward in time, the Renaissance, Reformation and Enlightenment all served to undermine these authorities: the King was killed and God had at least one foot in the grave. At the same time knowledge now became increasingly subject to unprecedented and sustained growth, hugely accelerated change and less certainty. This raised the question of how, in the absence of a divinely delegated knower and in the face of increased uncertainty, knowledge could be legitimated – *the* central problem for philosophy since Descartes.

One highly influential answer was to focus on the methods by which knowledge could be achieved. First, it should be noted that though knowledge became subject to accelerated change, this did not necessarily diminish belief in the *possibility* of absolute and universal truth which would hold for all people at all times and in all places; a monist conception of knowledge was not inimical to recognition of its instability and fallibility (preconditions for its progress). It was widely believed that for each question there was, waiting to be discovered, a single answer: truth rather than truths. What was radical was that the key to these monist truths lay not so much with the individual as with the method (Biagoli 1993, Shapin 1994).

This notion revived a Platonic view of knowledge, one which held 'that there are certain axiomatic truths, adamantine, unbreakable, from which it is possible by severe logic to deduce certain absolutely infallible conclusions' (Berlin 1999: 2). Crucial in the seventeenth and eighteenth centuries was the widely perceived burgeoning success and imitability of the natural sciences. The model of mathematics and, later, mechanics dominated conceptions of the means of placing knowledge – not only of nature but also of society, man (as was), values, morals, and politics – on a sure foundation. As under the *Ancien Régime*, knowledge formed a pyramid, with the linking together of diverse phenomena under as few laws as possible (cf. Bernstein 1996, 1999). What was different, however, was an emphasis above all else on the 'what' and the 'how', objects of study and procedures, and in particular observation and experiment:

> As the science of man is the only solid foundation for the other sciences, so, the only solid foundation we can give to this science itself must be laid on experience and observation. (Hume, 1739-40)

The royal road to wisdom, then, lay with procedure; knowledge itself, its organisation and procedures, would guarantee knowledge. For thinkers as diverse as Bacon, Spinoza, Helvétius, Saint-Simon, Comte, Bentham, Hobbes and many others, certainty of knowledge could be achieved through certainty of method. In an anti-humanist move, the infallible knower was thereby replaced by the infallible method – a transition from a warm world of bodies to a cold world of bodies of knowledge (cf. Gellner 1974a). The realm of the sacred shifted from a single Knower to the procedural means to a singular knowledge, a Copernican revolution of legitimation. Although the privileged procedure varied across thinkers – the application of universal reason, scientific method, introspection and doubt, for example – all shared a belief in the universal nature of this method. Anyone, it was claimed, could attain knowledge, provided they submit to the special method (Ward 1997); differences of spatial and temporal location among knowers were of less importance than the means by which they sought knowledge (Shapin 1988, Daston 1992). In this way specialised procedures offered a means of controlling the instability of knowledge – *who* is speaking makes no difference to whether or not what is being said is true, and though the speaker may change, the procedures remained stable and certain. This represented a fundamental shift of emphasis in the legitimation of knowledge: from strong boundaries and control over *who* can claim knowledge to strong boundaries and control over *what* can be claimed knowledge of and *how* – a move from knower to knowledge.

The Romantic Revolution

These notions of the proper basis of knowledge were not uncontested. In what Berlin describes as 'the greatest shift in the consciousness of the West that has occurred' (1999: 1), the 'romantic revolution' of the late eighteenth century saw a sustained critique of Enlightenment beliefs and a fundamental change in the legitimation of knowledge. Romanticism, howsoever defined, was less concerned with truth than with *belief*. It mattered less whether one's truth claims were 'scientific' or practically adequate or represented an advance in the state of knowledge than whether one believed in them wholeheartedly. Science, method, ideas, knowledge were thus secondary to the state of the mind of the knower;

what was admired was integrity, sincerity, dedication to an ideal, *whatever* the ideal (Berlin 1999). It mattered little what one claimed knowledge of or how, so long as one truly believed. In other words, intention was more important than effect, commitment more important than consequence. This influential shift in legitimation thus focused more on the character of the knower than the content of knowledge. Universal and singular truths, discovered and legitimated by public criteria were displaced by private turmoil and inner truths created by individuals as the key to insight. A new emphasis on the pluralist nature of knowledge took hold based on a sense of difference, emphasising dissimilarities rather than similarities, a celebration of the particularity and uniqueness of knowers and thus knowledge. Arising from this knower form of legitimation are a host of attributes typically associated with Romanticism (and which are worth comparing to cultural studies), including: confused teeming fullness and richness of life, multiplicity; the strange, exotic, mysterious, irrational; uniqueness, revolutionary change, pursuit of novelty, concern with the fleeting present, living in the now, rejection of knowledge past and future, exile and alienation, minorities rather than majorities... among many others (see Berlin 1999).

Summary

Taking this very brief and heuristic account as a whole, I have highlighted two principal ways in which knowledge has typically been legitimated. As shown in Table 1, the model for the *'Ancien Régime'* was of monist and stable knowledge and that of the 'reign of reason' monist and stable method, while that of Romanticism emphasised its instability and plurality. In the case of the '*Ancien Régime*' and Romanticism, the emphasis falls on *who* you are, the character, nature or dispositions of the actor; whereas Enlightenment ideas emphasise *what* the actor is claiming knowledge of and *how* they reach that knowledge. One foregrounds people, the other procedures: knower or knowledge modes of legitimation.

Table 1: Summary of dominant modes of legitimation

	Stability of knowledge	**Variety of 'truth(s)'**	**Forms of legitimation**
The *Ancien Régime*	stable	monist	Knower
The Enlightenment	managed instability	monist	knowledge
Romanticism	unstable	pluralist	knowers

Though this schematic account may appear as a pendulum swinging from one to another mode, both are always and everywhere co-present. They are, so to speak, two sides of the same coin – one face may predominate at any one time, but the other face is still there. Thus I am not suggesting abrupt and total transformations, as associated with Foucauldian notions of changes in episteme. The reader, should they wish, may find countless examples of, say, knowledge modes in Romanticism or knower modes in Enlightenment thought. What I am highlighting, however, are two forms of legitimation which have dominated at different times – the key difference is where *emphasis* is placed: knowledge or knower – and which have been realised under different social and intellectual conditions. Moreover, these are *self*-characterisations, espoused rather than enacted practices.[9]

The Legitimation of Cultural Studies

I now turn to consider how cultural studies today might fit into this heuristic schema. I can consider how cultural studies is legitimated only cursorily here (see Maton 2000a, 2000b), but wish to argue that in recent years there have been marked emphases on weak boundaries around and control over *what* and *how* legitimate cultural studies knowledge can be produced, and conversely strong boundaries and control over *who* can claim to be doing so.[10]

What and How – Knowledge

Perhaps the central theme of legitimation in cultural studies is non-disciplinarity. It has been described as 'multi-', 'inter-', 'post-', 'cross-', 'trans-', 'anti-', anything but 'disciplinary'. This follows a wider commitment to weakening

---

[9] Pulling tight a thread which weaves through the garment of history is dangerous, both for the author and the reader. The temptation is to scan critically for omissions and so read such an argument as if it aimed at comprehensiveness. The account offered here is not an intellectual history, but rather a theorisation of the *dominant* modes of belief regarding the basis of knowledge, illustrated schematically by historical examples. It is thus primarily heuristic, a starting point. Two further possible misreadings are, first, to elide modes of thinking about thought with the modes of thinking themselves; whether these self-characterisations accurately reflect actors' practices is not my concern here. Secondly, one may elide a focus on dominant patterns of thinking about the basis of knowledge with the marginalisation or devaluation of other beliefs and ideas. My aim here is not the rescue of forgotten or dominated modes of thought, but the analysis of those forms which are widely perceived as having been highly influential at various moments in time.

[10] Again, I should emphasise that the following summarises *self-characterisations* of cultural studies; enacted practices may be entirely different.

academic hierarchies and boundaries, between disciplines, official knowledge and everyday life, the teacher and the taught, high and low culture, and so forth. As 'undisciplined', cultural studies is proclaimed as freeing knowledge from the suffocating grip of specific procedures specialised to a delimited object of study. Methodological and ontological pluralism, with both 'culture' and 'studies' left undefined, free for redefinition or totalising (as in 'a whole way of life'), are declared legitimating attributes of the subject area. Indeed, commitment and sincerity often appear more important than purely 'intellectual' criteria – praise and critique focus on political intent, where the heart is rather than the contents of the head. Alongside this sits an anti-canonical position, valorising cultural studies as not only free from the restrictions of a canonic tradition but also actively undermining established canons, including any nascent traditions of its own. Thus one finds a propensity to recurrent rupture and renewal, with regular announcements of radical 'breaks' and the subject's rebirth which decentre past work and proclaim the originality and freshness of current ideas. Instead of cumulative development, the necessity and vitality of cultural studies is measured by the arrival of new 'voices' or 'post-' theories and a rapid turnover of 'hot' topics, themselves typically focused on the new and the now or, in Raymond Williams's terms, the 'emergent' rather than 'residual' aspects of culture and society.

Who – Knowers

In contrast to 'what' and 'how', questions of who can claim knowledge have typically been more strongly and explicitly defined. Cultural studies has been legitimated in terms of a radical educational and political project, associated with democratic and participatory forms of education, and portrayed as offering an oppositional pedagogy capable of giving voice to the experiences of marginalised social groups. In contrast to the 'simplistic' generalisations of theory and the detached observer, the importance of primary experience and the 'view from below' have been central to claims made for the subject area. This emphasis on 'giving voice to' dominated social groups underpins standard intellectual histories, which typically trace a movement from the experiences of working-class men through a feminist emphasis on the silenced voice of women to later interventions in terms of race and sexuality. Common to these is a critique of existing 'voices' for failing to represent a new 'voice', underpinned by (often tacit) notions of standpoint epistemology, where truth resides in the intersubjective social characteristics of the knower. Alongside the embracing of anti-foundationalist ideas, these positions celebrate difference, the irreducible particularity of experience, and the multiplicity of subjectivity, identity and truths. Central to the proclaimed *raison d'être* of cultural studies is thus its possession by what Blake called the 'holiness of the minute particular' and belief that knowledge resides in the unique knower.

Summary

This is, of course, an abbreviated caricature (as self-characterisations themselves often are), but sufficient to give a flavour for comparative purposes of how cultural studies is typically legitimated by many of its current proponents. According to this, cultural studies is not a static knowledge formation (like the *Ancien Régime*), but (unlike Enlightenment ideas) change is found less in the sustained growth of knowledge than in a rapid turnover and ongoing instability of approaches and voices. The form taken by its legitimation (like the *Ancien Régime*) stresses strong boundaries around and control over *who* can legitimately claim knowledge, and (like Romanticism) emphasises commitment and the unique particular. In opposition to Enlightenment legitimation, cultural studies leaves disciplinary boundaries, objects of study and procedures open and fluid – weak boundaries and control on what can be studied and how. In other words, the legitimation of cultural studies currently emphasises people rather than procedures – a knower mode of legitimation.

A Thought Experiment: Some Implications of Knower Legitimation

What implications might this mode of legitimation have for the position of British cultural studies in higher education? To begin to shed some light on this question I shall now run what scientists call a 'thought experiment' by taking one isolated feature of cultural studies – the knower mode of legitimation – and 'running' it by itself to see how it works and what implications it might have for cultural studies.[11] It cannot be overemphasised that this is not intended as a history or account of cultural studies; the aim is to show how the form taken by the legitimation of cultural studies may help shape the intellectual and institutional development of the subject area. To this extent, one might say that any resemblances to academic subjects, living or dead, are purely coincidental or, at least, interestingly contingent. It is thus worth bearing in mind here the contradictory pictures of cultural studies with which this article began.

[11] The following analysis draws upon sections of Maton (2000a, 2000b), which elaborate the intrinsic dynamic of knower modes.

The Proliferation and Fragmentation Process

For the sake of this experiment we begin with a situation where the dominant form of legitimation is that exemplified by Enlightenment conceptions of knowledge, something approximating to a positivist model. Using a knower-based form of legitimation, I critique this dominant notion of knowledge as silencing the voice of people such as myself. Until now, I claim, the production of knowledge has been monopolised by people with different inter-subjective characteristics to myself. These knowers, I argue, can know only from their own social and temporal location; their knowledge is true enough for them, but says little about, for or to knowers of my ilk.

Happily (for me), on the basis of this knower critique I carve out a space for myself within the intellectual field and higher education – my voice begins to be heard. Less happily, perhaps, I am now in the most vulnerable position to a similar form of critique. My position is underpinned by knower legitimation, a claim to privileged insight based on my subjective attributes, where 'truth' is defined as whatever is proclaimed by my 'voice', rather than on my knowledge of specialised procedures – a socialised rather than trained gaze. This knower category, however, could be said to itself conceal difference, silencing the voices of others. However low in the academic pecking order the position I managed to acquire, I am still now part of that order and susceptible to this critique and it is difficult to maintain a knower mode whilst denying to new voices that which I claim is denied to my own. It is, therefore, highly likely that, sooner or later, I will be subject to critique by a new knower, who would in turn themselves be subjected to knower critique by a newer knower. If these critiques were successful, then as each new voice is brought into the academic choir, the privileged 'knower' would become smaller; as more and more social categories are introduced, each new knower would be increasingly precisely defined.

So, for example, if I began by legitimating my practice and ideas on the basis of being a member of or giving voice to the (previously excluded) working class, then as new voices emerge (based, for example, on categories of gender, race and sexuality) which critique my ability to speak on their behalf, the basis of my knower claims may increasingly hyphenate: from 'the working class' to working-class-men, white-working-class-men, white-heterosexual-working-class-men and so forth. The multiplicities of subjectivity and identity mean that the potential categories for this process could be endless. Thus, my knower claims may become based on speaking for or giving voice to, say, Oxbridge-educated, white, heterosexual men of working-class origin currently seeking employment in higher education. Eventually one reaches simply me – 'I know because I am Karl Maton'. (Indeed, at this point one could introduce notions of the fragmentation of the self and talk of 'we'). It is easy to demonstrate (and to argue) that all categories conceal substantive difference to some degree. Once one knower category is made the basis of legitimation, then the likelihood is that this category will fragment, producing a proliferation of evermore hyphenated, smaller and smaller categories, each strongly differentiated from one another and each with its own representative or sponsor. Unlike notions of a neutral language to which everyone may stand in equal alienation, this form of legitimation argues for some and not others; it is exclusive (for each knower proclaims its own unique insight) rather than inclusive (cf. Moore and Muller 1999).

It is worth at this point returning to the structure of another form of knower legitimation, that of the *Ancien Régime* (see Figure 2), to which the process of proliferation and fragmentation exhibits rotational symmetry. Figure 2.1 shows the structure of papal and feudal hierarchies, where the authority to speak (and legitimacy of authorship) diminishes as one moves from the one to the many, from the single, divinely delegated knower at the top to the multitude at the bottom – from the sacred to the profane. Compare this to the process of proliferation and fragmentation over time I have been describing, which can be represented as Figure 2.2. So, to take cultural studies as an example, it might begin with the 'three kings' of Richard Hoggart, Raymond Williams and E.P.Thompson and the category of the working class, before dividing according to gender under the impact of feminist interventions in the 1970s, then dividing again according to race and later sexuality and so forth – a process of proliferation and fragmentation of knowers.

In the example I have been outlining, the hierarchy of legitimacy within this knowledge formation might look something like Figure 2.3., where the more hyphens one's knower category embraces, the more authoritative or authentic one's knowledge is claimed to be. Here the profane is the past and characterised by relatively less plurality. The development of a knower mode over time thereby comes to resemble, to adopt a slogan of the English Civil War, 'the old world turned upside down'. To this extent, it could be argued that this characteristic of cultural studies is not opposed to an *Ancien Régime*, but rather represents an inverted form of pre-Enlightenment ideas; Popes, Kings and cultural studies (in terms of legitimation) share more in common than one might have thought. Where legitimation is based on the valorisation of *dominated* knowers, then it would also represent the social world turned upside down; the hierarchy of legitimacy or relative status of knowledge claims within the academic subject inverts the hierarchy of social power found in wider society. Thus, in the case above, whilst my working-class credentials would (at first) be relatively valorised, later adjectives (white, heterosexual, Oxbridge-educated, etc.) would be of comparatively lower status. A subject area experiencing this process would thereby come to resemble a procession of the excluded.

Figure 2: The Rotational Symmetry of the 'Tree Diagram'

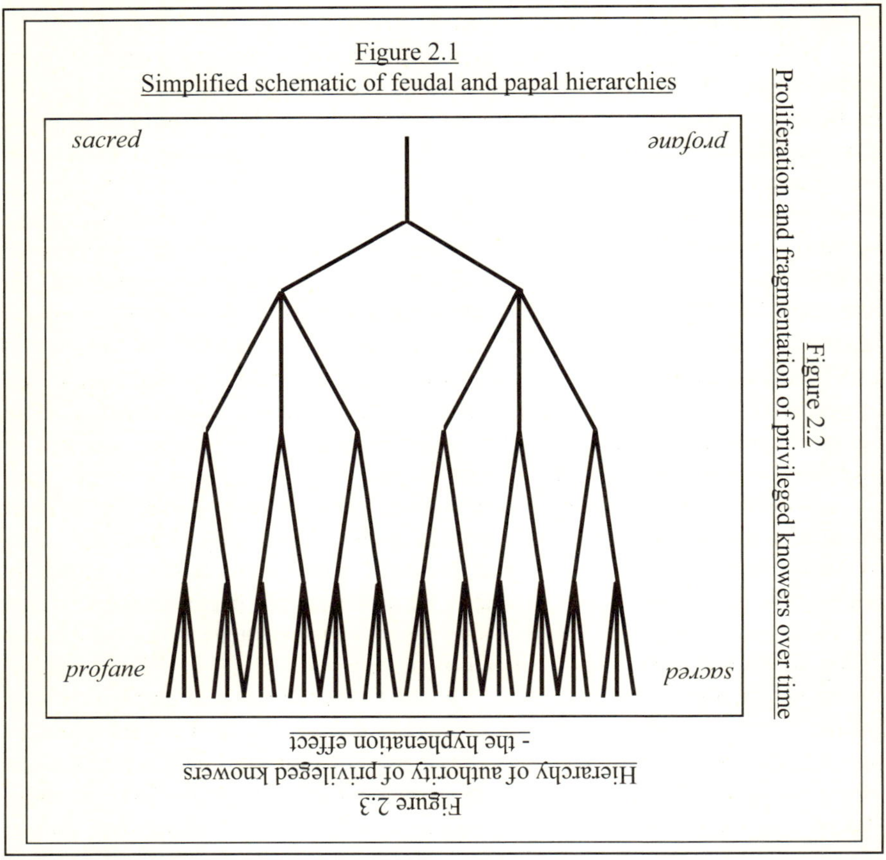

Intellectual Impacts

How might this process affect the intellectual and institutional positions of a subject area characterised by knower legitimation? In terms of intellectual development, two potential implications of this process are the fragmentation of objects of study and historical amnesia.

Towards narcissism

With proliferation and fragmentation of knowers, the focus of knowledge claims tends to get smaller as the social world is broken down into the incommensurable experiences of evermore specialised knowers. Thus, attempts at capturing social or cultural totalities would give way to thicker and thicker descriptions of smaller and smaller phenomena, fragmenting 'culture' into increasingly localized cultures. This itself generates pressures toward methodological individualism; approaches which claim to provide insight into these fragmenting categories might thereby come to assume increasing prominence. So, for example, one could witness a tendency to move from sociology towards social psychology, then psychology, and finally psychoanalysis. At this point, dialogue and translation become (in theory) impossible and there is little option but to retreat into autobiographical reflection, what Gellner (1992: 26) calls 'narcissism-hermeneuticism' – the search for certainty slips into solipsism. (Indeed, there would in fact be little point in writing at all, unless writing for an audience of one). Although each knower claim would highlight the claimant's relation to a wider social group, any attempts at connecting with such groups or movements would thereby become increasingly problematic – the gap between espoused and enacted political impact would widen, whilst vulnerability to accusations of self-obsession and social redundancy would increase.

Historical Amnesia

A second implication for the intellectual development of the subject area is historical amnesia (Maton & Moore 2000). I have mentioned that as proliferation and fragmentation takes place the past becomes the profane, a past of the dominant Other(s). This past tends to be dismissed with the emergence of the new knower. When it is the knower rather than the knowledge which is emphasised in claiming authority, then the focus becomes less critique of the message than shooting the messenger; it is not *what* has been said before that matters, it is *who* has said it. One sees this in the examples of Kings. Charles I, for example, faced the ultimate *ad hominem* argument in January 1649: his head was chopped off! Even then, the form taken by legitimation remained in place. In this case, Oliver Cromwell was first offered the Crown, then became *de facto* King, declaring in 1656: 'I could not refuse the power God put in my hands'. (Between 1327 and 1485 seven reigning monarchs of England were deposed; each time a rival claimant took over and the knower mode itself remained unquestioned). Although today the pen has replaced the sword, the principle remains the same: the past knower is deposed in favour of a new knower.

As this occurs, the intellectual past of the subject area is likely to become detached from its present and future. If knowledge is reducible to knowers, then new knowers bring new knowledge which existing voices are incapable of articulating. Existing knowledge cannot be integrated within the new discourse and must be displaced by the knowledge specialised to the new knower; as Bernstein puts it:

> Theories are less to be examined and explored at conceptual and empirical levels, but are to be assessed in terms of their underlying models of man and of society...

> The danger of "approach paradigms" [and knower modes] are that they may tend to witch-hunting and heresy-spotting; at the same time, they do provide a social basis for the creation of new – or the invigorating of old – sociological identities. (1977: 157, 158)

One would then witness a subject area perennially declaring radical breaks with the past. With each new knower, past work would be ostensibly abandoned, but then also reproduced from scratch – new messenger, same old message. If those disciplines which forget the past are likely to repeat it, then this might 'lead to a setting up of artificial obsolescence and rotation of fashion, characteristic of the consumer goods industry' (Gellner 1992: 46). In other words, the subject area would generate much sound and fury, signifying nothing – very little real 'news'. Intellectually, knower legitimation may thus lead to an energetic and vibrant knowledge formation, but one riven by fragmentation and exhibiting little discernible progress, a situation where, as Yeats put it,

> Things fall apart; the centre cannot hold;
> Mere anarchy is loosed upon the world...
> The best lack conviction, while the worst
> Are full of passionate intensity
> (Yeats 1919 'The second coming' 1.1-8).

Though the aim may be to bring as many voices into the choir as possible, the result may become a babble. If music is but organised noise, then the knower mode offers no common hymn sheet or conductor, no rules of method by which to achieve harmony for its range of voices, for each may sing what and how they wish.

Institutional Impact: Invisibility

In terms of institutional positions, the proliferation and fragmentation process leaves subject areas vulnerable and makes attempts to carve out sustained and discrete spaces within higher education problematic. Knower legitimation emphasises difference from rather than similarity with other knowers, encouraging struggles between different knowers and within specific knower categories. Questions arise, for example, as to whose is the *genuine* voice of the working class, which knower is the *real* working-class knower, leading to 'prolier than thou' legitimation struggles. Such struggles undermine the social bases for collective political action (such as through professional associations), including defence of the subject area from competing claims to status and resources. Moreover, knower modes are particularly vulnerable to utilitarian funding policies and attacks from without higher education questioning their purpose. One means of legitimating a discipline is to assert the significance of its object of study, but knower forms of legitimation focus instead on a subject of study, the previously silenced knower. The term 'previously' is key here, for this strategy depends on the voice being silenced and even proclaiming this leaves one open to counter-claims of being heard, undermining its force, and to further knower critique by a new voice.

Lacking an explicit strongly defined notion of what can and cannot be studied also leaves the subject area vulnerable to indiscriminate poaching of its actors and ideas. Instead of creating, for example, a named cultural studies department or course, one can add a module or staff member to existing institutional arrangements or adopt 'cultural' as a prefix without altering one's intellectual practices. Indeed, the fragmentation of knower modes makes them ideally suited to the marketisation and "pick'n'mix" modularisation of higher education. Such subject areas may thus, as Bernstein (1996: 177-8) puts it, 'reveal a suicidal tendency', resulting in a loss of original identity:

> Here, paradoxically, the [academic] subject shines with an invisible light in other knowledge structures when it may itself be dying.

Conclusion

What implications would this process of proliferation and fragmentation have for the position of cultural studies? On the one hand, it would leave cultural studies in an extremely precarious institutional and intellectual position, vulnerable to poaching by other forms of knowledge and possibly losing any sense of direction – the disciplinary map may swallow it whole without digesting its project. On the other hand, one could argue that cultural studies would thereby plant seeds in other disciplines, that culture is now being taken seriously by academia and 'a rose by any other name smells just as sweet'. One could additionally argue that a knower mode of legitimation represents a pragmatic and temporary strategy for carving out an initial space within higher education, regardless of any other implications. This may be true enough, but history teaches us that it is always difficult to decide when such strategies are redundant; they are habit-forming and, as illustrated above, the knower mode has a tendency to bite back.

These are the kinds of questions which have come to vex cultural studies. What I have done is to isolate *one* internal feature of cultural studies to show its potential implications for the subject's position in higher education. As I have emphasised, this is *not* the whole story, but it does show that any account of cultural studies – past, present or future – needs to address not only issues of agency or social structure but also the *internal* features of cultural studies as a knowledge formation. All too often, commitment and sincerity have been considered, at least tacitly, sufficient and questions of consequences and effects neglected. Where cultural studies has developed in directions not to one's liking, the temptation is to explain these in terms of external hindrance or lack of effort.

Both may indeed be true, but I am asking: what if the consequences of the stances we take lead to effects at odds with the ends we seek?

Although I have, somewhat provocatively, compared one aspect of cultural studies with papal infallibility and the divine right of kings, it is worth emphasising their differences. The most obvious is that whilst the knower mode of my thought experiment exhibits proliferation and fragmentation, the position of monarchs and Popes as privileged knowers have remained stable over relatively long periods of time. This highlights that the process is in no way inevitable. It is, rather, a power, tendency or disposition of knower modes of legitimation. Whether that tendency is realised depends on the empirical context. In practice, tendencies may be unexercised (because of a lack of enabling conditions), exercised unrealized (due to countervailing pressures), or realized unperceived (see Bhaskar 1975, 1979). In the case of 'popes and kings', the conditions for evoking this process are either absent or countered by other forces, such as social power and control in the form of the monopoly of violent coercion or the means of manufacturing consent. The structure of legitimacy was held in place at least partly by force; open questioning was largely forbidden and punishable in some cases by death – one could not have rival knowers. Thus, the tendency to proliferate and fragment is evident in feudal hierarchies when this countervailing pressure diminishes, such as when kingdoms break down into rivalrous fiefdoms under weak monarchs.

It is thus not the case that proliferation and fragmentation *must* result from adopting a knower mode of legitimation. The next task is to analyse the determinate conditions under which this tendency is either evoked and enabled or countered. This is to highlight the significance of social conditions and relations of power and the possibilities of agency in determining the ways in which specific academic subjects might develop. Knowing this tendency of the knower mode does not predict practices, but it does provide the basis for a slow reach again for control, as Raymond Williams put it, over their development – knowledge as power instead of a reduction of knowledge to power.

The future direction of cultural studies and its ability to change the disciplinary map thus depends not simply on commitment and effort, but also on understanding how the ways we describe ourselves have very real impacts on our own institutional and intellectual positions and thus what we are able to achieve. In effect, then, and *in this context*, I am reversing Karl Marx's eleventh thesis on Feuerbach to argue that:

> Thus far we've tried to *change* the world (or higher education or the disciplinary map) in various ways. The point, however, is to *understand* it, in order that we might know not only on behalf of whom, but *what* and *how* change may be effected.

This requires the modesty and maturity to accept that perhaps good intentions are not always enough and the intellectual honesty to consider analyses which may not always say what we would like to hear: a culture of consequence alongside one of commitment.

Bibliography:

Bennett, T. (1996) "Out in the open: Reflections on the history and practice of cultural studies", *Cultural Studies* 10:1, 133-153.

Berlin, I. (1999) *The Roots of Romanticism,* London: Chatto &Windus.

Berlin, I. (2000) *The Power of Ideas*, London: Chatto & Windus.

Bernstein, B. (1977) *Class, Codes and Control, Volume III: Towards a theory of educational transmissions*, London: Routledge & Kegan Paul.

Bernstein, B. (1990) *Class, Codes and Control, Volume IV: The structuring of pedagogic discourse*, London: Routledge.

Bernstein, B. (1996) *Pedagogy, Symbolic Control and Identity: Theory, research, critique* , London: Taylor & Francis.

Bernstein, B. (1999) "Vertical and horizontal discourse: an essay", *British Journal of Sociology of Education* 20: 2, 157-173.

Bhaskar, R. (1975) *A Realist Theory of Science*, London: Verso.

Bhaskar, R. (1979) *The Possibility of Naturalism*, Hemel Hempstead: Harvester Wheatsheaf.

Biagioli, M. (1993) *Galileo, Courier: The practice of science in the culture of absolutism*, Chicago: University of Chicago Press.

Bloch, M. (1962) *Feudal Society: The growth of ties of dependence,* London: Routledge.

Blundell, V., Shepherd, J., and Taylor, I., eds. (1993) *Relocating Cultural Studies: Developments in theory and research*, London: Routledge.

Bourdieu, P. (1988) *Homo Academicus*, Cambridge: Polity Press.

Bourdieu, P. (1991) "The peculiar history of scientific reason", *Sociological Forum* 6:1, 3-26.

Bourdieu, P. (1993) *The Field of Cultural Production*, Cambridge: Polity Press.

Burrell, J. (1683) *The Divine Right of Kings*, Cambridge: John Hayes.

Critchley, J. S. (1978) *Feudalism*, London: Allen and Unwin.

Daston, L. (1992) "Objectivity and the escape from perspective", *Social Studies of Science* 22, 597-618.

Gellner, E. (1974a) "The new idealism – cause and meaning in the social sciences", in: Giddens, A., ed. *Positivism and Sociology*, London: Heinemann.

Gellner, E. (1974b) *Legitimation of Belief*, Cambridge: Cambridge University Press.

Gellner, E. (1978) "Philosophy: The social context", in: Magee, B., ed. *Men of Ideas*, Oxford: Oxford University Press.

Gellner, E. (1992) *Postmodernism, Reason and Religion*, London: Routledge.

Golding, P. (2000) "What we need to know and why do we need to know it?" Paper presented at *The Future of the Media (and Media Research)*, ESRC Seminar, Stirling, January.

Hall, S. (1992) "Cultural studies and its theoretical legacies", in: Grossberg, L; Nelson C., and Treichler, P.A., eds. *Cultural Studies*, London: Routledge.

Hume, D. (1978 [1739-40]) *A Treatise of Human Nature*, Oxford: Clarendon Press.

Johnson, R. (1983) "What is cultural studies anyway?", *CCCS Stencilled Occasional Paper*, 74.

Maton, K. (1996) "Cultural studies in higher education: A framework for enquiry". Paper presented at *Teaching Culture and the Cultures of Teaching: An Interdisciplinary Conference*, Sussex, March.

Maton, K. (1999) "Extra curricular activity required: Pierre Bourdieu and the sociology of educational knowledge", in: Grenfell, M., and Kelly, M., eds. *Pierre Bourdieu: Language, culture and education,* Bern: Peter Lang.

Maton, K. (2000a) "Languages of legitimation: The structuring significance for intellectual fields of strategic knowledge claims", *British Journal of Sociology of Education*, 21: 2, June, 147-167.

Maton, K. (2000b) "Recovering pedagogic discourse: A Bernsteinian approach to the sociology of educational knowledge", *Linguistics & Education* 11: 1, October, 79-99.

Maton, K., and Moore, R. (2000) "Historical Amnesia: Victims of fashion and outbreaks of 'breaks' in the disciplinary map", Paper presented at *British Sociological Association Annual Conference 2000: Making Time – Marking Time*, University of York, April.

Miller, R.E. (1994) "'A moment of profound danger': British cultural studies away from the Centre", *Cultural Studies* 8: 3, 417-437.

Moore, R. (2000) "For knowledge: tradition, progressivism and progress in education – reconstructing the curriculum debate", *Cambridge Journal of Education*, 30: 1, 17-36.

Moore, R., and Maton, K. (2001) "Founding the Sociology of Knowledge: Basil Bernstein, intellectual fields and the epistemic device", in: Morais, A., Neves, I., Davies, B. and Daniels, H. eds. *Towards a Sociology of Pedagogy: The Contribution of Basil Bernstein to Research*, New York: Peter Lang.

Moore, R., and Muller, J. (1999) "The discourse of 'voice' and the problem of knowledge and identity in the sociology of education", *British Journal of Sociology of Education,* 20: 2, 189-206.

Morton, T. (1643) *The Necessity of Christian Subjection*, London: s.n.

Nelson, C., and Gaonkar, D. P., eds. (1996) *Disciplinarity and Dissent in Cultural Studies*, London: Routledge.

Norbrook, D. (1999) *Writing the English Republic: Poetry, rhetoric and politics, 1627-1660*, Cambridge: Cambridge University Press.

Popper, K. (1972) *Objective Knowledge*, Oxford: Oxford University Press.

Shapin, S. (1988) "The house of experiment in seventeenth-century England", *Iris* 79, 373-404.

Shapin, S. (1994) *A Social History of Truth: Civility and science in seventeenth-century England*, London: University of Chicago Press.

Striphas, T., ed. (1998) *The Institutionalisation of Cultural Studies: Cultural Studies*, 12:4.

Swartz, D. (1997) *Culture and Power*, Chicago: University of Chicago Press.

Ward, S. (1997) "Being objective about objectivity: The ironies of standpoint epistemological critiques of science", *Sociology* 31, 773-791.

'ALARMING AND CALMING. SACRED AND ACCURSED' – THE PROPER IMPROPRIETY OF INTERDISCIPLINARITY

PAUL BOWMAN

This work[1] addresses the question of cultural studies' aims, objectives, and methodological or paradigm orientations, from two apparently contradictory standpoints of (1) the institutional context of the discipline's location (its interdisciplinary situation of being both 'between' and 'across', as well as invading and transgressing other disciplines and their protocols and procedures); and (2) the 'quasi-transcendental' mode of deconstructive interrogation. The work is in one sense merely a reading of Derrida's *Dissemination*, and in particular 'Plato's Pharmacy'. But this reading is informed by more explicitly literal studies of hegemony, power/knowledge, and the politics and role of knowledge in culture and society, which considers the institution of cultural studies in relation to Derrida's arguments about structural overdetermination. So this work argues that cultural studies' aims, intentions, remit, and even and especially its public reception, can all be seen to be reaction formations, which, nevertheless, enable us to garner a clear sense of the strategic 'mission' of cultural studies, one which will be politically and pedagogically effective, and which clarifies the roles and orientations that cultural studies should have in order to impact positively (politically and ethically) on academia and therefore, in disseminated, deferred and referred ways, on the culture it claims merely to study.

> The liberty *of the question* (double genitive) must be stated and protected. A founded dwelling, a realized tradition of the question remaining a question. (Derrida 1978, 80)

In asking and trying to answer a question like 'what is cultural studies?' we would already – whether we knew it, wanted it, or not – be participating in an ultimately interminable reflection, one that is often deemed to be little more than an irritating digression away from more urgent and important matters. Yet this entirely academic question has an urgency and importance that is often overlooked, ignored or even denied. Indeed, even such *avoidance* has an urgency,

[1] An earlier, 'equivalent but different' version of this work – with a different orientation, argument, and conclusion, but with similar readings of the texts covered here – appeared in the *hot property* issue of the journal *parallax* (Taylor & Francis/Routledge, 2001, vol. 7, no. 2, 50-65), entitled "The proper-ties of cultural studies".

although it will never present itself as 'urgent' in the usual sense; for this 'urgency' devolves on the issues raised by the 'fact' that such an irritating question *won't go away*, and that *avoiding* this question (as if it had been adequately answered) is justified on the basis (or bias) of an obdurate insistence about the obviousness of what is 'obviously' urgent (and accordingly what should obviously be done in light of this obviousness). But, in asking and trying to answer the question 'what is cultural studies?' we would instantly have to call everything that is 'obvious' into question, for we will also be obliged along the way to re-pose the question as 'what is the *aim* of cultural studies?' Any answer to this will have to confront the question, 'what is the aim of this *academic* practice?', and, by extension, 'what, *as academics*, are we meant to be doing?' In fact, the question is tied to the very question of academic activity itself: the point and purpose of academic activity. And when *cultural studies* asks such questions, it touches on a particularly sensitive academic nerve: for the *way* cultural studies poses this question, and the position it occupies 'within' the university, reveal that 'cultural studies' (as 'subject' and 'object') exists at the point of an extremely painful injury (in the physical and legal senses of the word) 'within' the university.

In an 'obvious' sense, this much might easily be deduced from the febrile character of attacks on cultural studies. But this is a matter (of 'fact') that we will leave implicit and 'taken as read' here. For, rather than looking at the 'reception' given to cultural studies, we could do worse than take stock of an apparently paralysing, yet curiously ignored, set of conflicts right at the heart of cultural studies. For, what is its object, 'terrain', or 'field' of objects of its analysis, called *the cultural*? (see e.g. Hall 1996; Readings 1996). What, exactly, is cultural studies to study? The name 'cultural studies' gives little away, except a preliminary problem of specification, definition, demarcation and delimitation. This might justify its existence, to some extent: its object being the specification and elaboration of 'culture' or 'the cultural'. But couple this conundrum with another, that of the obligations specified for cultural studies by its founders (Hall 1996: 262ff), and note that this obligation is no less vague and even more euphemistic than its very first problem: namely that cultural studies should 'engage', 'confront', 'address', and even '*intervene*' in 'the cultural'. What in the world could that even *mean*, let alone *entail*? And furthermore, it has repeatedly been said that cultural studies *must not* merely take the position of a kibitzer or onlooker, from the safe, aloof, omniscient or sententious site of The University. Rather, as Stuart Hall said, in a 'retrospective' 'about' cultural studies (which can hardly be divorced from 'being' or 'doing' cultural studies itself; Derrida 1996: 22), that cultural studies, *to be cultural studies*, must never forget its ''worldly' vocation' (Hall 1996: 272): it has to be an academic practice tied to the problems, issues, and concerns of the 'world'; not merely to document, interpret or record them, but to *intervene*, take a stand, support, affect, work with, for, against and towards 'worldly', 'cultural' *things* (whatever any of this may mean, be, or entail).

Immediately, therefore, cultural studies is not 'neutral'. In saying it is to intervene, it is inevitable that many voices will denounce it as *biased.* But, what *is* its bias? In answering that question, one would have gone some way toward saying what it *is* and what it must seek to *do*. Yet, within cultural studies, there is little sign of any agreement as to how we should interpret 'our' vocation, what that vocation should be; or, where there may be some consensus about its premises and *telos*, there is little consensus about exactly *how* cultural studies should *do* what it is to do, which still amounts to asking what it is that it has to do; and therefore the question 'what is cultural studies?' remains. This is the same as to say that, whenever a 'cultural studies' academic presents a piece of work, of argument and analysis with a didactic 'message', this work, its 'message', will have been possible only on the basis of their advocation of a theoretical paradigm, that itself amounts to the imposition of a decision about what should be done and how.

The point here is at least twofold: First of all, the decision about who or what 'perspective' is 'right' also decides at the same time *what* one's aims should be and how one should therefore proceed. (The tautology here goes without saying.) And secondly, to note the fact that two people 'in' cultural studies may well advocate different paradigms[2] reveals that many disagreements, polemics, arguments, repudiations and *contretemps*, are predicated by a fundamental disagreement about the answer to the question 'what is cultural studies?' As Derrida has argued repeatedly, the decision about anything, if it is a decision, will also make a decision about the subject that is said to have 'made the decision'.[3] So, if we decide something like 'cultural studies should work to identify and combat the iniquities and injustices of capitalism', or something similar of 'patriarchy', 'ethnocentrism' or 'ideology', then 'our' identity, the identity of the subject of cultural studies, will also have been decided, at least provisionally, and this will reveal itself in terms of what will come to be seen to be the dominant paradigm, or ways of going about doing things, and indeed, *what* is done and *how* it is done. What orients disagreements – what actually enables any disagreement – arises as a result of fundamental differences in orientation: within cultural studies this amounts to different answers to the question 'what is cultural studies?' – a question that itself has different guises, such as: 'what should be done (as cultural studies)?' or, 'how are we to do it (to be cultural studies, and not something else)?' So, *this most abstract and irrelevant question is without doubt the most urgent*. For, what if the wrong decision has been made? What if

[2] Which is different from their holding different 'methodological preferences', because a 'paradigm' is an entire orientation, that will not just result in merely preferring one kind of analysis over another, but will rather determine *what* one is geared up to 'do' (prove, show, or teach) when using each method of academic practice.

[3] Derrida states this in rather more radical terms, and with more radical implications, but for our purposes, this understated reading will suffice. See, for instance, Derrida, in: Mouffe (1996: 84).

we are going about things in the wrong manner, a bad way, doing the wrong things, or doing the right things wrong? *Is* there 'a right thing to do'?

This latter question, which is inextricably bound up with the others, can be answered, I believe, by looking at the logic by which cultural studies was possible, and subsequently constructed, as a 'new' discipline. That is to say, we can see 'what' cultural studies 'is' by looking at how it was constituted and inscribed as an 'independent' academic subject. For, if we look at the history of, say, that which is called 'British' cultural studies, for instance, the overwhelming character of the initial (initialising) form of its initiation has the form of a *rejection*: a rejection of (1) the *ways* of going about doing (2) the *things* within (3) the *disciplines* of the university. In the spaces of literary studies, for instance, the legitimised range of valid (or 'appropriate') objects of study could be seen to be too eurocentric, and moreover, that the possibility of extending one's analysis *from* literature *to* the cultural (or anywhere else, for that matter) is automatically constrained by the fact that in departments of literature, one is only, chiefly, or primarily allowed to study literature. Even with concessions, such as syllabus expansion to include foreign or 'non-literary' literatures, one is constrained by the obligation to prioritise literature as the object of analysis. Within the human sciences, there is only so far that one can go in questioning the methodological presuppositions necessary for objectifying 'subjects' as statistics or other such formalisable data. Even when the considerations of criteria are made radically complex and inclusive, there will always be exclusion, regulation and homogenisation *in order for any order to be imposed at all* (Hunter 1999: 47ff). And, in disciplines where the establishment of valid data and calculation is the order of the day, those who reject the validity of what are imposed as being 'necessary methodological procedures' will thereby remove themselves from that discipline, its sanction, validation, and remit, because their actions will amount to an affront to the proper practices and procedures of that discipline. The same can be said for those who question *too much* the imposition of form on *history*, on the *psyche*, on the *anthropos* or *humanitas*, on the *deus*, the *logos*, the *machina*, the '*Ding an sich*', the *referent*; or indeed, even on the *question*: of how far and the directions one can take questions, the kinds of questions that are allowed, admitted, given credence, taken seriously, or taken beyond the limits that that discipline deems 'reasonable'.

For all discipline imposes enabling limits; that is, a set of conditions within which one can work, in a well policed, 'legitimate', 'correct', or 'proper', way. To transgress, ignore or refute these conditions is to question the validity of everything done within and in the name of that discipline. It is to move 'outside' of that space, to call it into question, and also to incur the wrath of its judgement, a judgement that will inevitably come from a position that agrees with the premises, hypotheses, and proper procedures, that have been transgressed. Of course, this is not to demonise discipline, for, as Thomas Kuhn was among the first to argue, a discipline will often radically revise itself in the light of certain developments, even when they are heretical to its stated rules, premises, and protocols. But, as Kuhn's argument also implies, such revision or revolution is never without *resistance*. For, in pulling the rug out from under a discipline's feet, or attacking its integrity, it will defend its present form and status quo. Discipline also imposes a hierarchy: authorities, experts, canons, guarantors, traditions, obligations, syllabi, modes of communication, pedagogy, reproduction, maintenance and self-preservation. All of these institute and reproduce what that discipline 'is', 'does', 'knows', and 'should be': its enabling limits. These limits are, of course, a form of exclusion, of regulation and policing, related to the 'common sense' of *all* identity-formation itself. As Derrida has argued,

> To keep the outside out. This is the inaugural gesture of "logic" itself, of good "sense" insofar as it accords with the self-identity of *that which is*: being is what it is, the outside is outside and the inside inside. (Derrida 1997: 128)

The founding or foundation of cultural studies amounted to a polemical rejection of many exclusions. Its 'rejection' was based on the political and ethical stakes of disciplinary exclusion. For, as has been said many times, in excluding so much that was related to the literary, but said to be not-proper-literature, the discipline of literary studies was imposing a hierarchy that was 'elitist', eurocentric, and patriarchal, at least. In producing and reproducing this canon (according to *and as* a paradigm) of proper or 'best' literature, the discipline also imposes definitions of 'culture', of value and orientation, that will themselves be aristocratic, eurocentric and patriarchal. Similarly, in opting for statistical kinds of analysis, the human sciences participate in a reduction of 'human agency' to putatively 'objective' knowledge (Mowitt 1992: 34-35) that is in no way 'natural', 'objective' or 'true', but always based on an interpretive bias, on reduction, exclusion, and censorship (that is itself always already politically tendential). The same can be said of the disciplinary regulation of questions of historiography by subordination to canonical versions of 'History', of questions of art to 'Art', of the theological to 'Theology', the potentially philosophical to 'Philosophy', and so on.

Cultural studies' rejection, then, was a *rejection of rejection*: an affirmation of inclusion. Not a rejection of the academic imperative 'to study' and 'to know', but rather a rejection of the biases of the current instituted ways in which this imperative had been imposed and perpetuated as *the proper* way to study *the proper* things. Already deconstruct*ive*, if not deconstruct*ion*, anything which does this will be accused of amounting to a process of *destruction*, for the foundation of cultural studies amounted to a polemical rejection that would necessarily often be perceived as a disrespectful, irreverent affront to the academic disciplines from which it differed by seeking to re-problematize 'as questions' the very things that the extant disciplines would have either *decided in a particular way* or else effaced, denied, or silenced as questions (in order to proceed: for these questions amount to potentially intractable 'methodological' questions of the political and ethical dimensions of what is to be included, what excluded, what valued and why, and what ignored as irrelevance – in short, a range of considerations that, were they to be taken on board at every step, may well scupper the possibility of even taking a step outside of such questioning. None of which is very helpful for a discipline that needs to proceed pragmatically along the route that defines it as *being* that discipline *itself*).

In one way, then, this impropriety of cultural studies is therefore proper.[4] But it is also inevitable that in stepping on the toes of the other disciplines in this way, by reopening the possibility of their own injuriousness, it will be deemed *disrespectful*. For reasons that I hope to demonstrate, cultural studies is *always already* going to lend itself to the role of 'hate object', as Lola Young once termed it, even and especially in the eyes of those it is apparently closest to (Young 1999: 3). This is a risk – more than a risk: *a structural inevitability* – that cultural studies should perhaps take on board: it will be hated, resented, belittled, ridiculed. In short, it will lend itself to the role of *scapegoat*. Moreover, if this state of affairs is indeed 'structural', then it cannot be entirely specific to 'cultural studies'. It is rather endemic to 'interdisciplinarity' itself.

I could easily now move on, to a section of argumentation through examples so as to justify 'properly' this assertion by piling up examples of cultural studies and other interdisciplines having been treated as 'hate objects' in different discursive situations. However, let us instead take it as read that we all already know this, and that we could all point to as many examples of scorn poured on cultural studies as such a 'proper' justification might be said to require. Instead, I propose that we move 'away' from cultural studies specifically, and also that we do not 'ask' or expect 'proper' cultural studies academics to furnish us with an explanatory account of the *structural* condition of interdisciplinarity within the institution. Just as we might be ill-advised to expect a politician to tell us everything we want to know about 'the political', so perhaps the annals of institutional cultural studies might not necessarily be the best place to look to find out all we want to know about disciplinarity and interdisciplinarity. Instead, perhaps we could start from a text that deals with the foundation or institution of the *structurality of structure itself*.

Discipline's Pharmacy: Kettles, Goats, Symptoms, and Gods

> The word "between" has no full meaning of its own. (Derrida 1997: 221)

Cultural studies is often said to be 'interdisciplinary'. But 'inter-disciplinary' can only properly be read doubly: to *be* interdisciplinary, to *do* interdisciplinary work, the interdisciplinary discipline will always be *more and less* than one

---

[4] 'Properly improper (uncanny, *unheimlich*)', see Derrida (1996: 29).

discipline.[5] *On the one hand*, the claim of interdisciplinarity signals an eminently pure academic activity, consisting, as it would seem, of a redoubling of academic effort, in order to *master* more than one discipline, to be hyper-academic, to *be* more and *do* more than 'single' disciplines themselves.[6] But, *on the other hand*, the 'interdiscipline' will be less, or at least other than, *improper in terms of*, each discipline it travels between.[7] To claim some multiple mastery or comprehension from a position that is 'exterior' (albeit 'exterior within', in the form of 'in between'), can only be met by the accusation that it is no mastery at all, especially and necessarily in the view of those disciplines that, it is claimed, have been 'comprehended' by this *other* view.

The 'inter-', the 'across', or 'between' is *at once* the most admirable and proper imperative of academia: to find out more, to find out all, or as much as possible, to increase scope and vision, to see more, to *know* more.[8] Yet it is, *as well*, the most contemptible and improper ('*the monstrous double*'; see Mowitt 1992: 39-40): for it trespasses, precociously, irreverently, and disrespectfully. The 'inter' is buried or interred deep *within* academia, and yet it remains *outside* each of its component parts, *less* than each, claiming to be *more*. Moreover, the term 'discipline', when applied as the designation of a specific 'discipline',

---

[5] Although, 'interdisciplinary' is often invoked as if it means 'antidisciplinary', which is a completely different matter, as 'inter' does not mean 'anti', nor does it mean 'less than', 'other than', nor free from 'discipline'.

[6] Stuart Hall argues, insists, as much in the essay from which we have been quoting, although by way of reference to Gramsci, and without touching on this kind of a reading. So, whether he might 'agree' with this reading of the structural situation of cultural studies is debatable, but he would agree with this reading of interdisciplinarity as hyper-academic in intent and character (Hall 1996: 267-268).

[7] How can one master more than one, more than one at a time, especially if 'being' does indeed always mean 'being with'? (See Derrida's *Politics of Friendship*, especially the opening readings of Aristotle.) Or, if one can master more than one, then how many, and what is the nature of that mastery, is it a *different* mastery to the master who masters only one? It surely cannot be *equivalent*... How can one, trained in one discipline, go on to master another, while still retaining a living, fresh mastery of the first (if indeed 'being with' or 'living with' always entails preferring certain friends, to the detriment of certain others)? The mastery of 'too much' or 'too many' may be deemed no mastery at all, especially by 'proper' masters of one 'proper' subject, or it may perhaps change the nature of 'mastery' – but could it possibly change or hope to change the *should-be-like* or the *ought-to-be-like* of mastery in the eyes of declared unities and their masters? Worse still, how can *one* disciple, especially one who has been trained exclusively/ostensibly, in the 'both' or 'several' that are claimed to comprise the interdiscipline, then go on to claim to 'comprehend' the others, when that disciple's training was not *properly* 'within' any of them (in their own terms), and was in actual fact 'outside' of them all, elsewhere, in the curious space of the interdiscipline itself?

[8] And this is arguably the first stage of the 'political' project of cultural studies. See Hall 1996, and his delineation of cultural studies as a project seeking to create Gramscian 'organic intellectuals'.

already specifies that *that* 'discipline' is part of a series or family, all united insofar as they are all *disciplines*; that is, all disciplines are what they are only by and through being united and subordinated to *discipline* – the discipline of (academic) disciplinarity. That which calls itself 'interdisciplinary' *doubles*, rather than *reduces*, its ties to discipline, because the identity of the interdiscipline is constructed explicitly *through* its relations with other disciplines. As such, it takes from them its identity. Yet it must, to legitimise its existence, produce 'the new', 'new knowledge'. Borrowing and returning, covering the same ground, but being obliged and desiring to cover it differently, standing *accused* of theft, irreverence, and exappropriation, whilst claiming and wishing to 'produce', 'improve', 'add', and 'alter', the interdiscipline cannot escape from a recourse to an overdetermined kettle-logic, which takes the form of: (1) The knowledge I am returning to you is brand new; (2) the holes were in it when you lent it to me; (3) you never lent me any knowledge anyway (Derrida 1997: 111). The interdiscipline is bound, doubly, to affirm and deny, to try to fulfill its debt repayment and to refute it. For, just like the disciplines it parasites and offends, or supplements and, in supplementing, subverts, it must, to be *a discipline*, or to have an identity 'of its own', keep its outside out and its inside in (Derrida 1997: 128), just like the others. This is the logic, the good sense, of all that lies before it, the logic of possession, identity, and non-contradiction, that determines the very 'gaze' of institutional legitimation in whose eyes the 'new' discipline must seek validation.

So one can see how the interdiscipline both reassures and upsets the academy. It at once promises to add a new dimension in its overall aim of omniscience; yet it threatens to rattle the order of things, to reorder and potentially disorder; it is both promise and threat. This double status arises in terms of the idea or ideal of the academy (of) itself (promising a new that threatens the old, a reordering that disorders) and also in terms of the extant hierarchy or status quo. We might say, 'Alarming and calming. Sacred and accursed'(Derrida 1997: 133). But, the 'gaze' of the academy is not *unified* itself, its decrees are not *univocal*, and so, whilst it must still be said that the interdiscipline will be subject to '*its*' gaze and decrees, and whilst the interdiscipline must seek legitimation and validity only in '*its*' or '*their*' terms (i.e., the university's), yet it will still, to a certain extent, 'lie outside ['its' – the other potentates/disciplines of the institution] field of effectiveness'. For no one else, no other discipline does, is, or knows, what the interdiscipline does, is, or knows; and accordingly it is no one else's business to pass judgement on the knowledge that is the interdiscipline's 'property'. But the interdiscipline, remember, has stepped on others' toes, stolen from them, meddled in their business, and is inevitably going to encounter *disdain* – so what will be the form of this first attack?

> What indeed would be the first thing a disdainful god would find to criticize in that which seems to lie outside his field of effectiveness? Its ineffectiveness, of course,

> its improductiveness, a productiveness that is only apparent, since it can only repeat what in truth is already there. (Derrida 1997: 134)

What, in truth, is already there, before the interdiscipline comes along to supplement it, badly, wrongly, arrogantly, impudently, offensively, rudely? That which it lies between: a status quo, an institution, its histories, values, priorities, truths and rectitude. If the interdiscipline lies between sciences, then it may have a hope of counter-verifying the verifiable allegations it encounters, or 'producing' products that will exonerate it and prove its use, worth, and scientificity. But, if the interdiscipline lies across, steps on the toes of (or *shoes*, since no institution is naked or natural; Derrida 1992: 31; see also Derrida 1987), and threatens to subvert the authority of the 'unproductive' disciplines, then to whom or what will it appeal for verification of its productiveness? In 'challenging' or accusing the *already unproductive* disciplines (the *not properly productive*: the 'discursive disciplines', those that are already parasitic kibitzers, producing nothing but their own discourse) – namely those that a utilitarian or capitalist orientation would already challenge or accuse (literature, philosophy, art, history, theology, the 'scientistic' disciplines: sociology, psychology, anthropology, etc.) – then the interdiscipline would not only find itself challenged by the 'productive' disciplines (whose worth, value and rectitude are ostensibly beyond question, and *held up as the ideal of knowledge itself*), it would also be challenged and accused by the unproductive.[9] Both polarities threaten to *symptomatize* the interdiscipline. The 'productive', by showing the universally condemnable interdiscipline to be a symptom of the uselessness of all such 'unproductive' disciplines; and the 'unproductive' disciplines, by claiming, 'look what we are not!' or 'you see how bad we could be!', appeals that are to be read 'you see how bad we could be / how good and worthy we really are! Accept us, condone us, validate us; were you to do so, we would willingly offer this sacrifice up to you!'

The interdiscipline will always already necessarily risk being experienced as a certain '*poisoner*' (*pharmakos*), 'contaminator', 'defiler', 'parasite', and, hence, *evil*, *bad*, or *corrupt/ing* element. Yet, this is an evil that has been 'included' – an 'outside' allowed 'inside', or perhaps a better word would be '*admitted*'. For its *admittance* will have been an *admission* premised and legitimised on the basis of a loophole-like contrary injunction, a paradox, contradiction, or double bind, in the categorical(ly) academic imperative, in the idea and ideal of the academy and of knowledge. The institution admits what promises to complete or further the cause of its 'guiding idea', that which appealed for admittance by invoking this idea. And yet, if the 'new', in 'furthering' and 'supplementing' the extant, denies, challenges or accuses the instituted institutional norm, disdains it, then it will be said to have gone off the

---

[9] For an excellent analysis of the function of notions of 'usefulness' and 'uselessness' within discourses, polemics and ideas of the university, see Robert Young's essay, 'The Idea of a Chrestomathic University', in: Rand 1992.

rails, to have been misled and to wish to mislead, to have deviated and be deviant, to be deemed 'sophist' – 'the man of non-presence and of non-truth' (Derrida 1997: 68). As such, the sophist, the poisoner, must be excluded, to preserve the integrity of the institution:

> The character of the *pharmakos* has been compared to a scapegoat. The *evil* and the *outside*, the expulsion of the evil, its exclusion out of the body (and out) of the city – these are the two major senses of the character and of the ritual. (Derrida 1997: 130)

As we have seen, the outside has been admitted into the body proper in the first place as both a gamble and an insurance policy: to admit the risk, to admit the possibility of either a good or a bad 'surprise': either the new subject will prove beneficial to power/knowledge, or else it will at least be *contained*. Either way, the point is to have *prepared* for the possibility of any order of surprise; to have *mastered* the surprise, before it has happened, to have *disciplined* the surprise, in advance, organised all the conditions of possibility for its 'character' if and when it emerges. In the event of the possibility of either a beneficial or a detrimental surprise for the 'inside' of the body proper, it has unquestionably dealt itself a 'stunning hand' (Derrida 1997: 157): inclusion of what may well need to be purged, should a 'crisis' arise (to 'keep the enemy closer'):

> These exclusions took place at critical moments (drought, plague, famine). *Decision* was then repeated. But the mastery of the critical instance requires that surprise be prepared for: by rules, by law, by the regularity of repetition, by fixing the date… (Derrida 1997: 133)

In times of crisis, the unity and integrity of the institution will have organised, in advance, the interpretation, the diagnosis and the prescription – a purgative proscription, to restore the proper:

> The city's body *proper*… reconstitutes its unity, closes around the security of its inner courts, gives back to itself the word that links it with itself within the confines of the agora, by violently excluding from its territory the representative of an external threat or aggression. That representative represents the otherness of the evil that comes to affect or infect the inside by unpredictably breaking into it. Yet the representative of the outside is nevertheless *constituted*, regularly granted its place by the community, chosen, kept, fed, etc., in the very heart of the inside. These parasites were as a matter of course domesticated by the living organism that housed them at its expense. "The Athenians regularly maintained a number of degraded and useless beings at the public expense; and when any calamity, such as plague, drought, or famine, befell the city, they sacrificed two of these outcasts as scapegoats." (Derrida 1997: 133)

The Anxiety of Inter-Disciplinarity

To break off from this reading of *Dissemination*, which would take more time and space than is available here, we should note that what amounts to a cataclysmic possibility for the interdiscipline is an unlikely 'event' which yet reveals the logic by which the university 'admits'. There is no univocal authority of or to the university to guarantee that such violent expulsions will take this form, although they *do* take place, and regularly, and the justifications or rationales of these exclusions invariably fit perfectly this scapegoat logic, the expulsion of the 'unproductive' *pharmakos*. But, instead of focusing on this dimension of the reading, we might note that, of the *character* of any new discipline, it must, despite any 'novelty', 'difference' or 'radicality', *inevitably* 'begin by repeating without knowing' (*ibid*: 75) the *form* of the disciplines it mimes in order to become equivalent with it. For, the recognition of something as actually *being* a discipline depends upon its recognisability as being *like* a discipline. Its relations with what it differs from will be "virtually but necessarily 'citational'" (*ibid*: 98). For, like all entities or identities, the interdiscipline, "always springing up from without, acting like the outside itself, will never have any definable virtue of its own" (*ibid*: 102). It does not set its own value, but rather "it is the King who will give it its value, who will set the price of what, in the act of receiving, he constitutes or institutes" (*ibid*: 76). Its value, its meaning, its force and law, are / come from / go to outside of itself: the outside it is inside as outside and other than. But, as we have noted, in the case of the 'transgression' that enables the interdiscipline, this disrespectful rejection may amount to being received or elaborated as a kind of parricide (*ibid*: 143). The interdiscipline might be deemed incorrectly and unjustly to be that which does not "know where [it] comes from or where [it] is going, ... [a] discourse with no guarantor... Uprooted, anonymous, unattached to any house or country, this almost insignificant signifier is at everyone's disposal, can be picked up by both the competent and the incompetent, by those who understand and know what to do with it, and by those who are completely unconcerned with it, and who, knowing nothing about it, can inflict all manner of impertinence upon it" (*ibid*: 144).

But, the discourse of interdisciplinarity, as with all speech, "always needs its father to attend to it, being quite unable to defend itself or attend to its own needs" (*ibid*: 77). The attending, if absent, father, is institutional legitimation itself. To secure such legitimation, the new must repeat the old, the laws of the extant, and "repetition is always submission to a law" (*ibid*: 123). But, who repeats and what is repeated? – "they repeat each other" (*ibid*: 169). In the *establishment* (verb and noun), the *institution through inscription*, of both the figure and configuration of 'father-figure' and 'son', it is actually this 'inscription' *itself* that "is thus the *production of the son* and at the same time the constitution of *structurality*" (*ibid*: 161). The constitution of this structurality follows a certain dominant pattern (we could say, a pattern that has become more than *hegemonic*: rather, a pattern that has become the *hegemon* itself; see Vitanza

1997: 422). The pattern of the constitution of *structurality itself* proceeds "According to a pattern that will dominate all of Western philosophy, [in which] good [academic] writing [and practice]... is opposed to bad writing... And the good one can be designated only through the metaphor of the bad one" (Derrida 1997: 149).

The good as opposed to the bad, the right versus the wrong, the should and the should not. A certain figure authorises this figuration, a figuration which remains to dominate the discourses of propriety, rectitude, seriousness, sobriety, and the proper property of the institution. There is 'knowledge' – *disciplined* 'knowledge' – proper, respectful, traditional, and so forth: knowledge that is 'legitimate'. And there is that which is a party to discipline, but dallies and plays, disrespectful, disjointed, improper – the 'false brother', the errant son, 'traitor, infidel and simulacrum'. The good son, 'the brother of the brother' is 'the legitimate one', figured "as *another sort of writing*: not merely as a knowing, living, animate discourse, but as an *inscription* of truth in the soul" (*ibid*: 149). The good brother, the rightful heir, is the father's stand-in (proxy, representative, metonymy, *logos*); such that, in the relation between the right and the wrong, "The name of the relation is the same as that of one of its terms" (*ibid*: 117). Here, I would argue, 'science', the scientific, scientificity: the idea and ideal of 'knowledge': omni-*science* (mastery, control, predication and prediction, repetition).

The Injury of Interdisciplinarity

Many may protest that we have left the questions of cultural studies, what it should be (like) and what it should do, by the wayside. But, we have not – preferring instead, in a possibly unorthodox, possibly predictable and entirely orthodox manner, to try to relate the putatively unorthodox to the orthodoxy that legitimates it and constitutes the fundamental 'conditions of possibility' for its emergence. Another point to make would be that 'deconstruction' has provided us with more than just a manner of questioning (to which it has often been reduced), and that if one looks at even the most supposedly 'obscure' of his 'philosophical' texts, one finds Derrida dealing with precisely the questions and problems that have dogged or enlivened cultural studies from the outset.[10] In addition, we have argued that the 'condition' that has been characterised as 'the anxiety of interdisciplinarity', which is 'felt' perhaps most pointedly 'within' interdisciplines themselves, is not isolated to or 'within' them exclusively: If it is a *symptom*, then it is a symptom of a *general condition*, permeating the 'body' of the university. This is what Derrida has called a 'being-ill' (Derrida 1992: 7), an

[10] Compare for example: "The question of knowing what can be called 'philosophy' has always been *the very question* of philosophy, its heart, its origin, its life-principle" (Derrida 1995: 411).

'anxiety', he has also elsewhere called a '*malaise*', that is 'getting worse' (Derrida 1995: 411).

This 'injury', can of course be tied to an experience of the *project* of 'the university' that 'today' consists in having opened up the fissure or wound which is the university's very constitutive incompletion – that incompletion which summons all academic desire, and which yet scuppers it at the outset (because it can never be completed, decisively, definitively). As we have suggested, the injury is also an *in-jury*, in the sense of being tied to the injurious, the un-just. The injustices instituted and rained down upon the 'proper', established, status quo of disciplines by upstart interdisciplines like cultural studies, and the 'proper' disciplines' own defence mechanisms of retaliation, is experienced as injuriousness by the interdisciplines, that see themselves as operating legitimately in the spaces identified as 'between', 'beyond' and 'outside' the extant disciplinary demarcations. So, where the interdiscipline will see itself as remaining committed to the enlightenment injunctions of academia, through and through, the traditional disciplines into whose terrain it intrudes as 'other' and yet familial, will see its different orientations and paradigms as unsettling and troubling. If this 'injury' is 'constitutive' and hence irremediable, is there at least some 'therapy' or 'strategy', that might help establish the *should* and the *must* of what cultural studies is to do? For, if we have indicated the 'structural situation' of cultural studies, in some measure, then what should be prescribed (and by what *pharmacist*?), as being what it should or must do?

In dialogue with Derrida and Kant's theorisation of the university, in the collection, *Logomachia: The Conflict of the Faculties*, Timothy Bahti poses the question: 'How healthy is the modern university…?' (Bahti, in: Rand 1992: 68). In his account, which is given form, or in-formed, and figured through the images of *leverage*, and of all the oscillations and conceptual difficulties involved in thinking through "the opposition of right and left [which] does not arise from a conceptual or logical determination, but only from a sensory topology that has to be referred to the subjective position of the human body" Derrida, in: Rand 1992: 31), and also through his experience of the therapy to repair a collapsed lung (based on leveraging the injured lung with the strength of the healthy lung at the other side, to redress the balance), the injury to or of the university is that of "an imbalance between wings or projects of the university, such as that one faculty or capacity – that of 'science'... – is being celebrated and enhanced from within the university, while another – the humanities – is being belittled and reprimanded from outside" (Bahti, in: Rand 1992: 70). Noting that Humboldt had anticipated the possibility of this situation arising, in advance, Bahti argues that this is a question of *value*, for:

> The university will itself profit, and will allow the surrounding, supporting society to profit in turn, if it enters into the valuation of high-tech, cutting-edge applications of science, while it is threatened with suffering loss, …if it does not know and value the 'humanistic' values it ought to maintain. This is an injury of values or of evaluation: one part of the academic body becomes the *locus* of a promise of greatly

> increased values, while another part suffers an attack against its ostensible undervaluing or devaluing of values. (*Ibid*: 70)

Bahti has no qualms about offering his own suggestion for, if not a 'remedy' or 'solution', which carry the resonance of dissolution and absolution,[11] then a 'therapy', itself surely interminable, for this injurious imbalance in which the sciences are discursively overvalued as both profitable and the source and resource of all values, and in which the 'humanities', the supposed guardians and knowers of 'values' are accused of neither knowing them, nor measuring up to them, and actually of destroying them. As he says, this therapy would "seek to vitalize the very issue of evaluation, of the production and ascertainment of values", in which the work of the humanities would consist of "asking anything claiming value or having value claimed for it to justify such evaluation" (Bahti, in: Rand 1992: 70-71). For, the 'injury' and 'therapy' might be described as the following: "'Where are the values?' is the question put to the humanities at the same moment that values are everywhere claimed for university sciences – this is the injury. The same question, 'Where are the values?' put forcefully and insistently back to the university by the humanities, is the leveraged therapy" (*ibid*: 71).

Yet, we should perhaps note that Bahti is emphatically speaking of *the humanities*. The case of contemporary *interdisciplinary* study '*within*' the humanities, stands apart, somewhat, or 'outside', what he judges to be true of the humanities as a whole. While he says: "Few of us could deny, I believe, that the curricula we offer our undergraduate and graduate students, and the scholarship we expect and accept from our graduate students and colleagues, is preponderantly the history of literature, the history of art, the history of culture and society"; this is not strictly true of cultural studies. However, what Bahti goes on to say might be read as a manifesto for a procedure, revision, or revaluation of what the 'humanities' *should* do, *en masse*, and in adhering or in agreeing to such a procedure they would thereby be subscribing to a major step already taken by cultural studies, and which, additionally, therefore, can also be read as a (countersigning, validating) *justification* of cultural studies in terms of what the entirety of the humanities *should* do, in order to counteract injury and in-jury and in order to 'strengthen' themselves. For Bahti continues, and we should cite this at length (even though such an overlong citation might be thought improper):

> The injury, then, is one in which one part of… the 'humanities', has become so empowered that the other part, once called philosophy and now perhaps awkwardly designated as method, theory and metacritical, nonpositive analysis, is threatened with usurpation and atrophy. What one might mean by 'philosophy' here is… inquiring rationally, judging freely, and doing both all the way down to the principles of inquiry, reason, judgement, and freedom…

---

[11] "Both *solutio* and *resolutio* have the sense of dissolution..." (Derrida 1998: 3).

> For all the activity devoted to historical knowledge – by which I mean the courses, the examinations, the papers and dissertations and submitted manuscripts – there would be the repeated occasion, on each such occasion, for these small and simple questions: How? Why? So what? That is, the present distribution which, for some century and a half, has favored historical knowledge over its philosophic judgement, need not be revamped or done away with (which is hardly realistic anyway), so much as used as the fulcrum for the corresponding questions of how and why one knows such knowledge, questions weakened to muteness but thereby given voice by virtue of their very other. My sense of injury within the 'humanities' leads me to insist, quietly but firmly, that all historical knowledge without an accompanying rationale for its constitution and existence is counterintellectual, and ultimately counterrational. My sense of a possible therapy suggests that each bit of historical knowledge, each occasion for its articulation and transmission, should become the occasion for inquiry into its methodology and teleology. Even to acknowledge, and to insist upon the acknowledgement, that history has a history, and that the history 'known' is not a substantial object but a subjectively constructed cognition, can be critical in this context. Put more polemically: no history of literature, no history of art, no history of society, without a philosophy of history, a method of historiography, an internal and external accounting. (Bahti, in: Rand 1992: 72-73)

We see here, then, an injury 'within' the university in the relations between the scientific faculties and the humanities. This is matched by an injury 'within' the humanities, between, on the one hand, the historical, empirical, 'positive' branch, and, on the other hand, the 'theoretical', 'philosophising' branch. That which is 'accursed' in the eyes of the instituted hegemony of power/knowledge, the theoreticism of interdisciplines like cultural studies is elevated, made 'sacred'. Such sacralisation is precisely what takes place in the institution of *any* and *every* 'knowledge' as *being knowledge* of an order that must be mediated and controlled by an institution of 'knowers', or in other words, a discipline, as René Girard has shown (cf. Mowitt 1992: 38-40). In thus privileging 'theory' or 'theorisation' over any given kind or object of knowledge, one would thus be sacralising or fetishising at least the open-ended fact that "knowing is essentially theoretical" (Godzich, in: Weber 1987: 163), which, although, it is still a fetishising, it is at least a kind of tie that does not bind (and blind) one to counter-intellectually placing an essential limit on thinking, as is entailed by being encumbered with a proper set of undisputable 'facts'. Even thinkers like Bill Readings, who relate the rise of cultural studies to the deconstructive and destructive work of global capitalism, find hope in the possibility of countering all irrational, unintellectual, prejudiced, or ideological adherence to tradition and superstition, in all guises, by way of fetishising and 'essentialising' the value of 'Thought' itself: theory.[12]

Disciplines, once instituted, have a tendency to present 'their' 'knowledge' as definitive, correct, and sacred. This is always through the imposition of a

---

[12] Cf. Stuart Hall: "Hence, there are no theoretical limits from which cultural studies can turn back" (Hall 1996: 267-268).

hierarchy, a hegemony, a canon, and an economy of values, that are exclusive, and always in some measure violent, unethical, and biased. They inevitably prefer to 'reduce' their 'theoretical' component and claim it is merely one part of their whole make-up. Yet it remains the constitutive 'part', that ill-deserves to be treated as a supplement. So perhaps the best thing for cultural studies to do remains to be unsure of what it is and what it should do, and hence to question everything, as much as is humanly possible; and this is practical, pragmatic, '*real'*, not 'just theoretical'. Just as theoretical as everything else, except more justly so, for theoreticism knows itself as such, and does not mask, masquerade, or misrecognise itself, or dissimulate its constructed character, as 'proper knowledge' has a tendency or predilection towards. Though always unsettling, risky, challenging, and inevitably open to denunciation for being 'just theory', to *think things as theory*, is perhaps to be most open to what is called the 'ethical' and the 'political', to interrogate every injunction about what one 'must' do or be (like), for:

> The best liberation from violence is a certain putting into question, which makes the search for an *archia* tremble... *an-archy*... (Derrida: 1978: 141)

Bibliography:

Derrida, Jacques (1978) "Violence and Metaphysics: Essay on the Thought of Emanuel Levinas", in: *Writing and Difference*, London: Routledge.

Derrida, Jacques (1987) *The Truth in Painting*, trans. G. Bennington and Ian McLeod, Chicago: Chicago Univ. Pr.

Derrida, Jacques (1995) *Points... Interviews, 1974-1994*, Stanford, Ca.: Stanford UP.

Derrida, Jacques (1996) *Monolingualism of the Other; or, The Prosthesis of Origin*, Stanford, Ca.: Stanford University Press.

Derrida, Jacques (1997) *Dissemination*, trans. B. Johnson, London: Athlone.

Derrida, Jacques (1997a) *Politics of Friendship*, trans. G. Collins, London: Verso.

Derrida, Jacques (1998) *Resistances of Psychoanalysis*, Stanford, Ca: Stanford UP.

Hall, Stuart (1996) "Cultural Studies and its theoretical legacies", in: *Stuart Hall: Critical Dialogues in Cultural Studies*, London: Routledge.

Hunter, Lynette (1999) "Rhetoric and Artificial Intelligence: Computing applications in the sciences and humanities", in: *Critiques of Knowing: Situated textualities in science, computing and the arts*, London: Routledge.

Mouffe, Chantal, ed. (1996) *Deconstruction and Pragmatism*, London: Routledge.

Mowitt, John (1992) *Text: The Genealogy of an Antidisciplinary Object*, Durham and London: Duke.

Rand, Richard, ed. (1992) *Logomachia*, Lincoln & London: University of Nebraska Press.

Readings, Bill (1996) *The University in Ruins*, London: Harvard UP.

Vitanza, Victor J. (1997) *Negation, Subjectivity, and the History of Rhetoric*, New York: SUNY.

Weber, Samuel, ed. (1987) *Institution and Interpretation*, Minneapolis: University of Minnesota Press.

'THEOR-ESE', OR THE PROTOCOLS OF THE ELDERS OF CULTURAL STUDIES

MALCOLM QUINN

This essay offers some ideas on what cultural studies is 'for'. While refuting the notion that cultural studies is simply 'for' culture, I offer some definitions of how its apparently transgressive and revolutionary position may be seen as being 'for' the academy. I offer the hypothesis that the 'out-reaching' and 'over-reaching' methodologies of cultural studies construct a fantasy space in which academics remain in charge of their own disciplinary and institutional boundaries, transgressing or redefining them at will. This fantasy arises in a contemporary situation in which academics are actually less and less able to define the limits and set the contours of their institutional and professional domains. It is in the light of this argument that I revisit some aspects of the 'Sokal Affair', and claim that Sokal's intervention, far from refuting the anti-disciplinary premises of cultural studies, rather affirmed the institutional necessity of tenured radicalism and licensed transgression.

Whether one prefers one's culture with a big C or small c, as abstract entity or embodied practice, all culture is reaction formation, and the extremity of that reaction is proportionate to the condition that culture cultivates. In this sense, Cultural Studies is also a cultural formation, but not in the way that its practitioners often think. There is still a strong attachment by cultural theorists to those models which examine the conditions 'for' cultural practice, including Cultural Studies. This is to ignore the possibility that the condition is what the practice itself is 'for'. In addressing the question of what Cultural Studies is for, this essay discusses some aspects of the 'Sokal affair', which, as is well known, began when the physicist Alan Sokal submitted a spoof cultural studies article "Transgressing the Boundaries: Towards a Hermeneutics of Quantum Gravity" to the cultural studies journal *Social Text*, edited by Bruce Robbins and Andrew Ross (Sokal 1996). It was accepted, published in *Social Text* 46/47 in Spring/Summer 1996 and subsequently revealed to be a 'hoax'. I am arguing that what the Sokal Affair revealed was not a 'crisis in Cultural Studies', but a crisis in academia which is normalised as cultural studies. That crisis, I shall argue, is a crisis of distinction; more specifically, a question of whether the distinction between academic and non-academic is one that academics can make for themselves.

I should also state up front that the Sokal Affair is a dead issue, which is precisely what is interesting about it. What one can say with certainty about this imbroglio is that nothing happened, or more accurately what was revealed was how nothing had already happened, and nothing was already happening. Cultural studies stages a permanent anti-institutional revolution which nonetheless guarantees the university's historical cultural 'mission'. Sokal's article, with its kernel of pure nonsense, was both the cultural 'other' which guarantees the progressive, anti-institutional aspect of cultural studies, and the 'obscure object' of study which guarantee institutional continuity. In other words, 'Transgressing the Boundaries' did for cultural studies what cultural studies does for the University, which is to confirm that the University still has the rights to an idea of culture, that academia's reactions can be traced back to academic formations, and not to those that lie beyond its control. To give an example which I will be returning to throughout, it's all very well if you can feel that the domination of the dominated or the otherness of the other is your responsibility, less comforting if, like Professor Bernard Porter of the Universities of Newcastle and Yale, you find your lecture notes posted on the internet without your say so (Porter 2000: 12-13). Porter said that this made him feel that "what I had been offering as personal interpretation, attached to me, had been transmuted into general, objective truth, a kind of impersonalised commodity" (*ibid*: 12).

I would argue, however, that the key issue here is not the alienation of the individual, but the *form of the translation* from particular to general, which affects both the individual academic and the University as a whole. Academia is losing the form of its translation from academic to non-academic, in fact it can be said that the non-academic is increasingly translating academia back to itself, much as Bernard Porter found himself 'translated' on the internet. Cultural Studies, with its core fantasy of anti-, post- or inter-disciplinarity, represents this translation, on academia's behalf, as a problem which has its origin in the culturally reactionary status of academics and their disciplines. In this way, for example, art history is preserved by being 'culturalised' as visual culture. Alan Sokal's article was as conservative a reaction to the threats posed to the integrity of academia as cultural studies is, mainly because it was a model of the type of reaction-formation that has made cultural studies necessary. Sokal's narcissistic illusion was that in cooking up cultural studies he was really doing something else, that his flattery had a double meaning. Cultural studies practitioners also think that they are doing one thing and something else, namely academic work which is also cultural, that is, work which is reflexively and democratically situated within the conditions of all types of cultural practice. I have claimed, however, that we should pay less attention to the conditions for cultural practices and think more about what conditions the practice is for, which does not allow for the privilege of a double meaning for what you do, but does allow you to think about how to model the articulation of particular and general in the move from academic to non-academic. It doesn't matter, in terms of content, what is considered academic and what is not, and people can keep shifting that boundary *ad nauseam,* but what does matter a great deal, as I have said, is whether the distinction between academic and non-academic is a distinction that academics can make for themselves. In the example quoted by Bernard Porter, this 'power of distinction' has been lost – Porter does not know whether he is in the lecture hall or on the internet, and can't do anything about it, since someone has already made that decision for him. This is less an issue of the 'means of production' of academic labour than an issue of whether academia can still be said to produce itself, or is being produced elsewhere. This is what the institutionalised versions of cultural studies are 'for' – to promote the 'double meaning' that academic work is both itself and cultural, and retain a fantasy of distinction through a discourse on transgression. Such a discourse, for example, would allow Bernard Porter to think that he put those lecture notes on the internet himself, as a gesture of anti-institutional subversion. The Sokal Affair was an interesting case, because illusion was countered by illusion – it seemed as if *Social Text* had been robbed of the power of distinction by accepting a piece of nonsense, whereas nothing had in fact been altered. Sokal thought that Cultural Studies was selling both the academic store and the 'Old Left' down the river, whereas for some time, cultural studies had been busy destroying disciplinarity and left politics 'in order to save them', as well as breeding its own set of eschatological fantasies about external threats to academia.

I will turn to these fantasies in a moment, but first I'd like to mention the origins of Sokal's hoax in the publication in the Spring of 1994 of Paul Gross and Norman Levitt's book *Higher Superstition: the Academic Left and its Quarrels with Science.* Gross was Professor of Mathematics at Rutgers University and Levitt Professor of Life Sciences at the University of Virginia, and their specific attacks on socio-culturally based studies of science by offending authors of what they termed the 'academic left' had emerged from the already established 'Culture Wars' on American campuses, conducted over the status and legitimacy of 'postmodern' theory and critique and the relevance or otherwise of the 'Western' literary canon. Gross and Levitt claim that Sokal, at first dismayed by their attack on the left and then converted by the realisation that "a once-vigorous intellectual tradition of radical dissent... [was] slipping into irrationality" (Gross and Levitt 1994: x) was inspired to compose "his delightful parody" and submit it to *Social Text,* in the winter of 1994; as they state "the joke arose from Sokal's reading of our book" (*ibid*: x).

'Transgressing the Boundaries' models itself on Gross and Levitt's 'recipe' for 'Theor-ese', described in all seriousness as constitutive of the 'contiguous ideological field' of their foe, 'the academic left', and it was taken all too literally by Sokal when constructing his interventionist device. In 1994, Gross and Levitt had argued that:

> Each practitioner assembles his or her arsenal from favourite polemical bits and pieces – a little Marxism to emphasise the twinship of science with economic exploitation, a little sexism to arraign the sexism of scientific practice, a little deconstruction to subvert the traditional reading of scientific theory, perhaps a bit of

> Afrocentrism to undermine the notion that scientific achievement is inevitably linked to European cultural values. (*Ibid*: 11)

Sokal assembled his own 'arsenal' according to this supposedly descriptive model of a postmodern ideology and rhetoric, more in imitation of Gross and Levitt's generative schema than of any existing example of a typical article in a Cultural Studies journal. The result was a kind of 'Protocols of the Elders of Zion', a forged text intended to confirm suspicion, arouse condemnation, and to establish the existence of the academic left as a conspiracy, a 'contiguous ideological field'. The paradoxes multiply, since it was Sokal's intention to reassert the value of the 'true' left by unmasking the 'false' one; but he had first to assemble the *ur*-text of the '*faux*-left' to accomplish this aim.

What needs to be clearly stated is that the paranoid fantasy of 'Theor-ese' had already arisen from within Cultural Studies, as a reaction to changes in the market for intellectual goods, and what the cultural theorist Meaghan Morris described, in her seminal essay "Banality in Cultural Studies" (Morris 1988: 17), as the economic 'boom' in certain ways of doing theory. It is worth examining Morris' criticisms of Cultural Studies in parallel with the universalising 'ideology' evoked by Gross and Levitt, since, in some respects, she anticipates their paranoid vision of an all-conquering and all-consuming template for textual production. Morris argued that:

> Sometimes reading magazines like *New Socialist* or *Marxism Today* from the last couple of years, flipping through *Cultural Studies*, or scanning the pop-theory pile in the bookshop, I get the feeling that somewhere in some English publisher's vault there is a master-disk from which thousands of versions of the same article about pleasure, resistance and the politics of consumption are being run off under different names with minor variations. (Morris 1988: 15)

This is a latter day version of Karl Marx's comment in *Capital* volume 1, that "the literary proletarian of Leipzig" who produced compendia on political economy by rote was a factory worker in all but name (Marx 1976: 1044). This literary proletarian is Marx's projection of his activity into the commodity, a fantasy scene in which *Capital* would be just another book on political economy, just as Bernard Porter's Professorship becomes a set of notes posted on a website. What was intriguing about Sokal was that he wanted to prove that this fantasy of extinction was true 'in' academia, rather than true 'for' academia – in other words, it was all the fault of Cultural Studies, which is a bit like blaming the person that takes out the trash in a building for its structural faults. Once Gross and Levitt had imagined and specified the characteristics of a powerful means for occupying cultural and disciplinary space Sokal made it happen, returning a text produced according to the dictates of an imagined 'master-disk' or perfect template to cultural studies, as proof that this fantasy 'actually existed'. The fantasy, precisely, was that of a supra-mobile, efficient, pan-disciplinary agency progressing across forbidden terrain ("Transgressing the Boundaries"). Whether that fantasy takes the form of a 'master disk', a 'contiguous ideological field' or a 'cultural totality', the Sokal Affair shows it informing concrete actions within a supposed 'post-disciplinary' situation. Before it was revealed as a hoax, Sokal's original article seemed to the editors of *Social Text*, Bruce Robbins and Andrew Ross, to be an example of science haltingly attempting to translate its terms into the language of Cultural Studies. For Sokal himself, that same 'postmodern' language was becoming universalised to the point where it had begun to encroach on the turf of the sciences. But this is not a 'Two Cultures' issue; 'Theor-ese' is a fantasy about how things appear and where they appear, not about what it is that appears.

As I have said, the important issue here is not one of content or the canon, but to return to Bernard Porter once again, an issue of whether you are still doing the quality control – an off the cuff and witty lecture gets written up as an eternal truth which can, presumably, be fed back to Professor Porter in an essay. This is not so much what is known as 'shrunken head syndrome', but rather 'expanded head syndrome', in which the process of commodification has made your musings and improvisations definitive. Alan Sokal was also worried about quality control – his text was hard-won, perfect nonsense, synthesising a set of general principles in the form of an article which also serves as a kind of 'master disk'. The ultimate instance of the modelling of academic production without academic input is in Andrew H. Bulhak's 'postmodernism generator' web site.[1] Bulhack

[1] The 'postmodernism generator' can be found at http://www.csse. monash.edu.au/community/postmodern.html. See also 'Postmodernism Disrobed – Richard Dawkins review of *Intellectual Impostures'*, in: *Nature* 394 (9.7.98), 141-143, reproduced at http://www.spacelab.net/~catail/posfmoderism [*sic*] _disrobed.htm (14.10.98). Dawkins refers to Sokal's complaint about not having 'the knack' to produce sentences with 'no meaning whatsoever': "If he were writing his parody today, he'd surely have been helped by a virtuoso piece of computer programming by Andrew Bulhak of Melbourne: the Postmodernism Generator... it will spontaneously generate for you, using faultless [*sic*] grammatical principles, a spanking new postmodern discourse, never before seen... it is a literally infinite source of randomly generated syntactically correct nonsense, distinguishable from the real thing only in being more fun to read. You could generate thousands of papers per day, each one unique and ready for publication, complete with numbered endnotes. Manuscripts should be submitted to the 'Editorial Collective' of *Social Text*, double-spaced and in triplicate" (*ibid*: 4-5). In his response to Dawkins' review, Sokal agrees that the 'postmodernism generator' is amusing, but asserts that it could not pass itself off as 'the real thing (i.e. pass the academic postmodernist version of the Turing test)'. Sokal's reference here is to the famous 'blind' test proposed by Alan Turing, who suggested that a computer could be described as intelligent if a human being could not distinguish its responses from those of another human. Sokal goes on to say that the program's 'local structure' of a few sentences at a time "is an inauthentic imitation of a certain postmodernist academic style, they don't have the global correlations characteristic of real academic articles (even postmodernist ones). It would be really interesting to know if the program could be improved in this respect." He concludes by stating firmly that articles in *Social Text* "do NOT resemble the output of the Postmodernism Generator"

uses a system for generating random text from recursive grammar as his 'master-disk'. Every time a link on the web site is opened, the 'Dada Engine' produces another few pages of gibberish using recognisable keywords, rhetoric and famous names. Bulhark's 'postmodernism generator' employs sophisticated mathematics to produce studiously dumb results. To argue, as he does, that his program simulates 'postmodern' writing seems manifestly false, something that even Alan Sokal has acknowledged (see footnote 1); what it does is simulate a mode of 'production without production', a magical means of making academic products without academia getting in the way. The monstrousness of 'Theor-ese' is the phantasmic supplement of academics not knowing in the slightest what the future holds for them in the global market. The nightmare is that the *nirvana* of free trade in knowledge across a self-consistent global culture might just happen; not just academic procedure without disciplinary assembly, but academic procedure without academic input, a production without production, that is, a production without site, without contingency and without the slightest hint of inconsistency. This is another materialisation of the pervasive fantasy that one is being 'produced elsewhere'.

"Transgressing the Boundaries" was simply another reminder that the multivocal, multidisciplinary cultural debate that academia wants to see itself as engaging in with is a fiction, and that what seems to guarantee the 'conversation' is a mute, unreadable and meaningless object no longer attached to the 'enculturation' of disciplinary orthodoxy but instead solely to a process of modernisation which is ultimately driven by extra-academic forces; new objects discovered by constantly updated modes of production for new markets such as 'science studies', as exemplified in the 'Science Wars' edition of *Social Text* in which the article appeared. Without the fantasy of progressive debate, and without the support of traditional disciplinary prohibitions (both of which are linked to notions of cultural autonomy and its roots in national self-definition) Cultural Studies is just another player on the market, and its status as a University subject is compromised by the realisation that it is prolonging the living death of the tradition of 'enculturation' whilst at the same time proclaiming its anti-essentialist and anti-traditionalist stance.

This paradox is usually summed up in the dismissive description of Cultural Studies practitioners as 'tenured radicals' but this phrase, with its insinuations of venality and cynical opportunism, fails to entertain the more disturbing possibility that the quasi-disciplinary, quasi-intellectual project of cultural studies may be one of the few remaining means of securing a difference between the University sector and the free market in knowledge goods, of retaining the connection between the institution and its historical devotion to ideals of knowledge for knowledge's sake. This suggests another way of seeing Sokal's carefully crafted

---

(Alan Sokal http://www.gakushuin.ac.jp/~881791/Alan.html (14.10.98), taken from Sokal's e-mail conversation with Hal Tasaki, Department of Physics, Gakushuin University on 9 July 1998).

nonsense as an aspect of the 'work' of Cultural Studies; both as the annihilating object of academic modernisation on the one hand, and as a distillation of the way in which Cultural Studies is useful to the idea of the University, that is, as the 'nonsensical object', the piece of the real which itself sustains the ideology of the University; as Donald A. Norman, president of UNext Learning Systems and professor emeritus at the University of California has succinctly put it: "the university has a narrow view of scholarship: the more irrelevant the discipline, the more it is prized" (Norman 1999: 14). Sokal, of course, saw his nonsense only in relation to empiricist sense, but, again, Sokal's article is to *Social Text* what *Social Text* is to the University, that is, both are the guarantee of an extension of life and the harbinger of a possible death. In this light, the 'Emperor's New Clothes' fable, which has been used by defenders of Sokal to underline the message that the editors of *Social Text* (as well as thinkers such as Lacan, Kriseva, Irigaray and Latour) have been exposed as charlatans, might be reconsidered in terms of the paradoxical role which 'post-disciplines' such as Cultural Studies, and Cultural Studies practitioners, occupy in the contemporary University; that is, as Emperors not without clothes but without a kingdom or a state, whose business it is, nonetheless, to declare their rule over statelessness and entropy, and thus maintain normativity not in crisis but *as* crisis, by means of a permanent anti-institutional revolution which underwrites the institution's historical links to 'culture'.

I'd like to conclude by offering an unintentional yet apposite commentary on the 'culturalist' double meaning of cultural studies (and the 'positivist' double meaning of Sokal's nonsense) as it appears in a reference to Hegel's model of a 'Language of Flattery' in Slavoj Zizek's *The Sublime Object of Ideology*. Zizek (1989: 211) says:

> the subject can pretend that his flattery is nothing but a simple feigning, accommodation to an external ritual which has nothing whatsoever to do with his innermost and sincere convictions. The problem is that as soon as he pretends to feign, he is already a victim of his own feigning: his true place is out there, in the empty external ritual, and what he takes for his innermost conviction is nothing but the narcissistic vanity of his null subjectivity.

The important point to make here is that both Sokal and the editors of *Social Text* have had to believe that their practices were internally doubled, that they were both one thing and something else, and not simply part of the same 'empty external ritual' sustaining academia's idea of itself. What the Sokal Affair has revealed instead is that this notion of a doubled practice (positivism and nonsense for Sokal, or the discipline and 'the wider culture' for *Social Text*) sustains an illusion of control over the relationship between the academic and the non-academic. As Bernard Porter's example shows, that illusion can be shattered without warning. As he says, "If I had known that my lectures were to be disseminated so widely, I would certainly have given them differently" (Porter

2000: 13). Were this to occur, where would Porter then draw the line between the academic and non-academic?

Bibliography:

Bulhark, Andrew "The postmodernism generator", http://www.csse.monash.edu.au/community/postmodern.html

Gross, Paul R. and Levitt, Norman (1994) *Higher Superstition: The Academic Left and its Quarrels with Science,* Baltimore and London: John Hopkins University Press.

Marx, Karl (1976) *Capital,* Volume I, intro. Ernest Mandel, trans. Ben Fowkes, Harmondswoth: Penguin.

Morris, Meaghan (1988) "Banality in Cultural Studies", *Discourse,* 10: 2 (Spring-Summer) 3-29.

Norman, Donald A. (1999) "Prepare For a Shock", *The Times Higher Education Supplement,* September 3 1999, 14.

Porter, Bernard (2000) "Take Note", *The Guardian Education* 7.3.2000, 12 -13.

Readings, Bill (1996) *The University In Ruins,* Cambridge, Ma. and London: Harvard University Press.

Sokal, Alan (1996) "Transgressing the Boundaries: Toward a Transformative Hermeneutics of Quantum Gravity", *Social Text* 46/47 (spring/summer), 217-52 (reproduced in Appendix A of Sokal and Bricmont 1998).

Sokal, Alan and Bricmont, Jean (1998) *Intellectual Impostures,* London: Profile Books.

Zizek, Slavoj (1989) *The Sublime Object of Ideology,* London: Verso.

CULTURAL STUDIES AS RHIZOME – RHIZOMES IN CULTURAL STUDIES

SIMON O'SULLIVAN

This essay reconfigures the question of cultural studies and interdisciplinarity using Deleuze's and Guattari's concepts. Proposed is a different *geometry* of cultural studies – a geometry in which *movement* takes precedence over stasis and definition. In order to theorise cultural studies as a plane of consistency – in contact and connection with other plateaus and 'peopled' by intense thresholds and haecceities – it is important not only to take into account cultural studies' relation to existing strata (Cultural studies as a line of flight) but also, and at the same time, its continuing stratification (institutionalisations) and future lines of flight (deterritorialisations away from and beyond cultural studies). Formulating the questions of interdisciplinarity and institutionalization in these terms allows for a more dynamic mapping of the relation between centers and margins (strata and movement) and opens up new ways of looking at ethical issues of deterritorialisation and subjectivity. In conclusion, a notion of cultural studies as *experimentation* is proposed – away from cultural studies as the 'interpretation of culture' and towards a *pragmatics* which allows for a mapping of connections between different objects and practices, events and assemblages.

It seems to me that there are a series of assumptions behind cultural studies – assumptions which themselves produce the problem – or anxiety – of interdisciplinarity. Perhaps the most pertinent assumption is that cultural studies has a position within the academy, that is to say, is itself a discipline, at least of sorts. No doubt cultural studies departments – and centres – have to fight their corner. There is a certain pragmatics at work here: departments need funding, etc. But there is also a project of demarcation at work. In defining their area of enquiry – albeit, if Derrida is on the syllabus, by delimiting what they are *not* – cultural studies departments achieve a vicarious victory against the anxiety of homelessness. Those working within cultural studies have to earn their bread: hence the proliferation of journals, conferences, readers, etc., aimed specifically, at least in one sense, at demarcating a space, a project, for cultural studies. And this anxiety is tied into questions of pedagogy: cultural studies has to be something that can be *taught*. As such it must have at least a semi- coherent area of inquiry or else it risks take over moves, merger threats from other disciplines, other departments. Hence the anxiety about interdisciplinarity.

But, I think, there is a more powerful assumption behind cultural studies, an assumption that can perhaps be summed up with one word: interpretation. For this is what cultural studies does: it *interprets* culture. As such, cultural studies has two albeit inter-linked areas of inquiry: the field of culture itself and the field of methodologies for interpreting that culture. Cultural studies has, to put it simply, an object of study. As such cultural studies does not differ, at least not structurally, from other more traditional and established disciplines. Its field may be larger – more complex – and its theoretical resources more fluid, but there seems nevertheless to be an assumption of a determinate relation between the two: find your object, your cultural phenomenon, and then *read* it. Cultural studies in this sense operates as a kind of colonisation. It panders to our desire to *understand* the world and to *make sense* of our experiences in that world. In this sense cultural studies partakes in what Lyotard once called the "fantasies of realism" (Lyotard 1984: 74).[1]

In the above, cultural studies can be thought of as part of the *strata* of the academia. Here cultural studies works as a mechanism to *organise* – and thus define – 'culture', and in doing so *organise* the subject. In this sense, and in common with other disciplines, cultural studies operates to fix knowledges. This is particularly the case with the kind of cultural studies which develops out of Marxian – and Frankfurt School – theory. That is, a cultural studies whose project is representational (*re*presents culture from a theoretical perspective). Or, conversely cultural studies as critique of representation (cultural studies as 'ideological critique'). It was of course Adorno who identified this first project as the work of the culture industry: the latter's tendrils reaching further and further into everyday life. And yet cultural studies can itself be understood as an industry (a peculiarly academic industry), mirroring the work of capitalism in its desire to *interpret* reality. The second project – ideological critique – is characteristic not just of the Frankfurt School but also of the deconstructionists and their associated allies (the 'signifier enthusiasts'). Here the work of cultural studies (understood as Critical Theory), involves an *attempt* at understanding the movement of capitalism (the workings of ideology – understood as *representation*), as well as an *intent* on locating resistances (hence the importance for Adorno, and others, of the work of art). But these resistances are, as deconstruction shows us, difficult to

[1] Lyotard 'defines' these fantasies as operating: "whenever the objective is to stabilise the referent, to arrange it according to a point of view which endows it with a recognizable meaning, to reproduce the syntax and vocabulary which enable the addressee to decipher images and sequences quickly, and so to arrive easily at the consciousness of his own identity as well as the approval which he thereby receives from others – since such structures of images and sequences constitute a communication code among them all. This is the way the effects of reality, or if one prefers, the fantasies of realism, multiply" (*ibid*). Hence, for Lyotard the importance of the artist and writer who counteract this 'reality effect'; who are precisely "working without rules in order to formulate the rules of what *will have been done*" (*ibid*: 81). In this essay I want to suggest that cultural studies might take on the role which Lyotard assigns to art.

articulate (they seem to be always already *articulated within* the dominant), hence, for Adorno at least, such sites are inevitably figured as *utopian*.[2]

Lyotard once remarked that the problem of this negative critique is that the thing critiqued (indeed, the act of critique itself) often, inevitably, ensnares the critic. The critique becomes defined, *determined* by, the object of criticism.[3] The 'sites of resistance' are, if you like, predetermined by that which they resist; no rules (the 'rules of representation') are broken. Cultural studies becomes in this sense complicit with the dominant reality; it works within certain spatial and temporal parameters. As Bataille might say it operates within 'mundane time' and on the human register.[4] Indeed it assumes – and reinforces – a certain notion of a subject (however fragmented) and a certain notion of an object (however expanded).

Could there be another way of understanding the work of cultural studies? One which replaces this fundamentally hermeneutic project with a heuristic one? Cultural studies as an 'experimental *milieu'*, as a project in which pragmatics, *getting things done*, replaces understanding. Cultural studies as an affirmative and strategic mapping of the possibilities of life. Indeed cultural studies as a kind of 'war machine' precisely *against* interpretation – and *against* representation.

In fact to a certain extent cultural studies has always had this parallel project. At the same time as demarcating territories it produces lines of flight, deterritorialisations into other *milieux*. Lines of flight which themselves become territorialised and subsequently new lines of flight. Cultural studies has, as all disciplines have, as well as its cops and its priests, its mavericks, its adventurers,

---

[2] "Art's utopia, the counter-factual yet-to-come is draped in Black, it goes on being a recollection of the possible with a critical edge against the real, as promised by its impossibility. Art is the promise of happiness, a promise that is constantly being broken" (Adorno 1984). As we shall see, Gilles Deleuze turns away from this emphasis on the possible versus the real, replacing them instead with the categories of the *virtual* and the *actual*. Such a reconfiguration involves a rethinking of the effectiveness of art (and of the aesthetic), understood as no longer a *promise* of 'another world', but rather as an *access point* into other worlds.

[3] Lyotard writes that the danger with negative critique is that "the thing criticised holds back and even consumes the one who criticises, as Sodom petrified Lot's wife" (1988a: 155).

[4] See for example Bataille's essay on *Prehistoric Painting: Lascaux or the Birth of Art* (1980). Here Bataille contrasts 'work time' (to do with *utility*; with being *human*) with 'sacred time', precisely a transgression of this norm (a move 'into' the natural – cosmic – realm). Bataille argues that the practice of cave painting (understood as ritual) involved a 'playful' activity aimed specifically at accessing another mode of being and a different temporal order – characterised as the 'marvelous': "We must finally admit that, in every ritual operation, the seeking after a specific end is never but one amongst a number of its operators' motives: these motives derive from the whole of reality, its religious and sensible (aesthetic) sides alike. In every case they imply what has always been art's purpose: to create a sensible reality whereby the ordinary world is modified in response to the desire for the extraordinary, for the marvellous" (*ibid*: 34).

its sorcerers. These figures are to be found in the margins, at the edge, in the no man's land between disciplines. For them cultural studies – intellectual work in general – is a project embarked on without preset rules and without predetermined objects. It is a 'voyage of discovery', a journey which itself produces the terrain it maps. Two such adventurers – we might call them philosophers (philosophy understood here as active concept creation) – are Gilles Deleuze and Felix Guattari.

Their project, at least as it appears in their second volume of *Capitalism and Schizophrenia*, *A Thousand Plateaus,* is not to *understand* the world (to understand culture) but rather to create the world differently; to overcome the "ontological iron curtain between being and things" rather then to reinforce it (Guattari 1995a: 8). Such a project involves less an object of study – indeed objects might themselves strategically disappear in such a project. Even less does it involve a reading, an interpretation of objects (that is, it has no clearly defined, fixed, subject either). Instead it involves a *pragmatics*, the creation of 'psychic tools' with which to reorder our 'selves' and our world. I want now to briefly map out how one of these concept-tools – the rhizome – operates, and how a 'rhizomatics' might help in reconfiguring the cultural studies project. In doing so I will also map the rhizome's 'rhizomatic' connections with other Deleuzian concepts and with other allies:

> 1 and 2. Principles of connection and heterogeneity: any point of a rhizome can be connected to anything and must be... A rhizome ceaselessly establishes connections between semiotic chains, organisations of power, and circumstances relevant to the arts, sciences, and social struggles. (Deleuze and Guattari 1988: 7)

The rhizome is anti-hierarchical and a-centred. No single organising principle predetermines the consistencies and compatibilities between the network of its elements. The rhizome precisely fosters transversal, even *alogical*, connections between heterogeneous events. No longer a field of culture distinct from nature, indeed, no longer a realm of theory distinct from its object; and no longer the work of politics separated from the practice of art. Instead we have a continuous open system, with multiple entrance ways, of contact and communication between different *milieux*. Cultural studies could be understood as precisely this programme of *geometry*. Here cultural studies becomes a *map* – a strategy for reconfiguring our experiences. Thinking cultural studies as rhizome involves an affirmation of the former's *inter*disciplinary, or even *trans*disciplinary function; it removes blockages and opens us up to other adventures, other voyages. Cultural studies, in this place, is very much a *pragmatic* programme. An escape root/route from fixity and stasis. A means with which to enter smooth space.[5]

---

[5] "Smooth space is filled by events or haecceities, far more than by formed and perceived things. It is a space of affects, more than one of properties" (Deleuze and Guattari 1988: 479).

And this implies not just a reorientation in the object but a reconfiguration of the subject as well. The rhizome is *out* there but also *in* here (indeed, the rhizome renders 'inner' and 'outer' – as ontological categories – redundant). Guattari calls this project *resingularisation*, and for him it is predominantly a material, pragmatic project. Here he is writing about his work with psychotics at La Borde clinic in France. The extract is taken from his book *Chaosmosis* in which Guattari outlines what he sees as a new *ethico-aesthetic* paradigm for thinking subjectivity:

> ...certain psychotic patients, coming from poor agricultural backgrounds, will be invited to take up plastic arts, drama, video, music, etc., whereas until then, these universes had been unknown to them. On the other hand, bureaucrats and intellectuals will find themselves attracted to material work, in the kitchen, garden, pottery, horse riding club. The important thing here is not only the confrontation with a new material of expression, but the constitution of complexes of subjectivation: multiple exchanges between individual-group-machine. These complexes actually offer people diverse possibilities for recomposing their existential corporeality, to get out of their repetitive impasses and, in a certain way, to resingularise themselves. Grafts of transference operate in this way, not issuing from ready-made dimensions of subjectivity crystallised into structural complexes, but from a creation which itself indicates a kind of aesthetic paradigm. One creates new modalities of subjectivity in the same way an artist creates new forms from a palette. (Guattari 1995: 6-7)

The possibility of making transversal connections between people and between people and things is, for Guattari, not so much a cure for psychosis, even less a reintegration of the psychotic into society (the re-oedipalisation enacted by psychoanalysis), rather it is a means by which individuals can reorganise, or *resingularise* themselves in a creative and affirmative manner. For Guattari, La Borde is a machinic assemblage – a space in which different complexes can aggregate together. Importantly, and like the rhizome, this assemblage is always opening up to an outside. The machine, the machinic assemblage, is not to be confused with, or reduced to the merely technical machine. Indeed the machinic assemblage can best be understood as a function, a fluid function of connectivity and deterritorialisation. In this sense the rituals of archaic societies (complexes of signifying and a-signifying functions) are as much machines as the city mega-machine. The rhizome too is in this sense machinic. Or the machine is rhizomatic. Both foster connections, both deterritorialise. And at stake in both is an 'overcoming' of the subject / object split. As Guattari writes elsewhere:

> The autopoietic and 'hypertextual' position of the machine thus possesses a pragmatic potential, which allows for a creative standpoint of machinic composition, occurring in the face of the ontological iron curtain which separates the subject on one side from things on the other. (Guattari 1995a: 12)

This is a kind of return to the project of cultural studies as outlined in my beginning; cultural studies as a strategy for ending alienation. But here this 'healing' (this *reconciliation*) of the split between subject and object is not utopian, not transcendent, but is instead reconfigured as *immanent*. An immanent aesthetics. A pragmatic programme of de- and re-subjectification.

Back to Deleuze and Guattari and to the rhizome:

> 3. Principle of multiplicity: it is only one when the multiple is effectively created as a substantive, 'multiplicity', that it ceases to have any relation to the One as subject or object, natural or spiritual reality, image and world... A multiplicity has neither subject nor object, only determinations, magnitudes, and dimensions. (Deleuze and Guattari 1988: 8)

Thinking cultural studies as multiplicity involves a re-mapping of the terrain of cultural studies; subject and object disappear replaced by 'determinations, magnitudes and dimensions', moments of intensity and lines of flight. Indeed, thinking cultural studies as rhizome implies a different kind of *strategic* individuation; not a different kind of *reading* but a *transformation*:

> What we're interested in, you see, are modes of individuation beyond those of things, persons or subjects: the individuation, say, of a time of day, of a region, a climate, a river or a wind, of an event. And maybe it's a mistake to believe in the existence of things, persons, or subjects. (Deleuze 1995: 26)

In this place, cultural studies creates the world differently. Like a kind of Science Fiction, we enter a world populated not by people and things but by events, *haecceities*, and intense thresholds. The human – as organised, signified, subjectified – disappears. Or at least becomes little more than a strategic position (a territory), a launch pad into other worlds.

How to think this multiplicity of which we are part without reducing it to the simple? How to think *an-original* complexity that does not arise – or return to – the One? For Deleuze and Guattari this must involve a subtraction: always, subtract the leader, the general. Always subtract the centre. Always *n-1*. Michel Serres, another ally in our rhizomatic project, attempts a similar task – thinking the multiple – in his book *Genesis*. Serres is particularly wary of the hegemony of the concept – that mechanism of classification which distributes and produces unities. For Serres, instead, a kind of *quasi-concept* is needed to think the work of the multiple:

> Time-as-weather, fire-as-heat are not concepts in the usual sense. Clock-time is such a concept, entropic time is, perhaps, another such, and temperature as well. A cloud is an aggregate, a nebulous set, a multiplicity whose exact definition escapes us, and whose local movements are beyond observation. A flame is an aggregate... that is even more nebulous. Heat and flame, cloud and wind, climate and turbulences, we could refer to them as concepts of multiplicities. (Serres 1995: 103)

Like Deleuze and Guattari, Serres attempts to individuate the world differently. To 'free' the multiplicity from the shelter of the unifying concept. For Serres the world is made up not from 'well formed' objects but by aggregates which require a different kind of thought altogether. Indeed, for Lyotard, yet another ally, thoughts are themselves cloud-like:

> Thoughts are not the fruits of the earth. They are not registered by areas, except out of human commodity. Thoughts are clouds. The periphery of thoughts is as immeasurable as the fractal lines of Benoit Mandelbrot. Thoughts are pushed and pulled at variable speeds. They are deep, although core and skin are of the same grain. Thoughts never stop changing their location one with the other. When you feel like you have penetrated far into their intimacy in analysing their so-called structure or genealogy or even post structure, it is actually too late or too soon. (Lyotard 1988b: 5)

Such a *rethinking* of thought involves a rethinking of the *cogito*; the 'mind' is no longer the *origin* of thought, but is a kind of threshold, or temporary turbulence, within a thought cloud-field. Here thought, thinking, is itself a multiplicity; *creative* thinking as such involves a reconnection with this nebulous realm (of potentialities) beyond (in fact, always parallel) to the subject.

Deleuze and Guattari likewise, at times, turn away from the concept and rethink thought. Hence the importance of science, involving *function* (we might say, involving a 'machinic mapping' of the world), and of art, involving *affects*.[6] When concepts are considered (in the philosophical project *per se*) they are understood creatively; active concept creation as a means of problem solving, precisely to 'get something done'. For example Deleuze's concept of *difference* – mapped out before his collaboration with Guattari. Here the world is no longer *thought* as being comprised of distinct entities – not even of aggregates of smaller and smaller parts. Instead a notion of *difference* becomes the condition of possibility for phenomena. But this difference is not that between already demarcated signifiers (it is not a semiotic) rather it is a *difference of intensity* (we might say a *difference of affect*):

> Every phenomenon refers to an inequality by which it is conditioned. Every diversity and every change refers to a difference which is its sufficient reason.

[6] See Deleuze and Guattari's *What is Philosophy?* (Deleuze and Guattari 1994). Brian Massumi has written an interesting, and instructive, essay on affect in relation to the human brain/body configuration (Massumi 1996). He demonstrates that affects – understood as a-signifying 'events' passing across the body – everywhere and always accompany (and in some senses determine) the more obvious (i.e. signifying and structuring) elements of subjectivity. In fact we might say, with Massumi, that the universe of affect (the universe of the *virtual*) often works to *interfere* with linguistic expression, and indeed the other 'subject constructing' mechanisms of late capitalism. Massumi, via Spinoza, gives this project of thinking affect a name: *ethics* (*ibid*: 222).

> Everything which happens and everything which appears is correlated with orders of differences: differences of level, temperature, pressure, tension, potential, *differences of intensity*. (Deleuze 1994: 222)

Such a reconceptualisation allows us to move from a signifying register to an a-signifying (an *affective*) one. The world – as multiplicity – is constituted by moments of, and differences in, intensity. Of course, to a certain extent this is not new. Indeed it may involve a return to a pre-theological, a *pagan*, mapping of the world. Deleuze has himself positioned his work in a genealogy of 'bastard' – or pagan – philosophers from Heraclitus to Nietzsche. A line of nomadic thought everywhere accompanying state philosophy as its mutant twin. Or of course we could turn away from the west to the east – and to the *immanent* philosophies/religions. Hinduism can be characterised as a multiplicity – a bewildering and muddling collection of deities with no apparent order or centre. Hence the apparent difficulty for the Western mind in grasping this system which is not a system. But in our *reading* of Hinduism this multiplicity is also reducible to the One. The different Gods are *understood* as fragments, specific incarnations, of the One. So much for the Western interpretation of this magical multiplicity. An interpretation which brings Hinduism closer to Christianity. In fact, with Deleuze we have something even further removed from such pantheist mythologies: the world as *conditioned* reality. In *this* world (our world seen differently) there are only conditions which produce other conditions. Here process (movement) replaces stasis (fixity) as the world's – and the subject's – *modus operandi*. We are closer to the Buddhist – or the Taoist here. No essences, indeed no theology (no 'representation'), but a 'fundamental' insubstantiality, impermanence, and interpenetration of all phenomena. The world as a vortex of energy; the world, and ourselves within that world, as a "region of fire" (Lyotard 1993: 13).

"Multiplicities are defined by the outside: by the abstract line, the line of flight or deterritorialisation according to which they change in nature and connect with other multiplicities" (Deleuze and Guattari 1988: 9). Cultural studies, as multiplicity is fluid. What it 'is' is defined by its outermost edge – its line of flight. As such cultural studies is a dynamic, open system. One that changes its nature as the number of its dimensions increase (as it crosses into other *plateaus*). Cultural studies as such does not name a discipline but rather a *function*. Cultural studies *is* a deterritorialisation from other disciplines, from academia, and inevitably from itself. For as soon as cultural studies becomes fixed (becomes a *discipline*) then the real work of cultural studies will be going on elsewhere.

> 4. Principle of asignifying rupture: against the oversignifying breaks separating structures or cutting across a single structure. A rhizome may be broken, shattered at a given spot, but it will start up again on one of its old lines, or on new lines... Every rhizome contains lines of segmentarity according to which it is stratified, territorialised, signified, attributed, etc., as well as lines of deterritorialisation down which it constantly flees. (Deleuze and Guattari 1988: 9)

Not the rhizome versus the root (no dualities); indeed it is the nature of the rhizome to be broken, it is the nature of the root to produce rhizomes. For in reality these two are entwined; the rhizome in the root and the root in the rhizome. Cultural studies, within the academia, may be ossified, may be *frozen*, but this does not mean we have to go elsewhere. Rather we *switch* registers: "A new rhizome may form in the heart of a tree, the hollow of a root, the crook of a branch. Or else it is a microscopic element of the root tree, a radicle, that gets rhizome production going" (*ibid*: 15).

Strategically this might mean that as well as looking to other *milieux* (Eastern philosophy, the new sciences, techno-culture, etc), and at *minor* literature (that which has been left outside the canon of cultural studies), we might also look to the redundancies within cultural studies: lines of flight from traditional representational paradigms – in fact suggested by those paradigms. And here we return to those issues I raised at the beginning. Cultural Studies as strata – but strata which contain within possibilities of destratification. For you do not get the one without the other. Cultural studies as a constant process, a constant movement, and also cultural studies as the interruption (the *freezing*) of this movement. Cultural studies as rhizome (always *between* disciplines), and then, rhizomes *in* cultural studies. In fact cultural studies inevitably produces the stratification of lines of flight (reinstalls the signifier) and yet, in so doing, prepares the ground, the territory, for future deterritorialisations.

Cultural studies here is a smooth *and* a striated space. A space of expansion, of experimentation, and also a space that is organised and classified; one does not come about without the other. Every nomad always has several base camps, temporary consolidations of territory depending on the seasons – territorialisations which produce deterritorialisations. Indeed cultural studies is not, and cannot be, a wild destratification. Such a line of flight is ultimately destructive. As Deleuze and Guattari say in another of their plateaus: "Staying stratified – organised, signified, subjected – is not the worse that can happen: the worse that can happen is if you throw the strata into demented or suicidal collapse, which brings them back down on us heavier than ever" (*ibid*: 161). Indeed:

> you have to keep enough of the organism for it to reform each dawn; and you have to keep small supplies of signifiance and subjectification, if only to turn them against their own systems when the circumstances demand it, when things, persons, even situations, force you to: and you have to keep small rations of subjectivity in sufficient quantities to enable you to respond to the dominant reality. (*Ibid*: 160)

The watch word in this project of deterritorialisation – this project of cultural studies – is caution. Always proceed with the smallest of doses. And always proceed from a consolidated territory.

> This is how it should be done: lodge yourself on a stratum, experiment with the opportunities it offers, find an advantageous point on it, find potential movements of deterritorialisation, possible lines of flight, experience them, produce flow conjunctions here and there, try out continuums of intensity segment by segment, have a small plot of new land at all times. It is through a meticulous relation with the strata that one succeeds in freeing lines of flight. (*Ibid*: 161)

This is not a programme of escapism. Even less the outline of a utopian metaphysics. Rather it is a call to arms *and* a call for attention to be focused on the actual, if only to unlock the potential becomings, the *virtualities* encapsulated within every moment. And this virtual is *not* some 'Other' place (not even an endlessly deferred one): "Indeed, the virtual must be defined as strictly a part of the real object – as though the object had one part of itself in the virtual into which it plunged as though into an objective dimension" (Deleuze 1994: 208-209). The virtual is another (temporal) dimension of the object – or rather, and following Bergson, the virtual is the 'completely determined structure' of the object, and the actual is but a 'part'. We only ever encounter this actual part ('reality'); the project of cultural studies might be to access the other (virtual) potentialities; in fact to actualise the virtual. And this is where the *inter*disciplinary nature of cultural studies once more becomes important. The inter is now between the actual and the virtual, for, as Brian Massumi asserts, it is "at the edge of the virtual, where it leaks into actual, that counts. For the seeping edge is where potential, actually is found" (1996: 236).

For Deleuze this actualisation of the virtual is a "genuine creation" (Deleuze 1994: 213). As such it is important that the virtual be differentiated from its 'near enemy': the *possible* (the utopian).

> The only danger in all this is that the virtual could be confused with the possible. The possible is opposed to the real; the process undergone by the possible is therefore 'realisation'. By contrast, the virtual is not opposed to the real; it possesses a full reality by itself. The process it undergoes is actualisation. It would be wrong to see only a verbal dispute here: it is a question of existence itself. (*Ibid*: 211)

Indeed, I would argue that the dominant model of cultural studies within the academy is precisely one based on the possible. Either the melancholy science (as Gillian Rose called it) of Adorno's utopian blinks or the equally melancholic, even pessimistic, endless deferral of the possible heralded by Derrida and de Man. Cultural studies which replaces the possible with the virtual becomes a much more affirmative project. Affirming the fullness of life (understood as endless creativity) rather than lamenting its lack.

In fact this project can take place from within the heart of the other. It is not as if a rhizomatic cultural studies looks elsewhere – it is based in the same terrain, albeit it thinks that terrain differently. For example cultural studies might still be involved in a kind of semiotic project – but it might think the sign differently (as signifying (ideological, psychoanalytical, etc.) but *also* as having asignifying functions), something Lyotard seems to hint at:

> First therefore, a different reaction, a different reception. We do not suppose, to begin with, that the signs… transport messages which are communicable in principle. We don't start off by saying to ourselves: someone or something is speaking to us here, so I must try to understand. To understand, to be intelligent, is not our overriding passion. We strive instead to be set in motion. Consequently our passion would sooner be the dance, as Nietzsche wanted, and as Cage and Cunningham want. (Lyotard 1993: 50)

Here the sign becomes an *intensity*, a trigger point for movement (a 'setting in motion'). Indeed the tensor can be understood as precisely the *affective* side of the sign. If *interpretation* still has a role it is in this sense: to reactivate the frozen event; to unravel the virtual pasts and virtual future (the potentialities) of the *sign* – the latter understood as 'meaningful' but *also* as *productive*. Interpretation is our confrontation with this bundle of energy, this *haecceity*; precisely a meeting, an encounter, between force fields.

> 5 and 6. Principle of cartography and decalcomania: a rhizome is not amenable to any structural or generative model. It is a stranger to any idea of genetic axis or deep structure...The rhizome is altogether different, *a map and not a tracing...* What distinguishes the map from the tracing is that it is entirely orientated towards an experimentation in contact with the real... The map is open and connectable in all of its dimensions; it is detachable, reversible, susceptible to constant modification. It can be torn, reversed, adapted to any kind of mounting, reworked by an individual, group, or social formation. It can be drawn on a wall, conceived of as a work of art, constructed as political action or meditation. (Deleuze and Guattari 1988: 12)

So, nothing precedes the making of the rhizome. The rhizome is not a *re*presentation. It does not trace, or *photograph*, something that came before. And this is not to put in operation an opposition. As Deleuze and Guattari say, maps can be traced and tracings can become maps. "It is a question of method: *the tracing should always be put back on the map*" (*ibid*: 13). Cultural studies here becomes programmatic and *diagrammatic*: "The diagrammatic or abstract machine does not function to represent, even something real, but rather constructs a real that is yet to come, a new type of reality" (*ibid*: 142).

Again this 'new type of reality' is not utopian, nor transcendent but *immanent* to this reality. Cultural studies in this sense is indeed an 'abstract machine'; a function of deterritorialisation operating from within already existing strata. In their conclusion to *A Thousand Plateaus* Deleuze and Guattari again outline the functioning of the 'abstract machine'. Their definition might equally apply to a 'rhizomatic' cultural studies:

> Abstract machines operate within concrete assemblages: They are defined by… the cutting edges of decoding and deterritorialisation. They draw these cutting edges.

> Therefore they make the territorial assemblage open onto something else, assemblages of another type, the molecular, the cosmic; they constitute becomings. Thus they are always singular and immanent.

And so what are the implications of all this for cultural studies – as it is practised today – and for 'interdisciplinarity'? Well, as regards the latter cultural studies *is* 'interdisciplinary' in the sense that it is *between disciplines*, it is what 'produces' these 'disciplines' – these bodies of knowledges – deterritorialisations. We might, in this sense – and to borrow a notion from Alain Badiou – understand cultural studies as an *event site*, "a point of exile where *it is possible* that something finally might happen" (Badiou 2000: 84-85). Less certain is what this project – of cultural studies – might look like; how to write this, how to teach it? Again, as regards the latter, cultural studies is a pragmatics. Students must be given the tools with which to create their own concepts (their own *quasi* concepts) and produce their own deterritorialisations. And it is at this point that the nature of pedagogy changes. No longer, or not only, imparting a body of knowledge, teaching a set of competences, but an encouragement to experiment, an encouragement to *in*competence. No longer producing specialists but providing 'tool boxes'.

And the practice, or the 'writing', of cultural studies itself is no longer an interpretation but becomes an experiment, an 'exploratory probe', an event amongst events. In such a project other media might equally be utilised (no more hegemony of the essay/article). Indeed cultural studies, in common with other creative practices, might involve taking up different materials from different *milieux*. At stake in these experiments is the accessing of other worlds. Not worlds 'beyond' this one (no transcendent, nor *utopian* principle) but worlds, 'incorporeal universes' as Guattari calls them, *virtual* and *immanent* in this one. Cultural studies might be a name for this work of *imagination*.

And in such a project our allies might not necessarily be within the Academy. Our allies will in fact be on the *outside*, or at least at the outermost edge. Indeed cultural studies is also about locating these allies, these anomalies that stalk the fringes. For these figures – these 'events' – these moments of intensity – are the border guides/guards, the access nodes into other worlds. A certain notion of politics might – strategically – disappear here (the 'subject' of politics himself disappears), indeed this project might be best characterised as *ethical*. In as much as it involves exploring the potential for becoming – the potential for self-overcoming. But this is not necessarily to disavow the political project, the work of representation and of representational critique. Rather it is to reconfigure these projects as 'molar', which, important though they might be, when focused on exclusively, efface the 'molecular' (understood as the realm of *affect*) of which they are constituted. As such the molecular – the rhizome – is a kind of guerrilla war against representation. A war with no winner and in which the taking of sides is always strategic and pragmatic. Cultural studies is the name of this project and the site within which this project takes place. Cultural studies as rhizome but also and always the burgeoning rhizomes within cultural studies.

Bibliography:

Adorno, Theodor (1984) *Aesthetic Theory*, London: Routledge.

Badiou, Alain (2000) *Deleuze: The Clamor of Being*, trans. Louise Burchill, Minnesota: University of Minnesota Press.

Bataille, Georges (1980) *Prehistoric Painting: Lascaux or the Birth of Art*, London: Macmillan.

Deleuze, Gilles (1994) *Difference and Repetition*, trans. Paul Patton, London: Athlone Press.

Deleuze, Gilles (1995) *Negotiations*, trans. Martin Joughin, New York: Columbia University Press.

Deleuze, Gilles and Felix Guattari (1988) *A Thousand Plateaus*, trans. Brian Massumi, London: Athlone Press.

Deleuze, Gilles and Felix Guattari (1994) *What is Philosophy?* Trans. Graham Burchell and Hugh Tomlinson, London: Verso.

Guattari, Felix (1995) *Chaosmosis: An Ethico-Aesthetic Paradigm*, trans. Paul Bains and Julian Pefanis, Sydney: Power Publications.

Guattari, Felix (1995a) "On Machines", in *Complexity: Architecture/ Art/Philosophy*, trans. Vivian Constantinopoulos, London: Academy Editions.

Lyotard, Jean-François (1984) "Appendix: Answering the Question: What is Postmodernism?" in *The Postmodern Condition*, trans. Geoff Bennington and Brian Massumi, Manchester: Manchester University Press.

Lyotard, Jean-François (1988a) "Beyond Representation", in *The Lyotard Reader*, ed. Andrew Benjamin, Oxford: Basil Blackwell.

Lyotard, Jean-François (1988b) *Peregrinations: Law, Form, Event*, New York: Columbia University Press.

Lyotard, Jean-François (1993) *Libidinal Economy*, trans. Iain Hamilton Grant, London: Athlone Press.

Massumi, Brian (1996) "The Autonomy of Affect", in *Deleuze: A Critical Reader*, ed. Paul Patton, Oxford: Blackwell.

Serres, Michel (1995) *Genesis*, trans. Genevieve James and James Nielson, Ann Arbor: University of Michigan Press.

Section B:

Anti-Disciplinary Objects and Practices

SPACE *BETWEEN* DISCIPLINES

NECDET TEYMUR

Disciplines assume the existence of their objects *and* define their unity. They *include* some phenomena and *exclude* others. They also define 'space(s)' (— a kind of *Lebenswelt*) for themselves, and by implication for those whom they leave out. These *disciplinary spaces* relate to concepts, theories, methods and departments. Fight for disciplinary territories is often no less vicious than that for land (— about which there are specialist practices and disciplines too!)

The concept(s) of *'space'* as used in environmental, architectural, urban or geographical discourses are in a different type of quandary. 'Space' is assumed to be the central object of a number of such fields, yet, as a concept, it encompasses almost *every-thing, every-where* and *every-time.* This results both in its confused functionality and in its limited rigour.

Notwithstanding the problem of what 'cultural studies' does, or does not, could or should encompass, an attempt to incorporate 'space' into its scope has, simultaneously, to tackle with the spatiality of disciplines and the extra-disciplinarity of space.

A (Disciplined) Introduction to Space

There are two key and one intermediate concepts in the title: a 'discipline' is a field on which I cannot claim more than an amateurish expertise. Space, as this paper will suggest, is a concept on which no one can truly claim to be an expert. As to the intermediate concept of 'between', it is in fact *the* concept which represents and embodies the whole problem and its possible resolutions.

With these disclaimers and claims, I will try to chart a brief trajectory of the emergence, formation and establishment of disciplines primarily in terms of the processes of inclusion and exclusion, and the creation of territories and 'others'. This will lead to the definition of the very spaces of these 'in's, 'out's and 'others' – in the first instance, in a metaphorical sense. These spaces will then be shown to be representing an interesting homology, even an overlap, with the common uses of the concept of 'space' in spatial and other discourses including cultural studies.

I will conclude by referring to the im/possible definition of the ubiquitous concept of 'space' in various disciplines and practices: (i) in the disciplines of *construction* (such as architecture, engineering, planning), (ii) in the disciplines of *explanation* (such as physics, astronomy, geography), (iii) in the disciplines of *representation* (such as visual arts, music, literature) and (iv) in the disciplines of *destruction* (such as military, diplomacy and commerce, and, strange though it may sound, occasionally, architecture, planning and construction). I will also refer to the traditional neglect of space in social sciences and what they and the discourse of space have both lost out as a result.

I will formulate a number of fundamental issues arising out of these observations, and introduce a set of concepts that can account for the *spatiality* of disciplines and the *extradisciplinarity* of space.

A Short History of Disciplines

First, a few statements of the obvious: to put it crudely, knowledge is a human, hence, social artifact. It comes about either as a side-product of our activities, or, as one that is the expected end-product. Once produced, knowledge is variously formulated, represented, recorded, used, and, also, owned. As a consequence of these processes, it is often classified, controlled, manipulated, bought and sold and, institutionalised. There is some, if not always a direct, link between the ownership of knowledge and that of its objects. Similarly, there might be some link between the territories dividing areas of knowledge and those dividing their objects. (Ironically, whilst the knowledge-producers are in deep concentration studying the universe, those who are not interested in knowledge tend to parcel up the universe!)

In the meantime, knowledge of different types emerges in different contexts (belief systems, sorcery, superstitions, skills, innovations, expertise, etc.) which come out and, variously, co-exist, compete, cancel out or transmutate with each other; or are superseded, suppressed or institutionalised. Religions, ideologies, branches, *écoles*, arts, sciences, paradigms, professions and disciplines are formed and named. Practitioners, experts, artisans, theoreticians, educators, etc. of these areas are formed. These divisions constitute the bases or the justifications for academic divisions, professional groupings, commercial associations, etc. They all generate their own rules, regulations, methods and, of course, areas of the universe *and* areas of knowledge on which they claim ownership, competence, jurisdiction and/or power. To protect what they own, they form solidarities, define common-purposes and invent defense mechanisms. The fight for epistemological (and institutional) territories is no less vicious than those for land!

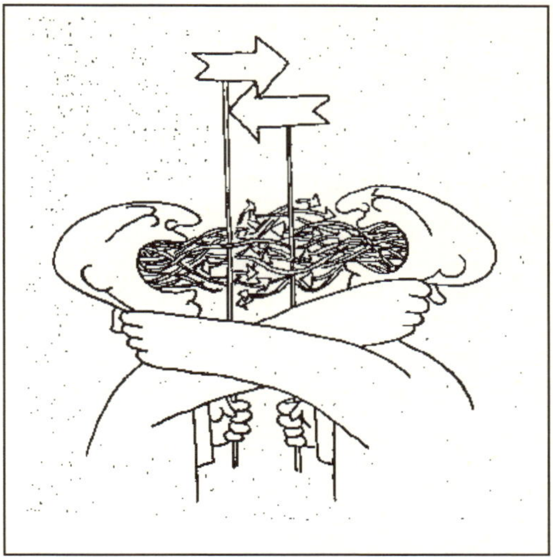

In the process, two important things happen: These formations (i) draw up boundaries for their knowledge; and (ii) (a) define their objects on the basis of the knowledge of these objects; and, (b) conversely, are defined by the limits of that knowledge and the perceived or imagined boundaries of those objects on which they claim jurisdiction (although they might often pretend to possess competencies beyond these limits).

These processes never stop, nor do they necessarily follow any chronological order. They may even follow a reverse chronology. Institutionalisation may be the motor of knowledge production as it could also be its follower, stimulant or suppressor…

The types of knowledge are defined by the contexts of the objects, the modes of their production and their use(s). Whether we like it or not, the traditional divisions of the mental and the manual (over which there has been much dispute), have corollaries at the level of knowledge and their social appropriation. There is, for example, a strong difference between 'disciplines' which primarily *produce* knowledge, and professions which primarily *use* it.[1] From this point of view, there are significant differences between physics and engineering, mathematics and accountancy, or history and architecture.

---

[1] For a discussion on the differences between *'professions'* and *'disciplines'*, see Teymur (1993).

Disciplinary Values and Others

Notwithstanding many other aspects, there are two significant outcomes in the formation of disciplines relevant to our discussion here: disciplinary values and disciplinary others;

1. *Disciplinary values:* Disciplines point out, isolate, frame or foreground certain objects or certain phenomena in the universe (or in nature, society, cities, etc.) and attribute to them significance, urgency, and hence, *value.* These objects are then made the objects of knowledge, hence, 'disciplinary objects'.

2. *Disciplinary others:* Disciplines also create *'others'* either by denying value to those which they deem unworthy of attention, or by excluding those already valued by other disciplines. (Obviously, there may also be objects not valued and accepted by any discipline. I call them 'outsider objects', their knowledge 'outsider knowledge' and their epistemology 'outsider epistemology'.) Therefore, in the process of creating their values and their objects disciplines negatively and/or positively create other values, other objects and other knowledges, hence, other disciplines.

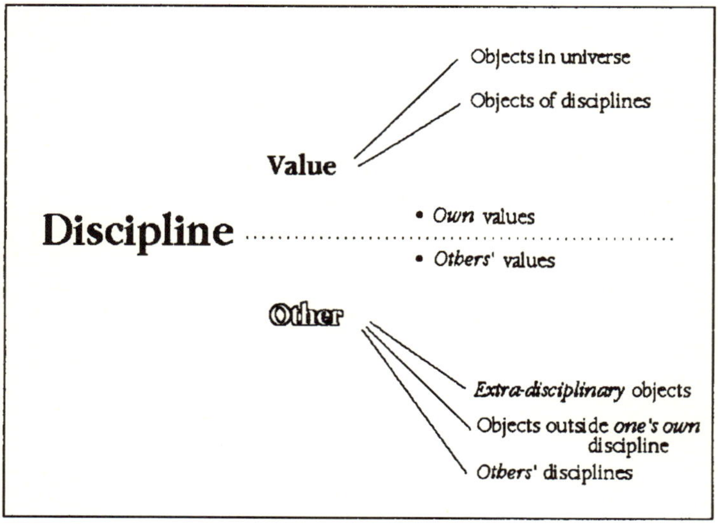

These operations result in, and reproduce, the very concept of 'discipline' both as a verb and behaviour *and* as social and epistemological formations. All those

'-logy's or '-ics's and their discourses provide frameworks within which things and words get safe homes and a voice.

In the meantime, various oppositions, even paradoxes, occur. Some disciplines may be defined primarily by what they exclude, and some, primarily by their own exclusion. Some may be defined by the very fact that their objects do not fit in any discipline, and some, by the fact that the objects could be in *any* and *many* disciplines.

Interdisciplinarity as Otherness

Seen from these points of view, it is not sufficient to see *interdisciplinarity* as a project of cooperative relationship between mutually exclusive formations. This applies to variations such as disciplinarity, pluri-disciplinarity, intra-disciplinarity, cross- disciplinarity, transdisciplinarity, etc., too. As a matter of fact, in the closely guarded territoriality of academic and scientific disciplines, interdisciplinarity is an area largely made up of 'othernesses'.

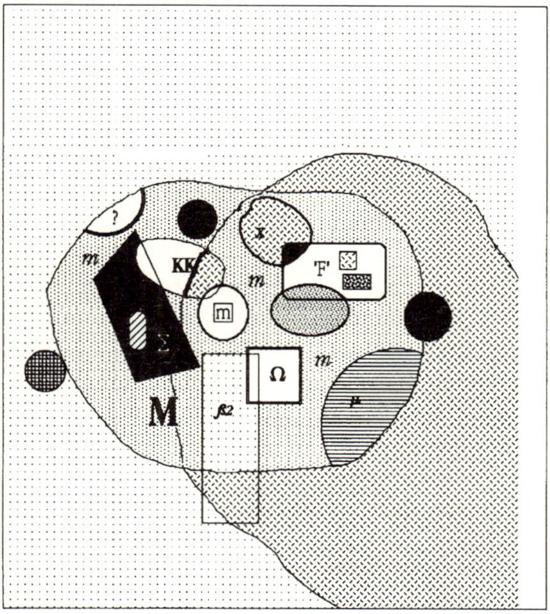

Interstool spaces ...

A typical field of interdisciplinarity (as distinct from those of disciplines) is precisely a field not so much of agreements, alliances or co-operative intentions as protected boundaries, walls and barbed wires. As distinct from the safe havens provided by institutionalised disciplines, the fields of interdisciplinarity are forever unsafe, if not always unsound.

The disciplinary wholes so defined could be likened to islands, packages and more commonly, to pigeon holes. However, to advance my thesis of interdisciplinarity in relation to the concept of space, I prefer to use the colloquial analogy of the *'stool'*.

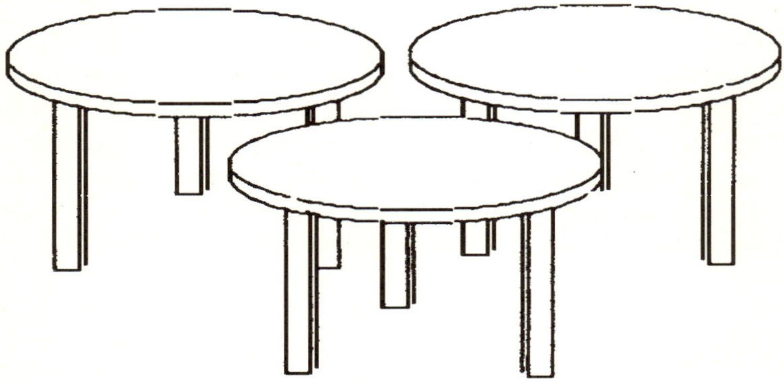

If disciplines can be described as 'stools', we can imagine these pieces of furniture (or facility, or tools) meeting the needs to support bodies. (In this context, I will restrain myself from extending this analogy to include ordinary chairs, university chairs, meeting chairs or Royal thrones!) In collectivities, there can be a variety of stools to meet the needs of different sitters – there could be height-adjustable stools or padded ones, some would be designed for bars, some for classrooms and some for pianists. Even when the stools are of the same kind, their locations in the room and the status (and the sizes) of sitters could vary. Therefore, stools can seldom form uniform patterns or even levels. As the seats of most stools, as distinct from most chairs, are of round shape, even when they are tightly laid out, they can never form a surface without holes and gaps. Those who try to sit on such a surface could not sit properly, place their legs anywhere, and their bottoms would necessarily touch more than one stool. And, those who happen to fall between these closely laid out stools, could not easily get out!

With this imaginary possibility in mind, we can extrapolate that there could be a series of relationship of *otherness* between those who sit on one stool, and those who sit on more than one, or between those who manage to sit on stools and those who fall between them. There could also be those who never manage to sit on any stool – now, or in the past. As the presence of gaps between stools is an inevitability, and as some either constantly fall into these gaps, or in fact reside there, these gaps should not be seen as absences of stools, but part of the universe of stools.[2] In other words, these gaps are not nothingness. (We can benefit from the wisdoms of Zen (Lao Tzu 1955: 63; or Rumi 1996)

Towards a New Concept of 'Interdisciplinarity'

The gaps between disciplinary territories, the fields that happen to be outside disciplinary boundaries, or, indeed, the spaces that cannot be accommodated by established disciplines are (just like those between the proverbial stools) neither nothing, nor voids. To be sure, the areas of knowledge that have not (yet) been institutionalised are not necessarily absences of knowledge, or ignorance, but are likely to be either different types of it, or raw ingredients of the knowledges to come. Hundreds of thousands of years of human history contain a wealth of experience, know-how, know-what, skills, techniques, technologies, sensibilities, representations, intuitions, beliefs, wisdom, etc. that cannot all easily be confined to the convenient '-logy' boxes. Nor should we expect any one discipline to account for what was not included in its formation in the first place. We therefore need alternative, if critical, modes of understanding both the interdisciplinary *structures* and inter- and intra-disciplinary *spaces* – *whether* formed by exclusion, or negligence, or incomprehension, or incapacity, or insularity, or inperception, etc.

In short, we need at once to recognise the impossibility of a comprehensive inclusion *and* the exciting possibilities of comprehending this vast uncharted territory. With this dual attitude I would state the obvious that:

1. No discipline is ever pure, free or original, hence, inclusive of all and exclusive of the others.

2. It should be possible to perceive and think of phenomena that do not happen to come under any one discipline.

3. We need a concept of discipline that does not deny the existence of non-scientific forms of knowledge as can be found in visual arts, literature, even religion.

4. Ignorance is not an absence of knowledge, but a form of it. Like knowledge, it is purposeful (see Teymur undated).

5. Not only the presence, but also the absence of knowledge and absence of disciplines has functionality (*ibid*).

---

[2] "Form is emptiness" cf. Blyth (1981: 91).

6. Interdisciplinarity is not simply a 'fruit salad' composed of a variety of (more or less compatible) disciplines. It could be imagined as a completely *new* fruit/discipline not reducible to the sum of its ingredients.

7. Disciplines are artifacts that have their own history (and geography), yet, despite all their efforts to value-out and to exclude others, they all include the elements of those that have been left out. In this sense, *all disciplines are necessarily intertextual and interdisciplinary.*[3]

Following on from the last preposition, if we can imagine all disciplines variously as the products of social, discursive, epistemological and practical processes, we might start recognising those objects and knowledges that remain *outside, between, under, among, etc.* them as equally social, discursive, epistemological and/or practical. These under-defined fields could then be described, for want of a better term, as *inter-disciplines* (with hyphen) as distinct from *interdiscipline* (without hyphen).

With this definition in mind, we can try to envisage a notion of disciplines that ignores neither other disciplines and their objects, problems, referents, discourses and knowledge, nor those bits of the universe that have not so far been (fully or wholly) accommodated by traditional disciplines. This way, disciplines would be the richer by not ignoring those that they have excluded during their formation. Rather than aspiring to be even purer, they would go for an 'impure' view of knowledge. Moreover, they would recognise that in all their purity, they in fact include parts of what they have excluded, if not always in flesh, then as negativity. And, they would be more responsible than either ignoring or labelling out the other, and would thus begin to consider the problems of the excluded *both* as *their* (i.e. their own) and *their* (i.e. the other's) problems. This would hopefully be the beginning of a strategy of *democratic epistemology.*

'Space – between the Stools or, the concept of the 'Inter-stool'

The notion of an interdisciplinarity that includes *both* the inside and the outside seems to need a different set of concepts. If, provisionally, we call *both* the gaps, the in-betweens, the excluded, the outsides, etc. *and* the insides, the bounded territories, the safe havens, and the stools themselves as *'space',* we can begin to imaginatively tackle the problematic concepts of 'disciplinarity' and 'space' together.

Recognising, as we did earlier, that there is no way the traditional stools could form an unbroken, uniform and continuous plane for sitting (at least, without losing their functionality as seats), the task therefore would become one

[3] For the concept of *'intertextuality'* proposed in the '60s by Julia Kristeva and others, see Worton and Still (1990).

of accounting for the stools as well as their gaps. The concepts of *space* (between) and the *Space* (that is) would start functioning both as metaphors and as real – in collaboration, and not of two outsides, or outsides and insides, or not indeed, poor representations of each other, or of something else, but as *one inclusive concept.* That this might go against the whole history of thought on specialisation of space and the territorial divisions of the sciences and the disciplines of space is precisely that which we are trying to problematise here. In this way, 'space' would define together both its disciplinary impossibility and its claim for a space amongst already mapped-out spaces of disciplines.

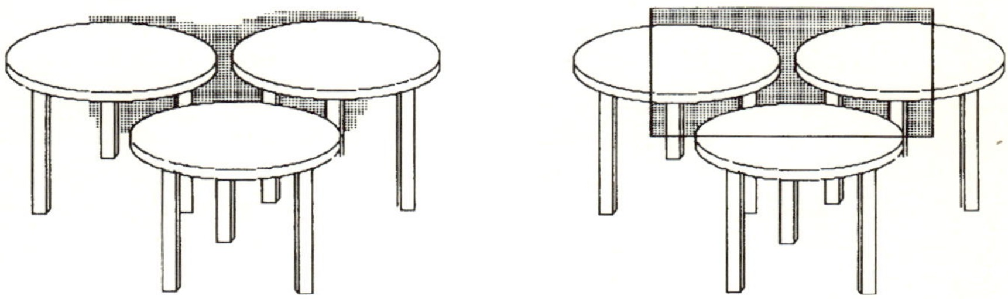

We know that nearly all practices, arts, institutions and disciplines have some concern with space. They obviously define 'it' differently, represent it differently and entertain different expectations from it. Geometry, mathematics, physics, astronomy, biology, ecology, geography, psychology, history, economics, law, geopolitics, etc. on the one hand, and architecture, urban planning, interior architecture, agriculture, landscape design, real estate development, estate agency and military on the other variously consider space as their (real / conceptual / discursive) objects. Secondly, all art forms, including painting, music and literature not only deal with, represent, use or occupy space in a number of guises, but many can be regarded as *spatial* constructs in their very constitution (could there be music without space and without time?)

It is not the mission of this article either to give an exhaustive etymology of the word or to present an historical survey of thought on space. There is little need to further support the observations being made here the basis of such an archaeology. Suffice it to say that both in academic and colloquial discourses synonyms, doubles, replacements, opposites, conflations of the physical phenomena, the word and the concept of space abound: nature, environment, volume, distance, site, void, emptiness, gap, place, room, (floor) area, enclosure, territory, field, locale, etc.

Similarly, few philosophers, few scientists of note and few artists of importance have ever ignored the problem of space. From Aristotle to de Chrico, from Ibn-i Khaldun to Newton, from Einstein to Escher, from Kant to Bach, from Lao Tzu to Le Corbusier, from Oriental miniature painters to Eisenstein, or from

Velasquez to Bill Gates, space has never ceased to puzzle and occupy the human mind and has never ceased to be the object of attention and desire.[4]

Therefore, it would not be an exaggeration to suggest that there are few other objects of discourse or discipline, or few concepts claimed and appropriated by so many practices that still occupy a consolidated space in our culture, only 'Nature', 'Environment' (see Teymur 1982) and 'Hu(–man)'[5] could probably be more widespread). The crucial question would be whether such a concept could justifiably be the object of scientific research and discourse (albeit in the traditional definitions of scientificity).

Secondly, leaving aside the terminological ambiguities, the physical, urban, architectural, geographical and perceptual space is itself so fluid and so *continuous* that it would not be inappropriate to suggest that space is an *omnipresence.* Just imagine the space in the room where you are. It is by no means confined by walls and ceiling. It flows under the table, into the cupboard and the (virtual or the real) emptiness in the computer. It flows out of the window into the house next door and into the city, or into the branches of the trees and continues to envelope the countryside, the neighbouring countries (whether in the EU or not), into tropical forests, to then sneak in the areas between and inside New York skyscrapers, the little gap between the Moon and the Earth, and between all the planets and suns, only to encompass the depths of the oceans and your favourite holiday hide-outs and the inside of the percolators in Italian Cafes.

It should not be deduced from this (imaginary) continuity that space and spatial phenomena are passive frames or innocent backgrounds to life events. They, most specifically, cities, houses, roads, parks or fields, are phenomena that could and do affect almost every aspect of life in an infinite number of ways. They could make human beings feel 'at home' in this World, or be alienated from it (see Teymur 1996b). It would not be an overstatement to say that there can be no 'culture' without space.

What kind of knowledge would this simultaneously continuous, fluent, omnipresent and universal phenomenon that is both big and small, thick and thin and confined and infinite be the knowledge of? Can there be a discipline to accommodate all this on its own; or many disciplines that can encompass all between themselves? What would be the 'values' and the 'others' of any such discipline(s)? While trying to understand this impossible phenomenon, what other than our present disciplines, tools, paradigms and discourses could we be relying on? In other words, leaving aside the possibility of managing, controlling and planning this infinity, what is the extent to which we can understand space in both its universal unboundedness and its local specificities on their own or in their ('glocal') relationships?

---

[4] For a comprehensive survey of the development of the concept of *'space'*, see Harvey (1969).

[5] For the definitions and models of 'man', see for example Simon (1957) and the work of Ernst Cassirer. See also Tekeli (1998).

‘The Symmetry of Ignorance’*:* ‘Epistemological Minimalism Maximalism’*, and a new concept of* ‘Space’

If we take space as the central object, we can see in operation a *‘symmetry of ignorance’* with traditional social sciences on one side and the practices and disciplines of space on the other. Until very recently, social sciences have largely ignored space when it could and should have been an inevitable dimension, a dependent and independent variable, a determinant and determined level and a structural necessity of social, cultural and political analyses. Obviously, there were exceptions such as developmental psychology (which however reduced space to children’s surroundings), anthropology (which looked at the (so-called) primitive villages where kinship patterns could be related to spatial organisation), or geography (where physical and social branches only recently combined forces to try to explain cities, regions, etc.)

Space practices such as architecture, planning and civil engineering treated space variously as form, volume, floor area, plot of land, distance, but seldom as a socially constructed system. They thus ignored society as a spatial phenomenon *and* space as a social one (see Hillier and Hanson 1984 and Markus 1993). I would suggest that both camps were the losers in this symmetry.

The spatial professions take space primarily as the object of problems to be solved. They reduce it variously to volume, floor area or equally ambiguous ‘built environment’. Technological variables are reduced to construction, economic relations to costing and cultural ones to users or clients. When professions are performing their functions, they are bound by fairly inflexible legal, temporal, financial and spatial constraints. They are expected to solve the problems and to do the job, within given limits and by the deadlines set by their clients (see Teymur 1992a). In fulfilling these functions, they are bound to use the minimum necessary knowledge to successfully fulfil their contracts. I call this *‘professional minimalism’* (or, *‘epistemological minimalism’).* This is in contrast with the sciences and, in a different sense, arts which have the aim of developing knowledge and creativity indefinitely – both qualitatively and quantitatively. I call this *‘epistemological maximalism’* (Teymur 1993, 1996a). It is possible to attribute the discomfort that the professional disciplines have in universities to the conflicts of maximalist knowledge and minimalist professionalism as reflected in their respective attitudes and tempo in educational contexts. Yet, although professionals are primarily a sociological, and sciences an epistemological, phenomenon, in fact they are connected with each other in their differences. There is no better case than that of ‘space’, as it is variously appropriated by a large number of disciplines and/or practices (see Lefebvre 1991, and Harvey 1996).

Towards an 'Interspatiality' *that is* 'Interdisciplinary', 'Interframable' *and* 'Glocal'

When we start seeing space as social, and society as spatial, this complex relationship can by no means be comprehended within the boundaries of single traditional disciplines, departments, schools or '-logy's. Instead, we need to develop some *new* concepts, theories and methods of analysis – if not, a new discipline altogether. This departure, however requires some pre-conditions:

1. An *interdisciplinary discipline:* similar to the proposed 'new fruit' as distinct from 'fruit salad', a new intertextual domain of knowledge that does not exclude those that have been left out.

2. *Interframability:* disciplines, practices and discourses define themselves, and operate, by 'framing' themselves. When it is space that is in question, the framing operation should be characterised by what I propose to call *'interframe',* hence, through *'interframability'* (see Teymur undated).

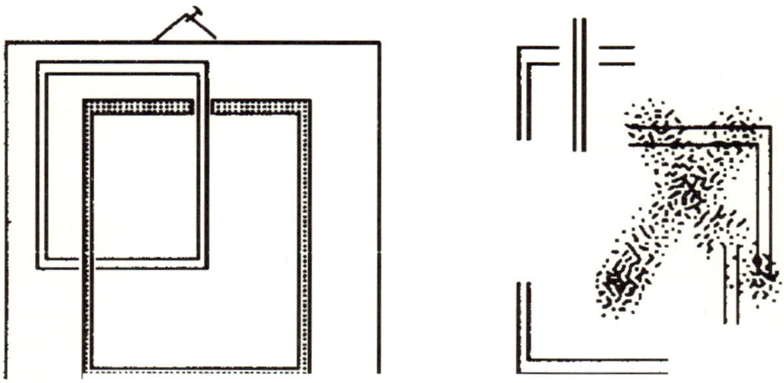

3. *Space-between-disciplines:* we need to develop a concept of *'space-between-disciplines'* as space is dealt with by a number of disciplines without being covered by any single one.

4. *Glocalism:* neither of the opposing concepts of the *local* and the *global* is adequate to cover the omnipresent, multi-local, non-localisable, trans-global, virtual, etc. space. Space, as many other socio-cultural phenomena, has therefore to be defined as *'glocal'* (see Teymur 1992b: 39-48).

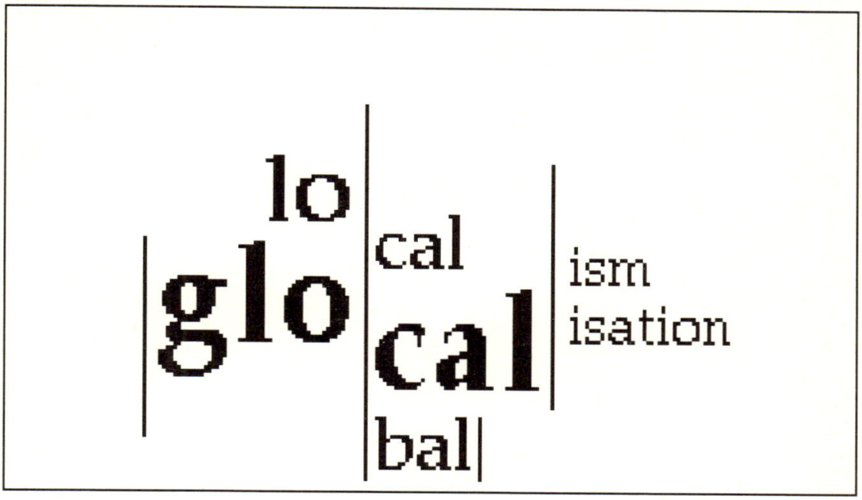

5. *Interspatiality:* as almost no spatial object, phenomena or event is entirely unique in either physical, perceptual or operational terms, a pluralist concept of *interspace,* hence *interspatiality* has to be developed.

6. *Interculturality of space:* spatial phenomena are never entirely or narrowly culture-specific. They cross geographical, social, generational, even temporal, boundaries. They manifest themselves as co-presence, as background, as determinant, as the mortar, or as the subject matter of cultural practices. Space is necessarily *intercultural.*

7. *Interlinguality, interdiscourse and intermedia of space:* The traditional modes of expression are often no match for the interdisciplinary, multi-media and multi-representational presence of spatial phenomena. No amount of, say, drawings, diagrams, writing, figures, photographs, film, painting, etc. can claim to give anything like the comprehensive account of them. A discourse of space that is itself interdiscourse, intermedia and, if necessary, interlingual should be constituted. This might have an additional spin-off for mono-media disciplines. (After all, why should social sciences be largely literary with some added statistics, or architecture be graphical with a lot of pseudo-philosophical accompaniment?)

8. A new *'software ethics':* It is necessary to balance the Western-generated and -dominated hardware culture with a *new* software culture. The existing correspondence between the hard- and the soft-ware halves of the said culture is based on the assumption that the world is an engineering problem.

> The corollary for our discussion here is that space as represented and designed by CAD programmes is treated primarily as a plot of land to be divided up, fenced off, bought, sold and built upon. The interspatial, glocal, intercultural and intermedia space that we have been describing would surely need a more liberated software than that provided by ArchiCAD. This software culture would be literally soft. It would not condone the dominant urban culture that is divisive, cut-throat, racist, militarist and consumerist that invariably makes space as the prime object of violence at almost every level of everyday life.

And extensions...

If and when we manage to enter and to entertain a discourse of space that cannot be constricted by professional, commercial, national or academic territorial instincts, we may begin to see the incredible combination of the mysterious undefinability of space on the one hand, and its concrete materiality on the other. This would start enabling us to comprehend the closeness of such facts of life as environmental pollution, urban land, tele-visual tribe or the internet community, ethical foreign policy, the Millennium Dome, the housing policy and the academy; and to develop an ethics that is just, integrated and sustainable.

When the so-called 'death of the grand narratives' is declared daily almost as a matter of ritual, space can indeed be an alternative focus to the oppositions between the grand and the small as well as the permanence and contingency. Both space and society can thus be understood socio-spatially. The conceptual expansion proposed here could at one and the same time open our eyes but might also blind us. But, it is a risk worth taking.

This should be seen as more than an academic project. This 'project' promises an ideal of 'spatial democracy' that would aim to annul the instinct of us and them, that results in the geographical or academic spaces guarded by barbed wires, guard dogs, closed-circuit TVs or university departments. This space would not be an object of technical practice, nor a topic for more papers, books and seminars; it would be an evidence to the possibility of life *between* disciplines, stools and spaces.

Knowledge and love are two things which do not diminish by sharing. Limiting these through institutionalised disciplines might look like an inevitable fact of civilisation. Yet, an *interspatial disciplinarity* could hopefully construct a shared and sharing culture.

Bibliography:

Blyth, R.H. (1981) *Haiku*, Volume One, Tokyo: Hokuseido Press.

Harvey, D. (1969) *Explanation in Geography*, London: Edward Arnold.

Harvey, D. (1996) *Justice, Nature and the Geography of Difference*, Oxford: Blackwell.

Hillier, B. and J. Hanson, (1984) *Social Logic of Space,* Cambridge: CUP.

Lao Tzu (1955) *The Way of Life (Tao Te Ching)*, New York: Mentor.

Lefebvre, H. (1991) *Production of Space*, Oxford: Blackwell.

Markus, T. A. (1993) *Buildings and Power*, London, Routledge.

Rumi, Maulana J. (1996) *Mathnawi, 5 vols,* ed. R.A. Nicholson, London: Adam Publishers.

Simon, H. A. (1957) *Models of Man*, New York: J. Wiley & Sons.

Tekeli, I. (1998) "Disiplinler ve farkl› insan modelleri", in: *Sosyal Bilimleri Yeniden Düflünmek*, Istanbul: Metis, 13-33.

Teymur, N. (n.d.) "Framing the Frames", in: Erzen, J. N., ed., *Art and Taboos,* Ankara: Sanart, 157-60.

Teymur, N. (1982) *Environmental Discourse, — a critical analysis of 'environmentalism' in architecture, planning, design, ecology, social sciences and the media,* London: Question Press.

Teymur, N. (1992a) "'The city lost under a pile of Architecture' — learning beyond the limits of architectural approach to the city", in: van Duin, L., ed., *Research as it relates to architectural teaching,* Delft: TUD, 144-49.

Teymur, N. (1992b) *Architectural Education*, London: Question Press.

Teymur, N. (1993) "Learning Housing Designing: the homeless design education", in Bulos, M. and Teymur, N., eds., *Housing: Design Research Education*, Aldershot: Avebury, 3-27.

Teymur, N. (1996a) "Epistemological Maximalism vs. Professional Minimalism", in: Foque, R., ed., *Doctorates in Design and Architecture*, Volume Two, TUD: Delft, 101-105.

Teymur, N. (1996b) "Housing as the Other", in: Komut, E., ed., *Housing Question of the Others,* Ankara: Chamber of Architects Publications, 3-21.

Worton, M. and J. Still, eds., (1990) *Intertextuality: Theories and Practices,* Manchester, Manchester UP.

BIBLIOGRAPHIC BOUNDARIES AND FORGOTTEN CANONS

ANDREW CARLIN

Taking sociology as its working exemplar, this essay explores the bibliographic precedents of 'substantive' topics and bibliographic bases of 'cultural disciplines'.

This essay argues that the changeable focus of sociology towards reified, substantive topics, e.g. the sociology of begging, the sociologies of space and time, occurs at the expense of extant corpora of literature. As 'new' topics attain increased profiles within the discipline, sociologists disattend previously published works which are not recognised as relevant to their projects-at-hand.

The tendency within sociology to reify topics has implications for research. Rather than developing a more inclusive discipline, reifications of subject-areas exclude bodies of literature. Furthermore, neglected works have addressed those issues which sociologists who subscribe to changing fashions regard as 'innovative' topics of inquiry. Some modern theoretical developments are unacknowledged rewordings of existing sociological works, which are no longer fixtures on course reading-lists.

Introduction

In this essay[1] I shall remark upon bibliographies and "disciplinary boundaries" (see Carlin 1999a: 61). I take textual artefacts (bibliographies, footnotes, textbooks) as data for study because they are loci of disciplinary boundaries and, therefore, of interdisciplinary bases. Whilst there exists a discipline dedicated to the study of bibliography, it does not subject bibliographies to textual analysis. By interrogating bibliographies as iterative rather than inert texts we can examine phenomena such as disciplinary boundaries and the "ownership" of subject-matter – what Charles Page referred to as "restricted scholarly territories" (Page 1959: 584). This analytic attitude reveals the entailments of bibliographies. To paraphrase Graham Watson, I am treating bibliographies "as *texts in which are embodied the interpretive practices* whereby [scholars] realise their disciplinary boundaries" (Watson 1984:352; emphasis supplied). I suggest, then, that bibliographies are sites of interdisciplinarity.

Interdisciplinarity is the practical accomplishment of analysts *via* the selection of methods and disciplinary conventions. An analytic gain of interdisciplinarity is to bring conceptual and epistemological assumptions of

[1] I would like to thank Robert C. Hanson and Rodney Watson for their comments.

individual disciplines into sharper relief (Watson 1987: 285-286). Whilst the election of "disciplinary interactions" (Smith 1992: 261) may constitute an "interdisciplinary field", it remains the case that the articulation of disciplinary work is the logical prior of interdisciplinary work. In order to *do* interdisciplinarity we have to trade upon disciplinary work. Henceforth, this essay facilitates considerations of interdisciplinarity predicated upon the logical grammar of individual disciplines. Furthermore, as I shall outline, disciplinary work is manifest through its "discipline-specific" (Garfinkel 1996) bibliographies. As such, bibliographies can be treated as discipline-specific documents.

The locations for bibliographies under consideration are in works from 'substantive' fields and textbook presentations of sociology. Following Lynch and Bogen (1997: 482), I take textbooks to be "part of a stable, highly standardised, widely disseminated disciplinary pedagogy". Moreover, within textbooks there are to be found attempts to delineate the discipline and its subject matter.[2] Hence, I shall elaborate on the synoptic nature of textbooks, and the 'editor's work' in assembling a collection.

There is no mystery to my method: for those concerned with such matters as parameters and criteria for selection, the textbooks used here were simply within arm's reach. The generic nature of these observations may be surmised from the ready accessibility of materials; phenomena discussed here are locatable among library collections elsewhere. Among the sources for my arguments are the works of the analytical sociologist, Pitirim A. Sorokin. A consequence of the materials used is to assess the provenance of the programme of interdisciplinarity.

Textbooks and 'Textbook Definitions'

> The vogue for fashionable ideas in sociology is fickle. Sociologists eagerly latch onto what appear to be new bodies of thought; they toy with them for a while (organising symposia to discuss their significance for the discipline, giving over special editions of the discipline's journals to them, and proliferating texts that debate their merits), but then, often as not, sociology moves on.
> (Button 1991: 1)

Button illustrates how the "business of sociology" is flexible; flexible in terms of adapting to suit the needs of its practitioners, who introduce "new moves" in the discipline. 'New moves' in sociology do not challenge the discipline but are

---

[2] Through detailed description of "sociological emphasis" in textbook accounts, Hobbs shows "that the content, emphases, and unadmitted conceptual framework of 'textbook sociology' are *professionally unacceptable* and require modification" (1951: 3; emphasis added). In focusing on the field of the sociology of scientific knowledge (SSK), both as a *lacuna* in and contradictory feature of sociology-textbook presentations of science, Lynch and Bogen (1997) note how sociology textbooks are "asociological".

absorbed by it; 'new moves' actively maintain "the stable properties of the discipline's foundations" (Button 1991: 1). Button's remarks on 'new moves' cohere with Kuhn's (1962) notion of "normal science": 'new moves' do not precipitate revolutions within the discipline, but constitute additive fields predicated upon the presuppositions of the discipline as normal science.

There is a linguistic basis for these observations, which is the arrogation of words with ordinary, natural meanings by sociology; this is coterminous with the mapping of competitive "professional sociological" meanings onto these words (Rose 1960). That is, words, which already carry meanings, are re-appropriated for sociological purposes. In this way, we can see how the waxing and waning of fashionable topics in sociology are *worded entities*. Issues discussed in sociological literature are subject to preservation and transformation, whereby an extant issue is articulated differently at different times (for example, the re-wording of 'social exclusion' as 'marginality'). As Hughes (1961: 554) remarked, "An idea does not always keep the same name – especially in sociology." So there are not just new topics and new ideas, but new wordings of topics and ideas.

We can use Sharrock's (1974) notions of "ownership" and category-bound knowledge in discussing conceptual work and disciplinary work. In his seminal paper, Sharrock demonstrates how bodies of knowledge are seen to "belong" to particular collectivities. Descriptions of knowledge "specify the relationship which that corpus has to the constituency" (Sharrock 1974: 49). Using Evans-Pritchard's example of Baka medicine and Zande medicine, Sharrock shows how the naming of a corpus of knowledge in relation to a category makes the "ownership" of that knowledge procedurally available. We can apply Sharrock's observations to the iteration and reiteration of concepts for and topics of sociology as "sociological concepts", i.e. how analysts word and re-word "the business of sociology", or re-appropriate and redefine previously identified phenomena (Helm 1982: 156). With "interstitial" exceptions (Sorokin 1931; Teymur, chapter 6 in this volume), the study of certain phenomena is perceived to be "owned" by certain disciplines.

As the source materials used in this essay demonstrate, the programme of interdisciplinarity can be regarded as another instance of a 'new move', between and within disciplines. Button suggests that 'new moves' readily constitute what becomes known as "social theory today". We can even compare textbooks titled *Modern Social Theory*. For all the 'new moves' in sociology, a notable feature of the "modern social theory" of 1968 and 1992 is how similar it all is; Percy S. Cohen and Ian Craib (respectively) present readers with a stable and durable discipline – a discipline that is, to borrow Garfinkel's phrase, "invariant to the exigencies" of its adherents and detractors alike. From their opening chapters ("The nature of sociological theory" – Cohen [1968: 1-17]; "What's wrong with theory and why we still need it" – Craib [1992: 3-13]), readers are impressed by the uniformity of textbook presentations.[3] Even the opening gambit of the

---

[3] The textbook formula is contrasted with the original monograph by Sorokin (1929).

respective first chapters ("The word 'theory'" – Cohen [1968: 1]; "The very word 'theory'" – Craib [1992: 3]) is predicated upon the same presuppositions: that 'theory' is a polysemous term[4]; which, therefore, means different things to different people; that the word 'theory' can be off-putting for some; and that theories may be more complex than they appear due to the elaborate use of jargon. There is a similitude between discussions of theories concerning structure and action; cosmetic differences in Craib's text include the attention to the work of Jürgen Habermas, postmodernism, structuration theory and reflexivity. These advances constitute 'new moves' *within* the discipline rather than respecifications *of* the discipline.

There is a formulaic concern within textbooks to present the ubiquitous "Word About Sociology Itself" (MacIver and Page 1950: v-vi). This is, typically, a prefatory statement to define the subject-matter of sociology, and to differentiate sociology from other disciplines (Broom and Selznick 1955: 3-6; Coser and Rosenberg 1972: 1-16; Johnson 1961: 2-6). The contrast set used to determinate the subject is a familiar litany of disciplines: anthropology, economics, history, psychology. Hobbs dissents from the uniform view of sociology as a discipline with its own subject matter, arguing that "sociology, as presented in textbooks, is largely made up of residues – aspects of behaviour and society which are not included in other disciplines" (Hobbs 1951: 175).[5] Departures from what Lynch and Bogen (*op. cit.*) identify as the "standard" or idealised conception include 'specialised' volumes (Berger and Luckmann 1967: 207ff.; Connerton 1976: 11-39; Rao 1974: 1-17). Worsley *et al.* include a selection of readings within their edited collection on "Sociology as a Discipline" (1970: 15-66).

Bell and Vogel attempt to draw together an interdisciplinary slice of material on a substantive topic, the family, "without regard to the boundaries of academic disciplines" (1960: v). They try to collect and organise bodies of work, thematically related both by the substantive topic of study and theoretical orientation – Functional Analysis. However, it is this very unifying paradigm of the studies they select that makes this collection not so much interdisciplinary, but one that resides in the 'comfort-zone' that Button identifies as the "business of sociology".

As both Button and Watson independently argue, ethnomethodology – to take a case in point – "is not just another sociology" (G. Watson 1992: xxi). This means that ethnomethodology cannot be added to a list of sociologies. It does not fit into this 'comfort-zone'; it cannot be incorporated into 'mainstream'

[4] For diachronic and etymological analyses of 'theory', see Rose (1994). For an earlier, extended discussion of these developments, see Rose (1985).

[5] He goes on to assert that "sociology consists of a picking up of loose ends which have been ignored by other disciplines" (Hobbs 1951: 175). This point requires elaboration, however: Sorokin (1931) argues that sociology also consists of its *approach* to phenomena, which distinguishes it from other disciplines.

sociology; it cannot be used to address mainstream concerns *in the same way as* 'new moves' which take their place within the sociological Pantheon.

Watson (1984) took the defining of disciplinary boundaries as a topic for study. He examined the boundaries between social and cultural anthropology, and how they are achieved. The boundaries of a discipline are analysts' achievements. This is the case *a fortiori* when the analytic work of a discipline is parasitic upon members' work. In his seminal article on the ordinary language foundations of sociological concepts, which Ball (1970: 330) referred to as "an undeservedly neglected paper", Rose (1960) demonstrates that the terminology of sociology is based upon everyday terminology:

> The original sociological designations of society were of course not devised by *professional* social scientists. Indeed, almost all of the established technical vocabulary of sociology has been taken over from the common stock of words in ordinary languages, and there is hardly a widely-received sociological term that was not long ago assigned a *non-professional* and yet clearly sociological meaning. (Rose 1960: 196; emphasis added)

In assembling a collection of readings for students, Coser and Rosenberg (1972) provide, as the first chapter, a "Definition of the Field". But they *have* to provide a definition of the field because the field they define assumes a competitive relation with members' ordinary definitions:

> Culture, as used by American anthropologists, is of course a technical term which must not be confused with the more limited concept of ordinary language and of history and literature. (Kluckhohn 1972: 42)

Robert K. Merton recognised that functional analysis rendered itself a hostage to fortune *via* the inconsistent usage of terminology. In his book *Social Theory and Social Structure*, Merton (1957: 74ff) identifies the varied vocabularies of sociology, and delimits the use of the word 'function' within functional analysis. Earlier, Hornell Hart (1953) had reviewed over 100 papers on operationalism, in which the word 'operation' was inconsistently defined by different authors.

'Originality' and the Bibliographic Basis of 'Forgotten Canons'

Sorokin wrote an extensive and detailed series of critiques of various tendencies within sociology – *Fads and Foibles in Modern Sociology and Related Sciences* (Sorokin 1958). Whilst this book carries many serious messages for the social sciences, cultural studies and the programme of interdisciplinarity, the first chapter – "Amnesia and New Columbuses" – has particular relevance here.

Sorokin demonstrates how, time and again, entire bodies of sociological research are forgotten (or deliberately omitted) by authors who *claim* to have discovered new sociological territories.[6] Sorokin carefully documents those instances where:

> the indexes of their books list none, or very few, of the thinkers of preceding centuries, in contrast to a long list of 'researchers' belonging to the author's 'Mutual Back-Patting Insurance Company'. (Sorokin 1958: 4)

Sorokin's arguments are not confined to the non-attribution of ideas – as Ellsworth Faris (1953) comments on Talcott Parsons; and Newton (1999: 422, 435-436) suggests by comparing the 'new' theories of Anthony Giddens with the relatively forgotten writings of Norbert Elias. Here, Newton provides another example of the re-wording of existing theories as 'novel' contributions to sociological thought. Sorokin, in great detail, goes on to argue that "'modern discoveries' were made long ago; and in the works of the previous thinkers they were, if anything, analysed better, understood more adequately, and formulated even more precisely" (Sorokin 1958: 7) than contemporary sociologists reveal. Howard Becker recalls how, during his graduate education at the University of Chicago, Louis Wirth told students that "originality was the product of a faulty memory" (1986: 136).

However, what Sorokin describes was to happen to his own work. In the foreword to *Social and Cultural Mobility* (Sorokin 1959), he acknowledges the currency and wording of concepts "even by those who use them without any reference to my volume". We may also note the omission of Sorokin's work in articles purportedly about the sociologies of time and space. Both these substantive topics illustrate Button's arguments on 'new moments' in sociology – through the proliferation of journal articles and inception of dedicated journals. Yet the contributions to the sociologies of space and time routinely neglect Sorokin's works, *Sociocultural Causality, Space, Time*, published in 1943; his co-authored article with Merton (1937); and two volumes of his monumental *Social and Cultural Dynamics*, which date back even further.[7]

The constitutive practices of literature reviewing – the activities of information retrieval – are dependent upon establishing some correspondence between search parameters: titles, keywords, abstracts, etc (Carlin 1999b). Given the nature of keywords and controlled vocabularies, it is difficult to appreciate how Piper, in her (1996) essay on passing, failed to retrieve Watson's (1970) recognition of heterogeneous ethnic categories in (purportedly) ethnically homogenous institutions in South Africa. Whilst the practices of information

---

6 Robert Park was accused of not acknowledging his predecessors, until the graduate accuser "noted the dates of original publication, and wondered why his favourite authors had not acknowledged *their* debt to Park" (Hughes 1964: 19; emphasis added).

7 I am not claiming that Sorokin was the founder of the sociologies of time or space; Émile Durkheim, for example, acknowledged the importance of the classification and representation of time in his study *The Elementary Forms of the Religious Life*, originally published in 1912. Cf. Sorokin's own bibliographies for further references.

retrieval *may* direct researchers to Roth's (1963) work on timetables for tuberculosis patients in a sanatorium, such contingent research activities – that is, the reliance upon matching search-terms – miss the timetables and spatial arrangements of convicts (Wieder 1974), convicts and staff in selection-board meetings (Atkinson 1967), and delinquent children in residential care (Polsky 1962). More seriously, perhaps, the sociologies of space and time have still to pick up on Seeley's (1956) ethnographic study of a Toronto housing estate, which includes extensive studies of the rhythms and patterns of its residents.

I am neither trying to be adversarial, nor pedantic, but to highlight the issues of *relevance* and *salience* between and within bibliographic boundaries. Topicalising relevance demonstrates the deleterious nature of reading-lists, the development of sociology in its propositional forms ('the sociology *of*...') and the emergence of sub-fields – 'new' topics of study. Seeley's work is of relevance to research projects outside urban planning and the sociology of the city: if sociologists *chose* to re-read *Crestwood Heights*, they would find it of central relevance to the sociologies of space and time. As it is, Seeley does not find a place on course reading-lists. Course directors face *ipso facto* deadlines to reinstate texts such as *Crestwood Heights* within the canon. Due to neglect (where 'neglect' is measured by records of use and borrower statistics, and is visually available to the librarian from the last date-of-issue stamp inside the front cover), books are being withdrawn, i.e. discarded by university libraries on the grounds that they are superfluous to requirements.[8] It would be an irony indeed if *Crestwood Heights* was withdrawn in order to make room for 'new' texts on time and space.

Disciplinary boundaries and the "ownership" of subject-areas inhibit the study of begging practices, considerations of which are found under miscellaneous subject areas, e.g. sociology and social policy, the overlap between studies on begging, homelessness and poverty. Compiling a literature review for a study on begging (Carlin, Evergeti and Murtagh 1999) identifies, what Garfinkel found in his studies of the discovering sciences, "a gap in the literature" (Garfinkel and Wieder 1992: 188). This literature review highlights the requirements of interdisciplinarity, as I found literature relevant to a sociology of begging from across disciplinary boundaries.

Works which, regrettably, are no longer fixtures on course reading-lists provide detailed and extensive material on beggars and begging. I found works from that branch of sociology known as symbolic interactionism[9] to be rich in

---

[8] "Requirements" are twofold: academic requirements, as indicated by lecturers' recommendations and inclusion on course outlines; and library requirements, the pressure to find space to shelve and store books.

[9] In terms of "ownership", distinct forms of sociology are associated with symbolic interactionism, e.g. "Chicago School" and "Iowa School". Thus the type of sociology that the category-description "symbolic interactionism" stands proxy for is indexical. I am referring to the Blumer/Wirth ethnographic tradition commonly described as "Chicago School sociology".

their descriptions of beggars and begging and "noticeably absent" (Schegloff 1972: 388-389) from bibliographies in contemporary sociological accounts (Dean 1999). I was particularly struck by the relevance of historical accounts of journeys to Jerusalem and the Holy Land: a whole corpus of literature, readily available and relevant to sociologists, just waiting to be read.

A further point raised by the begging projects cited above is the status of materials consulted during the production of a literature review. Literature reviews are assembled objects (Carlin 1999b), in that corpora of literature are cumulatively retrieved according to the analyst's changing state of knowledge, *ad hoc* judgements *apropos* the relevance of materials to the problem at hand, and the contingencies of retrieval themselves (references which are returned by search engines according to search parameters, delays in receipt of inter-library loans, etc.). However, the practices of assembling corpora of literature – search-tools do not discriminate between disciplines, paradigms or epistemologies – potentiate the inclusion of logically incompatible source materials. The programme of interdisciplinarity risks the creation of "category mistakes" in its studies *ab initio*, through the conflation of different language games within the literature-reviewing process. Park (1967 [1925]: 123) appreciated this danger in a *caveat* for readers, that he discusses "two volumes so different in content and point of view in the same general category" (namely magic and mentality). However, his solution to the problem was to avoid analytic precision in favour of a "broad definition" of a category. The breadth of category-definition as an activity for all practical purposes is apparent in glosses produced by editors, to which I shall now turn in the following section.

'The Editor's Work'

A locus of 'establishing boundaries' and 'boundary maintenance' is the introduction to the textbook or the edited collection. Let me call this the 'editor's work': the onus is on the editor to provide coherence to the collection – a coherence achieved *via* the appeal to disciplinary boundaries.

Indeed, we could suggest that it is the responsibility of the editor to provide readers with a framework with which to read the collection. Turner (1974: 7) is explicit about the editor's work in his collection of readings on ethnomethodology: "The subsuming of these works under that rubric is my responsibility". It is incumbent upon the editor to provide coherence to the articles. Also, in putting out a call-for-papers and deciding which papers are accepted for publication, the editor is able to define a field as broadly or as narrowly as they wish. So the editor's work may impact upon interdisciplinarity: in the case of Laver and Hutcheson's collection (1972: 11), a wide definition of conversation facilitates the inclusion of papers from a variety of disciplines. Between editors there remains a difference in emphasis: whilst sociolinguistics, according to Pride and Holmes (1972: 7), "has been established as a distinct discipline for some years", Giglioli (1972: 8) asserts that its "interdisciplinary approach makes the substantive boundaries of sociolinguistics somewhat imprecise". In so doing, and in the case of Watson and Seiler (1992), the editor is able to identify and highlight "disputes about emerging disciplinary boundaries" (G. Watson 1992: xvii). Indeed, *Text in Context* constitutes a debate between (potentially irreconcilable) positions within the cognate disciplines ethnomethodology and conversation analysis (CA), *apropos* the requirement for and/or desirability of ethnographic background for the analysis of textual materials.

As an instance of the 'editor's work', we can examine the attempts to incorporate CA into the linguistic discipline pragmatics, *via* a practice of re-referencing or 're-bibliographicising'. *Re-bibliographicising* – compiling a bibliography anew – enables Schegloff *et al* (1996: 16ff.) to identify "convergences" between CA and linguistics. For those familiar with CA as a respecification of both sociology *and* linguistics, motives for this incorporationist project (the absorption of CA as another 'new move' in sociology and linguistics) become "inferentially available".

But herewith the reflexive relation of texts and bibliographies: the body of the text provides the relevance of references – *via* citations or suggestions for further reading – and these references, in turn, mutually elaborate the body of the text. For example, the references in Musgrave's *Sociology of Education* have an achieved relatedness to the sociology of education. Likewise, the contributions to Merton, Broom and Cottrell's (1959) edited collection inform and elaborate the references and further readings on substantive topics, such as the sociology *of* law, the sociology *of* medicine, the sociology *of* occupations, etc. Inspecting Alberione's (1962) text, we can see how, through the judicious work of citation – assembling a bibliography 'sympathetic' to arguments – that sociology can be presented as a Christian discipline. Thus, marshalling bibliographic items in this way can be regarded as a "standard device" for what Glaser and Strauss (1968: 228ff) – in terms of supportive quotations, "dramatic segments" and "telling phrases" – call "conveying credibility".

What I am arguing is that bibliographies *per se* are 'corpus-formative' documents – they define a field of study. Bibliographies, as textual artefacts, manifest the determination of a field *via* the practices of assembling bibliographies.[10] Such definitional privilege is arrogated by analysts, who discern relevance to a field in certain texts – but not others. I suggest that this is not a satisfactory state of affairs, because such determinations of relevance are made

[10] This determination is manifest through "noticeable absences" in bibliographies, too: on reading a discussion on, for example, politeness phenomena, we may observe that Norbert Elias' work is absent from the bibliography. Such a scenario is mooted by Rescher (1998: 92), who notes that even when particular references "one would normally expect to be taken into account" are missing from the bibliography, "[t]hey are prominent there through their invisibility." As I shall argue below, exclusions (and inclusions) in bibliographies make certain inferences procedurally available.

with the assumption that the relevance of any particular reference to a field is predicated upon its use within the field, or upon the analyst's awareness of its contents. From the examples discussed throughout this essay, this is an inadequate estimation of relevance. Furthermore, the *de facto* division of labour within sociology, produced by substantive fields of study, potentiates the analysis not just of disciplinary boundaries but *intra*-disciplinary boundaries.

This corpus-formative nature of bibliographies points towards the reflexivity of bibliographies as discipline-specific documents. Garfinkel and Sacks originally articulated the ethnomethodological notion of reflexivity in relation to descriptions: "a description [...] in the ways it may be a constituent part of the circumstances it describes, in endless ways and unavoidably, elaborates those circumstances and is elaborated by them" (1970: 338). We may also remark upon the reflexive relation between the corpus-formative nature of references and what Garfinkel (1996) terms "corpus status". The corpus status of material elaborates the corpus-formative character of its use; while at the same time the material draws its corpus status from the corpus-formative aspect of the bibliography.

Between and within discipline-specific corpora of literature, works are afforded different corpus status. Hence, the methodological implications of Sudnow's (1972) paper, for the sociology of time and visual sociology, may go unappreciated. The methodological and generic relevance of Mehan's (1978) paper on classroom interaction to linguists and sociologists may not be appreciated due to its placement in a specialist journal, where "specialist" refers to a journal's corpus status within specific academic communities. Likewise, analysts, for projects on temporality, may miss an empirical study of temporal accounts as produced by members (Button 1990).

Each of the above examples highlights the issues of corpus status and the perceived relevance of materials: a core journal for one scholar is of little interest to another. Howard Becker's discussion of publishing research is relevant here, as these materials are, *mutatis mutandis*, "published in a place where [members interested in a particular topic] would be unlikely to see it" (Becker 1971: 268).

Bibliographies and references listed under the heading "Suggestions for further reading" are, in Harvey Sacks' terms, "inferentially rich". Craib's textbook *Modern Social Theory*, is unremittingly hostile towards ethnomethodology; the level of animus within the text is reflected in the suggestions for further reading. Craib (1992: 110) recommends a paper (Atkinson 1988) that ethnomethodologists regard as an ill-informed attack on ethnomethodology as "A useful summary" of the area. This indicates the *pro tempore* nature of bibliographies, as Craib cites Atkinson without addressing Garfinkel's later statements on ethnomethodology (e.g. 1988), which were available to him at the time of writing. He refers to Aaron Cicourel as being "one of the most interesting ethnomethodologists" (Craib 1992: 105), even when Cicourel disaffiliated himself and his work from ethnomethodology; he refers to Cicourel's *Cognitive Sociology* as a classic text in ethnomethodology when, in its mentalistic emphasis on interpretation, there is little discernibly ethnomethodological about it; and regards Cicourel's work as the definitive corpus of ethnomethodological research.[11] From the readings Craib uses, and the further reading he recommends, one can infer his position *vis-à-vis* ethnomethodology. We should consider also whether an introductory textbook is the appropriate place to express such deeply-held opinions: quite simply, is it fair upon students? Although ethnomethodologists can easily defend themselves against the criticisms he advances, it places the onus on beginning students of social theory to extricate themselves from the conflation of education and vituperation.

According to 'textbook' writer Joseph Fichter, the student of sociology "is likely to be confused by certain contributions to sociological literature that go far beyond the field of sociology" (Fichter 1957: 6). Sociology is, and always has been, an "interdisciplinary discipline", albeit one which has "gradually purified itself of its analogous interpretations" (Fichter 1957: 7). For 'textbook' sociology, the sociologist must be cognisant of other disciplines insofar as sociologists deem them to be *relevant* to sociology. Biology, geography, history, philosophy, psychology: for 'textbook' sociology, the sociologist can pick and mix from this *smorgasbord* of disciplines what Fichter calls "prerequisites of knowledge" (1957: 7). However, Fichter's prerequisites of knowledge from these "auxiliary disciplines" (Fichter 1957: 8) – heredity, climate, behaviour patterns – the sociologist takes on trust. So the interdisciplinary programme of 'textbook' sociology is nullified through "methodological irony" (Anderson and Sharrock 1981; Watson 1998) – in Fichter's textbook, the "facts" of any discipline, when incorporated into sociology, are transformed into "assumptions" (Fichter 1957: 8). This is a discipline-specific example of Sharrock's analogy of "ownership", whereby a corpus of knowledge is preserved but its status (the ascription of category ownership) is transformed.

The 'suggested readings' sections of textbooks engage with the realisation of interdisciplinarity. For all Fichter's interdisciplinary zeal, nearly all of his 'recommendations for further reading' are sociological.

Discussion

Whether Cultural Studies constitutes the attempt to reinvent wheels, or invent different kinds of wheels with different kinds of spokes, its bibliographic bases and boundaries are not exempt from scrutiny in terms of disciplinary provenance and the history of ideas. Like Hughes (1961: 555), I am wary of synoptic glosses provided by textbooks. We should direct students towards the 'natural history' of

---

[11] For a critical assessment of Cicourel's work *vis-à-vis* the ethnomethodological programme, with particular reference to rules and rule-following, see Coulter (1974: 114-116).

concepts and theoretical precursors. Furthermore, we should be aware how phenomena are perceived to be 'owned' by disciplines, and re-worded over time – an awareness to be used in the preparation of course outlines and assembling reading lists.[12] As the above examples on begging, time, and space demonstrate, in order to produce adequate surveys of literature, analysts should not limit themselves to bibliographic databases[13] and keyword searches, bibliographic boundaries or discipline-specific materials.

A possible 'solution' to the 'problem' of "restricted scholarly territories" as practised by sociologists is to learn from the topical inquiries of the relatively forgotten sociologist, Pitirim A. Sorokin. He demonstrates a formal approach to subject-areas, disregarded by current, substantive fields. As his Harvard colleague, Talcott Parsons, remarked, "good general theory in the field of human action, no matter how firmly grounded in one discipline, is inevitably interdisciplinary theory" (1959: 37). For example, in an extensive and wide-ranging essay, Sorokin and Hanson assemble "a vast body of evidence" (1974: 99) relevant to a particular topic – namely, "creative love". News reports, case-studies, vignettes, analyses and bibliographic references are collected together without regard to the disciplinary provenance of materials. We could classify their study for different practical purposes: as a demonstration of formal sociology, a forerunner to grounded theory (Glaser and Strauss 1968),[14] or an instantiation of interdisciplinarity *in action*.

At the same time, we should learn from Becker's (1986: 144) approach to doing research: he describes how he collects various theoretical "modules" from extant works. These modules are concepts advanced by other authors, which may be useful to apply in his own inquiries. This is "one good reason to know the literature: so that you will know what pieces are available and not waste time doing what has already been done" (Becker 1986: 142). Alternatively, we could adopt a methodological policy of "ethnomethodological indifference" (Garfinkel and Sacks 1970), by focusing inquiry on the topic of study, not the disciplinary provenance of bibliographic items. Regardless of disciplinary boundaries, what is *relevant* to the inquiry is a candidate for inclusion *in* the inquiry.

---

[12] Ruitenbeek (Ogburn 1966: ix) suggests that "at a time when students especially are reluctant to study the fundamental works in their area of interest, but prefer to read extracts assembled for them, that the original works be made available". Doctoral candidates, encouraged to use the most up-to-date research in their theses, become aware that in terms of theoretical and descriptive adequacy, recently published sources do not necessarily supersede existing works.

[13] Bibliographic databases stored on CD-ROMs offer users choices between searching e.g. 'Arts and Humanities' or 'Social Sciences'; i.e. bibliographic boundaries are defined in media exogenous to the project at hand.

[14] Originally published in 1953 by The Julian Press, it makes no sense in chronological terms to characterise Sorokin and Hanson's study as either "Goffmanesque" or "Grounded Theory", for it predates such ascriptions.

In working towards interdisciplinarity researchers should remember the *caveats* proposed by Willard Waller: we should be careful not to import wholesale the ideologies and vagaries of disciplines – including their "self-contradictions and illogicalities" (Waller 1936: 932). Interdisciplinarity works both ways: it is not just a matter of taking the most useful pieces of disciplinary tools to suit a researcher's needs in an *ad hoc* manner; interdisciplinarity also involves learning from other discipline's mistakes.[15] Researchers committed to interdisciplinarity should expect critique from other disciplines when they make moves which are deemed inappropriate to the phenomena of study.

Disciplines are not necessarily complementary. It is of crucial importance to ensure that the programme of interdisciplinarity involves the realisation of cognate forms of inquiry. That is, when doing interdisciplinary work we should avoid the creation of "category-mistakes", which result from analysts making moves between incompatible "language games". Concepts may be used coherently within disciplines, but attempts to apply a concept outside the terms of its own category, e.g. between disciplines, undermines its logical coherence. Watson illustrates this using the following metaphor: "[in terms of interdisciplinarity] analytic practices cannot be conflated any more than the games of football and tennis be conflated to produce a 'supergame'" (Watson 1992: 11). I am referring here to the ordinary language philosophy of Gilbert Ryle (1966), and the analytic philosophy of Ludwig Wittgenstein (1958). Each individual discipline has its own logical grammar; disciplines constitute different "forms of life".[16] Appreciating the endogenous 'rules' of disciplines is crucial to the realisation of any meaningful programme of interdisciplinarity.

As Florian Znaniecki remarked,

> It is all very well to cultivate the borderlands between the special sciences, but each science should first cultivate properly its *own* field by its own methods. (Znaniecki 1940: 1; emphasis added)

Bibliography:

Alberione, J. (1962) *Fundamentals of Christian Sociology,* Boston, Mass: St. Paul.

Anderson, D.C., and Sharrock, W.W. (1981) "Irony as a methodological theory: A sketch of four sociological variations", *Poetics Today* 4, 565-579.

[15] Although analysis of the study of personal pronouns in linguistics and sociology demonstrates how the 'same mistakes' may be made by practitioners from different disciplines (Watson 1987: 265).

[16] Bjelić (1992) explicates differences between disciplines in terms of *Lebenswelt* pairs, namely scientific demonstration and the *in situ* work of demonstrating.

Atkinson, J.M. (1967) *The Selection of Prisoners for the Hostel Scheme: A Study of a Selection Board,* London: Home Office Research Unit.

Atkinson, P. (1988) "Ethnomethodology: a critical review", *Annual Review of Sociology* 441-465.

Ball, D.W. (1970) "The problematics of respectability", in: Douglas, J.D., ed. *Deviance and Respectability,* New York, NY: Basic Books.

Becker, H.S. (1971) "Problems in the publication of field studies", in: Vidich, A.J., Bensman, J. and Stein, M.R., eds. *Reflections on Community Studies,* New York: Harper Torchbooks.

Becker, H.S. (1986) *Writing for Social Scientists,* Chicago and London: University of Chicago Press.

Bell, N.W. and Vogel, E.F. (1960) *A Modern Introduction to The Family,* New York: The Free Press.

Berger, P.L. and Luckmann, T. (1967) *The Social Construction of Reality,* London: Penguin.

Bjelić, D. (1992) "The praxiological validity of natural scientific practices as a criterion for identifying their unique social-object character: The case of the 'authentication' of Goethe's morphological theorem", *Qualitative Sociology* 15, 221-245.

Broom, L. and Selznick, P. (1955) *Sociology: A Text with Adapted Readings,* Evanston, Illinois: Row, Peterson and Company.

Button, G. (1990) "On members' time", in: Conein, B., de Fornel, M., Quéré, L., eds. *Les Formes de la Conversation*, Vol. 1, Paris: CNET.

Button, G., ed. (1991) *Ethnomethodology and the Human Sciences,* Cambridge: Cambridge University Press.

Carlin, A.P. (1999a) "The works of Edward Rose: a bibliography", *Ethnographic Studies* 4, 61-77.

Carlin, A.P. (1999b) "Literature reviews as 'assembled objects': An ethnographic case-study", *5th Postgraduate Education Discussion Group Conference*, Keele University, November 27 1999.

Carlin, A.P., Evergeti, V. and Murtagh, G.M. (1999) "Visible identities at work: preliminary observations on categorisations and 'street performers' in 'Cathedral Square'", *British Sociological Association Annual Conference*, University of Glasgow, April 6-9.

Cicourel, A.V. (1973) *Cognitive Sociology,* Harmondsworth: Penguin.

Cohen, P.S. (1968) *Modern Social Theory,* London: Heinemann.

Connerton, P., ed. (1976) *Critical Sociology: Selected Readings,* Harmondsworth: Penguin.

Coser, L.A. and Rosenberg, B., eds. (1972) *Sociological Theory: A Book of Readings,* London: Macmillan.

Coulter, J. (1974) "The ethnomethodological programme in contemporary sociology", *The Human Context* 6, 103-122.

Craib, I. (1992) *Modern Social Theory,* New York: Harvester Wheatsheaf.

Dean, H., ed. (1999) *Begging and Street Level Economic Activity*, Bristol: Polity.

Faris, E. (1953) "Review of Talcott Parsons *The Social System* (1951; Glencoe, Illinois: The Free Press)", *American Sociological Review* 18, 103-106.

Fichter, J.H. (1957) *Sociology,* Chicago and London: University of Chicago Press.

Garfinkel, H. (1988) "Evidence for locally produced, naturally accountable phenomena of order*, logic, reason, meaning, method, etc. in and as of the essential quiddity of immortal ordinary society (I of IV): An announcement of studies", *Sociological Theory* 6, 103-109.

Garfinkel, H. (1996) "Ethnomethodology's program", *Social Psychology Quarterly* 59, 5-21.

Garfinkel, H. and Sacks, H. (1970) "On formal structures of practical actions", in: McKinney, J.C. and Tiryakian, E.A., eds. *Theoretical Sociology: Perspectives and Developments,* New York, NY: Appleton-Century-Crofts.

Garfinkel, H. and Wieder, D.L. (1992) "Two incommensurable, asymmetrically alternate technologies of social analysis", in: Watson and Seiler (1992).

Giglioli, P.P., ed. (1972) *Language and Social Context: Selected Readings,* Harmondsworth: Penguin.

Glaser, B.G. and Strauss, A.L. (1968) *The Discovery of Grounded Theory,* London: Weidenfeld and Nicholson.

Hart, H. (1953) "Toward an operational definition of the term 'operation'", *American Sociological Review* 18, 612-617.

Helm, D.T. (1982) "Talk's form: Comments on Goffman's *Forms of Talk*", *Human Studies* 5, 147-157.

Hobbs, A.H. (1951) *The Claims of Sociology: A Critique of Textbooks*, Harrisburg, Pennsylvania: Telegraph.

Hughes, E.C. (1961) "Tarde's *Psychologie Économique*: An unknown classic by a forgotten sociologist", *American Journal of Sociology* 6, 553-559.

Hughes, E.C. (1964) "Robert Park", *New Society* 118 (31 December), 18-19.

Johnson, H.M. (1961) *Sociology: A Systematic Introduction,* London: Routledge and Kegan Paul.

Kluckhohn, C. (1972) "The study of culture", in: Coser and Rosenberg (1972).

Kuhn, T.S. (1962) *The Structure of Scientific Revolutions,* Chicago and London: University of Chicago Press.

Laver, J. and Hutcheson, S., eds. (1972) *Communication in Face to Face Interaction,* Harmondsworth: Penguin.

Lynch, M. and Bogen, D. (1997) "Sociology's asociological 'core': An examination of textbook sociology in light of the sociology of scientific knowledge", *American Sociological Review* 62, 481-493.

MacIver, R.M. and Page, C.H. (1950) *Society: An Introductory Analysis,* London: Macmillan.

Mehan, H. (1978) "Structuring school structure", *Harvard Educational Review* 48, 32-64.

Merton, R.K. (1957) *Social Theory and Social Structure,* New York: The Free Press.
Merton, R.K., Broom, L., Cottrell, L.S. (1959) *Sociology Today: Problems and Prospects,* New York: Basic Books.
Musgrave, P.W. (1965) *The Sociology of Education,* London: Methuen.
Newton, T. (1999) "Power, subjectivity and British industrial and organisational sociology: The relevance of the work of Norbert Elias", *Sociology* 33, 411-440.
Ogburn, W.F. (1966) *Social Change,* New York: Delta.
Page, C.H. (1959) "Sociology as a teaching enterprise", in: Merton, Broom and Cottrell (1959).
Park, R.E. (1967 [1925]) "Magic, mentality and city life", in: Park, R.E., Burgess, E.W., McKenzie, R.D., eds. *The City,* Chicago and London: University of Chicago Press.
Parsons, T. (1959) "General theory in sociology", in: Merton, Broom and Cottrell (1959).
Piper, A. (1996) "Passing for white, passing for black", in: Ginsburg, E.K., ed *Passing and the Fictions of Identity,* Durham and London: Duke University Press.
Polsky, H.W. (1962) *Cottage 6: The Social System of Delinquent Boys in Residential Treatment,* New York: John Wiley and Sons.
Pride, J.B. and Holmes, J., eds. (1972) *Sociolinguistics: Selected Readings,* Harmondsworth: Penguin.
Rao, M.S.A., ed. (1974) *Urban Sociology in India: Reader and Source Book,* New Delhi: Orient Longman.
Rescher, N. (1998) "The significance of silence", *European Review* 6, 91-95.
Rose, E. (1960) "The English record of a natural sociology", *American Sociological Review* 25, 193-208.
Rose, E. (1985) "Changes of theory" *56th Annual Meeting of the Pacific Sociological Association*, Albequerque, New Mexico, April 18.
Rose, E. (1994) "The theoric construction in the Ethno-Inquiries", *Studies In Symbolic Interaction* 16, 37-62.
Roth, J.A. (1963) *Timetables,* Indianapolis, NY: Bobbs-Merrill Co.
Ryle, G. (1966) *The Concept of Mind* Harmondsworth: Penguin.
Schegloff, E.A. (1972) "Sequencing in conversational openings", in: Laver and Hutcheson (1972).
Schegloff, E.A., Ochs, E. and Thompson, S.A. (1996) "Introduction", in: Ochs, E., Schegloff, E.A. and Thompson, S.A., eds. *Interaction and Grammar,* Cambridge: Cambridge University Press.
Seeley, J.R., Sim, R.A., Loosley, E.W. (1956) *Crestwood Heights: A Study of the Culture of Suburban Life,* Toronto, Canada: University of Toronto Press.
Sharrock, W.W. (1974) "On owning knowledge", in: Turner (1974).
Smith, L.C. (1992) "Interdisciplinarity: Approaches to understanding library and information science as an interdisciplinary field", in: Vakkari, P. and

Cronin, B., eds. *Conceptions of Library and Information Science,* London: Taylor Graham.

Sorokin, P.A. (1929) "Some contrasts between European and American sociology", *Social Forces* 8, 57-62.

Sorokin, P.A. (1931) "Sociology as a science", *Social Forces* 10, 20-27.

Sorokin, P.A. (1937-41) *Social and Cultural Dynamics*, Four vols., New York: American Book Co.

Sorokin, P.A. (1943) *Sociocultural Causality, Space, Time,* Durham, NC: Duke University Press.

Sorokin, P.A. (1958) *Fads and Foibles in Modern Sociology and Related Sciences,* London: Mayflower.

Sorokin, P.A. (1959) *Social and Cultural Mobility,* New York: The Free Press.

Sorokin, P.A. and Hanson, R.C. (1974) "The power of creative love", in: Montagu, A., ed. *The Meaning of Love,* Westport, Connecticut: Greenwood Press.

Sorokin, P.A. and Merton, R.K. (1937) "Social time: A methodological and functional analysis", *American Journal of Sociology* 42, 615-629.

Sudnow, D. (1972) "Temporal parameters of interpersonal observation", in: Sudnow, D., ed. *Studies in Social Interaction,* New York: The Free Press.

Turner, R., ed. (1974) *Ethnomethodology: Selected Readings,* Harmondsworth: Penguin.

Waller, W. (1936) "Social problems and the mores", *American Sociological Review* 1, 922-933.

Watson, G. (1970) *Passing for White: A Study of Racial Assimilation in a South African School,* London: Tavistock.

Watson, G. (1984) "The social construction of boundaries between social and cultural anthropology in Britain and North America", *Journal of Anthropological Research* 40, 351-366.

Watson, G. (1992) "Introduction", in: Watson and Seiler (1992).

Watson, G. and Seiler, R.M., eds. (1992) *Text in Context: Contributions to Ethnomethodology*, Newbury Park, USA: Sage.

Watson, R. (1987) "Interdisciplinary considerations in the analysis of pro-terms", in: Button, G. and Lee, J.R.E., eds. *Talk and Social Organisation,* Clevedon, UK: Multilingual Matters.

Watson, R. (1992) "The understanding of language use in everyday life: Is there a common ground?", in: Watson and Seiler (1992).

Watson, R. (1998) "Ethnomethodology, consciousness and self", *Journal of Consciousness Studies* 5, 202-223.

Wieder, D.L. (1974) *Language and Social Reality,* The Hague: Mouton.

Wittgenstein, L. (1958) *Philosophical Investigations,* Oxford: Basil Blackwell.

Worsley, P., Mitchell, J.C., Martin, P., Morgan, D.H.J., Pons, V., Sharrock, W.W., Ward, R., eds. (1970) *Modern Sociology: Selected Readings,* Harmondsworth: Penguin.

Znaniecki, F. (1940) *The Social Role of the Man of Knowledge,* Columbia: Columbia University Press.

READING PHONOGRAPHY, INSCRIBING INTERDISCIPLINARITY

DUNCAN CAMPBELL

This essay examines some of the methodological problems associated with the analysis of popular music in an academic context. As it is currently conceived, interdisciplinary thought tends to reduce the specificity of its object by subordinating it to the demands of already-constituted methods and disciplines. I argue that, in the case of popular music, a productive interdisciplinarity would instead recognize the primary importance of the act of musical inscription, or *phonography* – the technological processes of recording and sound manipulation – for its analysis. Popular music's fascination with the phenomenality of sound, from Elvis Presley through dub reggae and on to 'post-rock' and contemporary electronic music cannot be thought in terms of existing disciplinary methods. Instead, doing justice to the object calls for new intersections between disciplines and new ways of thinking the spaces between traditional disciplines that popular music inhabits.

trajectory of a word tossed like a screeching phonograph record
(Dada manifesto, quoted in Cormack 1998: 199-200)

I

Despite the rhetoric of interdisciplinarity that seems to be everywhere in the humanities today, there can be no doubt that what Derrida terms 'ways of proceeding, socio-institutional practices, a certain style of writing' (Derrida 1983: 35-36) appropriate to particular disciplines have not disappeared. Indeed, while the Sokal hoax brought the question of interdisciplinarity to the fore, what it demonstrated was not only the incommensurable difference between 'ways of proceeding' in the sciences and (in the case of *Social Text*) the social sciences, but perhaps the impossibility of the traditional concept of interdisciplinarity. The mutual incomprehension and mistrust between both sides in the debate centred on the questions of disciplinary competence and methodology, that is, the authority of non-scientists to intervene in 'scientific' debates, and the legitimacy of the interdisciplinary usage of scientific theories. Stripped of what one could call their 'empirical foundation', such theories become no more than 'models' or 'metaphors' for interpretation; likewise, extracted from their context, the abuses of science that Sokal and Bricmont endlessly cite become an excuse for a wholesale dismissal of post-structuralist thought (Sokal and Bricmont 1998). The interaction between two disciplines, two 'ways of proceeding' becomes an interdisciplinary argument in which each side can think the other only in terms of caricatures by reducing the specificity of the other discipline, fighting over already-constituted borderlines and, finally, demonstrating that despite its rhetoric, interdisciplinary thought at present appears to re-inscribe disciplinary borders in such a way that, once more, they cannot be transgressed.

Interdisciplinarity in this sense proceeds 'outward' from pre-existing disciplines; yet, as Derrida suggests (with regard to philosophy), while there remains 'the necessity of discipline, of something specifically philosophical, that we should not dissolve philosophy into other disciplines [...] we need at the same time interdisciplinarity, crossing the borders, establishing new themes, new problems, new ways, new approaches' (Derrida, in: Caputo 1997: 7; see also Derrida 1995: 109-114). This 'crossing the borders' in an attempt to go beyond traditional disciplinary legitimation is, however, 'not simply interdisciplinarity' in its accepted sense: 'interdisciplinarity implies that you have given, identifiable competencies – say, a legal theorist, an architect, a philosopher, a literary critic – and that they work together on a specific, identifiable object. That's interdisciplinarity' (Derrida, in: Caputo 1997: 7). Resistance to the institutional framing of disciplines also resists the traditional sense of interdisciplinarity, which 'confirms (rather than deconstructing) disciplinarity by establishing lines of communication among already constituted disciplines' (*ibid*: 67). Putting the traditional concept of interdisciplinarity in question means rethinking the intersections between disciplines, their 'lines of communication', so that interdisciplinarity begins to occupy a borderline, a space (and time) of intersection *between* disciplines; interdisciplinary thought must begin to work on the gaps and spaces, the objects that do not fit disciplinary thought as such, that are not legitimated by current disciplinary practices. Deconstruction would perhaps be an example of an interdisciplinarity that occupies a contested space within the academy precisely because of its borderline status, its differantial relationship to, for example, 'philosophy' or 'literature'. The 'intersection' of deconstruction would therefore be interdisciplinary, if only we could agree what deconstruction actually *was* and if we could agree whether it was a method, an operation, merely a person (derrideconstruction?), or even a country. Perhaps deconstruction is interdisciplinary because of this refusal of definition, of conceptual closure, its perpetual placing of disciplines and concepts under erasure; despite the eloquent attempts of Rodolphe Gasché, for example, to rescue deconstruction for philosophy, the intersection of deconstruction and literature certainly opened literary studies to methods of reading that constituted the object as it proceeded, that did not apply pre-existing conceptual schemata to texts and did not reduce those texts it read to immaterial phantoms of meaning (see Gasché 1979).

The threat of deconstruction to the discipline, the institution, of literary criticism is summarised by Paul de Man in an essay from the late-1960s: de Man writes that 'the main critical approaches of the last decades were all founded on the implicit assumption that literature is an autonomous activity of the mind, a distinctive way of being in the world to be understood in terms of its own purposes and intentions' (de Man 1983: 21). Without wishing to rehearse this debate again, the consequence of what one could term the theoretical 'expansion' of literary studies was 'a radical questioning of the autonomy of literature as an aesthetic activity' (*ibid*) and the importation of concepts, methods and theoretical principles from outside the supposedly autonomous literary field. The importation of these concepts, vastly productive as they have been in their dismantling of a literary criticism based on aesthetic appreciation tempered by a moral sensibility, has also led to a tendency to explain literature away as merely the product of external factors, and to reduce it to one among many signifying practices. Literary studies has become interdisciplinary as a matter of course, as for example when Antony Easthope suggests that literary criticism is nothing more than a branch of that general semiotics which would be a 'new paradigm, the study of signifying practice' (Easthope 1991: 129), and yet the result of this expansion has been the erasure of the specificity of the literary, the expansion of literary studies into (in extreme cases) everything *but* literature. However, the question 'what is literature?' still remains; despite this interdisciplinarity, literature *remains* as something other, a gesture of inscription that cannot be reduced, as Derrida suggests:

> [w]hat is literature? And first of all what is it 'to write'? How is it that the very fact of writing can disturb the question 'what is?' and even 'what does it mean?' To say this in other words – and here is the *saying otherwise* that was of importance to me – when and how does an inscription become literature and what takes place when it does? (Derrida 1983: 37-38)

This question has still not been answered, indeed, it is still taking place, it is still being thought *otherwise* in a movement that is not exhausted by a conceptual structure, but that returns again and again to the 'literary ruse of the inscription' in order to pose, ceaselessly, the question 'what is literature?' (*ibid*: 38). Perhaps, therefore, it would be necessary to think of interdisciplinarity in this context in different terms, as a way of dealing with a 'specificity' of the literary inscription that cannot be thought within traditional disciplinary boundaries, certainly not merely within the discipline of 'literary studies'. This would necessarily be a 'productive interdisciplinarity', working on an object excluded from literary studies in the traditional sense, that recognises the remainder of the literary inscription which cannot be reduced or erased in favour of a 'transcendental' reading of whatever kind.

Inscription, thought generally, would be that material support that is the condition of possibility for systems of signification, as well as the literal act of marking, of making the sign in a sense that is 'more general than the simple empirical operation of graphical inscription in a suitable medium' (Johnson 1993: 22). Inscription is not merely a question of writing; in its most extensive sense, it is the mark of the relationship *between* matter and 'signification', *between* the sensible and intelligible. There is no transcendental idea *before* inscription that is capable of 'making meaning absolutely precede writing'; inscription therefore demonstrates 'the necessity of the medium of inscription, without which there would be no possibility of signification', as well as the necessity of thinking inscription between the sensible and the intelligible, as Derrida's reading of the *khora* so patiently traces, marks within the text of Plato (and reinscribes a motif that was already operative in/as *Dissemination;* Derrida 1978: 10 and Johnson 1993: 95).[1] Inscription leaves behind (how could it do otherwise?) a residue that cannot be assimilated or thought in terms of either meaning and communication, or as pure 'matter' that is dead, inert and passive. Smuggled into literary criticism in the guise of philosophical critique, 'inscription' as an operator opens the way to reconceptualization of the relationship between the sensible and the intelligible, between the two senses of sense, that is, as the meaning of the body and the body of meaning. The literary text – precisely because of this gesture of inscription that makes it possible – cannot be reduced to pure immaterial, spiritual meaning; what remains is always the body of meaning, the residue, the remainder beyond 'meaning' that itself *produces* the possibility of meaning. Literature *remains*, not as some immaterial phantom of pure meaning, nor as a meaningless noise, but as a material inscription, between the sensible and the intelligible, irreducible to either. It is this remainder that calls for an interdisciplinary response.

II

What I'd like to try and do in the rest of the article is to begin to rethink the question of inscription in relation to music (to 'popular' music in particular) and to argue for the necessity of an interdisciplinary reading of music that takes the matter of musical inscription as its starting point, rather than subordinating music to already-constituted methods and disciplines. Music (at least in its 'modern' form) begins from the operation of inscription; specifically, it begins with Edison's commissioning in 1877 of 'an apparatus that would etch acoustic vibrations onto a rotating cylinder covered with tinfoil' (Kittler 1999: 21). The

[1] As Derrida's reading of the Platonic *khora* shows, once the question of matter is opened, inscription becomes a metaphor for the ontological, a materiality that gets everywhere, to such an extent that *khoral* matter cannot be contained, restricted, disciplined (Derrida 1995a: 89-127); Caputo suggests *khora* figures 'an anonymous, pre-subjective substratum [...] within which the various unities of meaning, the various subjects and objects, presences and absences are constituted' (Caputo 1997: 143). For Jean-Luc Nancy, 'the Subject has no other locus, but in this aisthetic locus it neither finds nor constructs itself'; this question of inscriptive materiality necessitates a rethinking of subjectivity in terms of 'a new, unheard-of "science" of "sense" and "sensation" (but without sacrificing anything to romantic ineffability)' (Nancy 1993: 214).

radical effects of this inscription have been traced by Friedrich Kittler in his book *Gramophone, Film, Typewriter*, where he suggests that the phonograph becomes

> the only suitable model for visualizing the brain or memory [...] it alone can combine the two actions indispensable to any universal machine [...] writing and reading, storing and scanning, recording and replaying. In principle [...] it is one and the same stylus that engraves and later traces the phonographic groove. (*ibid*: 33)

For Kittler, 'all concepts of trace [...] are based on Edison's simple idea. The trace preceding all writing [...] is simply a gramophone needle. Paving a way and retracing a path coincide' (*ibid*). While an inscriptive model of the mind has been common since at least Plato, even in its most radical formulation in Freud it remains to a large extent legitimated by its resemblance to the literary text (see Carruthers 1990; and Derrida 1978: 196-231). With the phonographic model, inscription is separated from its empirical resemblance to writing so that the '*psychoanalytic graphology*' (Derrida 1978: 231) suggested by Derrida with regard to Freud will have already been breached by the *phonographic*, by the sense of inscription in its most radical form.

I mention this here merely to indicate the importance of the phonographic inscription in thinking about music, as popular music – in 'modern' forms at least – depends on technologies of mechanical reproduction for both its production and consumption. There would be no popular music without the phonographic inscription (whatever kind of subjectivity that inscription implies). While I find the blanket term 'popular music' not just patronising, but downright stupid in its opposition of the 'serious' (jazz, classical, whatever) to the popular (and hence ephemeral), there seems little option but to use it to mark a music that is 'non-classical', that is, music that takes place outside the institution, the discipline of the classical, or the accepted canon of classical taste and performance. It might be difficult to argue that many of the examples I will use are 'popular' in any demographic sense; nevertheless, I will use the terms 'music', 'popular music' and the 'non-classical' interchangeably to denote music that interests me because of its gesture of inscription. Of course, I wouldn't argue that all popular music (all non-classical music, all music) exploits its gesture of inscription in the manner I shall be suggesting; perhaps this is merely an indication of the problematic status of popular music within the academy: we lack any accepted vocabulary for discussing music. The music I want to discuss in this article produces an interdisciplinary response *because* of its gesture of inscription as well as refusing the codes of all those other disciplines from musicology to sociology which have been used to explain away the act of musical inscription within the academy. Of course, any criticism will borrow concepts, ideas, metaphors from other disciplines, but in this case this borrowing is necessitated by the musical inscription, which is something that can't be accounted for in traditional classifications, that can only be thought by an interdisciplinarity that takes *phonography* – the act of musical inscription – as its starting point.

The uncertain place of popular music in the academy is mirrored in the definitely uncertain status of the musical (or sonic) inscription in the history of philosophical aesthetics. For Kant, music 'speaks by means of mere sensations without concepts, and so, does not, like poetry, leave behind it any food for reflection' (Kant 1952: §53, 193). He continues, 'music, then, since it plays merely with sensations, has the lowest place among the fine arts' (*ibid*: §53, 195). Hegel, on the other hand, claims that 'music forms the centre of the romantic arts' as 'the point of transition between abstract spatial sensuousness, such as painting employs, and the abstract spirituality of poetry', a 'centre' that is, however, subordinated to the teleological movement of the Concept (Hegel 1993: 95). Even a discourse such as Heidegger's, which does not explicitly claim to order and classify the arts according to their relationship to a guiding concept, reduces sound to a mere indicative transparency, determined by something other than itself:

> what we 'first' hear is never noises or complexes of sounds, but the creaking waggon, the motor-cycle. We hear the column on the march, the north wind, the woodpecker tapping, the fire crackling. It requires a very artificial and complicated frame of mind to 'hear' a 'pure noise'. (Heidegger 1962: 207)

This comes as no surprise, considering the foundation of philosophical aesthetics as a discipline: Baumgarten claims that it is the task of logic to guide the 'lower cognitive faculty [...] in the sensate cognition of things'; thus '*things known*' (*noeta*) are the objects of logic, while '*things perceived*' (*aestheta*) are the objects of the inferior faculty, 'the science of perception, or *aesthetic*' (Baumgarten 1954: 77, 78). In Baumgarten's work, 'the sensible is to be lifted to the dignity of knowledge and impregnated with a special form of knowledge, and in this way subjected to rational treatment,' so that aesthetics 'too is ruled by an inner law. Even though this law does not coincide with the law of reason, it constitutes an analogue of reason' (Cassirer 1951: 340, 346). Sense-perception is subordinated to the reason that must order and guide it. For Marc Froment-Meurice, this demonstrates the paradox of any discipline which describes itself as an aesthetics:

> The sensible and material are the support for the ladder leading beyond (and above) toward the super-sensible (idea, concept, and today, value) [...] If the *aistheton* names the sensible not for itself but already in opposition and subordination to what gives sense to the sensible – *namely* the idea, which is never sensible – then the name "aesthetics" reveals its metaphysical origin (Froment-Meurice 1998: 180)

The aesthetic will be disciplined by the concept, by the law of reason and as such will be in effect erased from consideration; the goal of a musical aesthetics will be to account for music in terms of the rational and the conceptual, however fractured or indeterminate that relationship may well be seen to be. The 'sensuousness' of music will be above all a question of 'putting the imagination into a play which is at once free and adapted to the understanding' (*ibid*: 195), so that the matter of musical inscription is determined from above by a metaphysical discipline.

While this version of musical aesthetics is most relevant to classical music, what of popular music? What happens to the particularity of the musical sensation, the sensuousness of which Hegel writes? Despite the vast proliferation of readings of popular music that treat it 'seriously', either as another branch of cultural studies or as a discipline in its own right, the gesture of phonographic inscription is still reduced, placed as secondary to other disciplines which determine its form and function. Popular music is thought of as a sociological phenomenon, a debased classical music, a literary-critical narrative (personal, political, and so on), always determined from the outside by a *disciplinarity* that pays no attention to the status of the musical inscription; the multiple disciplinary codes of reading popular music – whether they are sociological, musicological, poetical, phenomenological, psychological, political – mirror the classical subordination of aesthetics to logic (or, in a more general sense, to philosophy). The sensuous particularity of music disappears in the face of external determination. To take Adorno's critique of jazz as an example that needs refuting, once again, popular music is neither simply a debased form of high culture, nor a pacifier produced by the military-industrial-entertainment complex; neither, though, is it necessarily a source of anti-hegemonic resistance as some 'cultural studies' readings seem to suggest.[2] While it is true that popular music is particularly subject to appropriation and reterritorialisation, or what Adorno would call 'the triumph of invested capital' (Adorno and Horkheimer 1979: 124) – for every Elvis a Cliff Richard, every Sex Pistols a Stranglers, every Nirvana a Blink 182, every LFO a Madison Avenue (ad nauseam) – this does not erase the (for want of a better word) *experience* of sensuous particularity, the sensation of the musical object. This, of course, is what Adorno's reading of popular music (and popular culture in general) attempts to do. In Adorno and Horkheimer's writing, 'invested capital' determines popular music down to the last note as part of a structure of repetition in which individual songs and records are no more than 'calculated mutations which serve all the more strongly to confirm the validity of the system' (*ibid*: 129). Resistance to the system is possible only through the conceptual seriousness of high modernism which may well be able to escape (if only negatively) that dominion of the commodity form which totally determines the inscription of popular music.

And yet, something always escapes, always *remains*; what a 'reductive' interdisciplinarity seeks to do is to reduce the musical inscription to a question of reference, to reconnect the inscription of music to its referent – to *any* referent that explains it and therefore erases the necessity to account for the inscription of music: the socio-political conditions of its production and reception, the

---

[2] Simon Reynolds (1998) has traced the movements in rave culture between utopian visions and commercial reterritorialization in his excellent *Energy Flash: A Journey Through Rave Music and Dance Culture.*

expression of an experience, the technical inadequacy of performers and composers, and so on – whereas the act of musical inscription is, I would argue, a radical *suspension* of reference. This is not to say we have entered a realm of free-floating signifiers, but that the musical inscription is not a simple referent, easily available to analysis, and neither does it refer *simply* to anything in particular; as with literary inscription, there is 'a *suspended* relation to meaning and reference' in the sense of '*suspense*, but also *dependence*, condition, conditionality' (Derrida, in: Attridge 1992: 48).

III

From the wax cylinder to MP3, the non-classical has been fascinated by the gesture of inscription, the process of recording. Despite what David Toop writes about the movement of 'turning the recording studio from its documentary origins to a virtual chamber of wonders', the phonographic inscription is virtual from the start (Toop 1995: 111). This virtuality is the

> structural possibility of being weaned from the referent or from the signified (hence from communication and from its context) [which] seems to me to make every mark, including those which are oral, a grapheme in general; which is to say [...] the non-present *remainder* [*restance*] of a differential mark cut off from its putative 'production' or origin. And I shall even extend this law to all 'experience' in general if it is conceded that there is no experience consisting of *pure* presence but only of chains of differential marks. (Derrida 1988: 10)

The recorded acoustic event is detached from its documentary context to the extent that even the supposedly 'pure' documentary performance of a Robert Johnson is an effect of the gramophone: the click and buzz of the strings against the frets, the bump of the sleeve on the body of the guitar, the crackle of the tube microphone (the marks of documentary authority) are precisely those things which are non-musical, accidental, dispensable. The phonograph cannot distinguish between meaning and noise, between the two senses of sense: 'the phonograph does not hear as do ears that have been trained immediately to filter voices, words, and sounds out of noise; it registers acoustic events as such' (Kittler 1999: 23). The 'acoustic event' is detached from its documentary context; it becomes a virtual event suspended from reference to the 'natural', the 'live', the 'spontaneous', the 'authentic', those virtues demanded of popular music that its very gesture of inscription *refuses*.

Despite the rock'n'roll myth of spontaneity, rock'n'roll's emphasis on the record as its basic unit has always meant that *phonography* – the art of recorded sound – came to the fore. The outline of this history is already well-known, from the 'slapback', that Sam Phillips used to record Elvis at the Sun studio (a 'home-made echo device that was created by running the original recording signal through a second Ampex machine [...] thereby achieving an almost sibilant phased effect' (Guralnick 1995: 103) which affects the grain of Elvis Presley's voice) to the master narrative of sonic experimentation, which runs through Phil Spector's monolithic wall of sound that was like nothing on earth ('Be My Baby' as inter-planetary love-song?), Brian Wilson's painstaking layering of textures on *Pet Sounds*, the Beatles spending endless nights excavating the history of rock and roll, utilising/developing new technologies (multitrack recording, electronic effects, the mellotron) and creating a drug-fuelled combinatorial science of sound.[3] In a version of this history, outlined by Simon Reynolds in *Energy Flash*, the recording techniques of the late 1960s and psychedelia in particular emphasised the fascination with inscription: psychedelia 'departed from the naturalistic model of recording (documenting the band in performance) and used multitracking, overdubbing, reversing, echo and other sonic processes to create sounds that could never be achieved by a band playing in real-time' (Reynolds 1998: 364). For Reynolds, 'sampladelia' – the combinatorial possibilities of digital recording and editing used primarily in dance music – is a 'radical break with the ideals of real-time interactive playing and natural acoustic space that still govern most music-making' (*ibid*: 365) and which intensifies the non-natural recording techniques of the 1960s through the creation of a 'fictitious psycho-acoustic space [as well as] timbres and textures and sound-shapes to which no ready real-world referents attach themselves' (*ibid*: 367).

However, this narrative suggests that the suspension of reference is purely a question of the intentional manipulation of sound, of the studio used as a tool to produce virtual effects. I'd argue that *all* recorded music, whether it realises it or not, whether it manipulates it or not, is a virtual inscription, and that virtuality is the structural condition of possibility of recorded music. Suspended from its origin, its referent, non-classical music occupies an uncertain space, 'between' origin and reception, between two phonographic systems (the record player and the mind), detached from both, an inscription which produces effects and affects that cannot be pinned down. I should also emphasise here that by 'virtuality' I don't just mean digitalisation. Digitalisation may well be the most extensive form of virtuality, as can be seen in cinema, for example, where '[c]omputer-generated imagery [...] may invoke the existence of a real object, but there is no guarantee that such an object ever existed [...] its use is practically a guarantee that the object *never* existed' (Romney 1999: 189). In his article 'Million-Dollar Graffiti: Notes from the Digital Domain', Jonathan Romney argues, with regard to digital technology in film, that digitalisation is a means of reducing what he calls the 'unquantifiable surplus' of the filmic inscription that escapes the control of reference, where 'the object refuses to be brought to heel' (Romney 1999: 197). Digitalisation, in this sense, is 'a foolproof method of disciplining the rebelliousness of things' (*ibid*). Romney calls for a new use of CGI and digital

[3] See The Beach Boys (1996) *The Pet Sounds Sessions*; on the Beatles, in addition to the vast range of bootleg studio working tapes, see Mark Lewisohn (1988) *The Beatles: Recording Sessions, The Official Abbey Road Studio Session Notes, 1962–1970*.

technology, 'not just scrawled across a film's surface, but stitched into its workings, distressing it from the inside' (*ibid*: 203).

Similarly, digital technology in music can also be used to control, domesticate and above all to discipline the waywardness of the musical inscription, rather than extending the fascination with inscription. This reduction of inscription is a disciplining that attempts to return the phonographic to a mythology of authenticity and presence, to reduce the noises of all kinds that infect the inscription. Digitalisation allows the production of 'authentic' instrumental sounds without any extraneous noise, the 'cleaning-up' of sound and the manipulation of sounds in order to reduce the inscription to a 'pure' expression of authorial consciousness in a desire to reconnect to an illusory presence that guarantees authenticity. Instead of celebrating the virtuality of inscription, the myth of soul is recreated technologically; a pre-recorded performance is interrupted with a 'present' vocal line: 'Boyzone – live on *Top of the Pops*', as if the 'live' performance itself were not always a technical construct. Even the voice, that most 'natural' of instruments is wired through a network of membranes, skins, technologies that produce it, vibrations from the diaphragm to the microphone, the inscriptions that mark out those intervals determined as 'melodic' or 'harmonic' within different traditions and so on. As Frances Dyson writes,

> the 'originary voice', no matter how pure, is bound to a certain hermeneutics; prior to any utterance, it is already a metaphor, and already caught within particular circuits, switchboards or 'machines' which both literally and figuratively encode, transmit and give meaning to vocal acts. (Dyson)

The reduction of the inscription to a matter of authentic expression is mirrored in the traditional literary-critical analysis of the song as text. In this case, 'text' does not have any connotations of radical textuality or inscription; it is merely an analysis that treats the lyrics as expression in the most banal sense, that reduces the sound to the song and makes music into a vehicle for the obvious sense of meaning provided by the lyrics. This reduction once more turns music into merely an indication of something else; it subordinates it to all those other narratological, poetic and social-realist concerns whose main aim is to find the 'authentic' experience that has resulted in the song's expression. In true literary-critical form, the high point of this kind of reading took place in the high/low culture debate and became reduced (again) to the question 'Dylan or Keats?'. The criterion of 'value' in this debate was purely lyrical, another manifestation of the obsession with the singer-songwriter as late-twentieth century romantic poet, the bearer of 'truth'. In the terms of this debate, music only has meaning when read through an already-constituted discipline, when the terms of that debate (and perhaps that discipline itself) were already outdated. Instead of Dylan versus Keats, why not Keats versus Miles Davis, 'Hyperion' versus *Dark Magus*?

Music has always been just as much a question of verticality (sound, noise, harmonics) as it has been a question of horizontality (song, lyrics, melody);

thinking of music in terms of inscription emphasises this other dimension, the dimension of the matter of sound. What both the unwillingness to acknowledge the technology of inscription and the reduction of the sound to the song do is to foreground the meaning of bodies, of materiality, rather than think in terms of the body of meaning, the act of inscription that makes meaning itself possible in the first place and that produces effects of meaning and reference, without being reducible to either. Recent forms of this obsession with inscription can be seen in the music Stefan Betke makes under the name 'Pole', where the malfunction of the pole filter infects each track as hisses and crackles from which melodies emerge and disappear, where 'songs' seem to be constructed from the noises erased in the digital process in an unstable hybrid of analogue and digital, a low-rent viral mutation of dub (Pole 1998, 1998, and 2000). Music is refigured as interference, the 'glitch' in the machine, the clicks and cuts of inscription that both constitute and interrupt the work of sense, computer bugs that mutate algorithms in digital processors and so on (Young 2000: 52-56). Similarly, this fascination is exhibited in the genre Simon Reynolds named 'post-rock', with its use of 'rock instrumentation for non-rock purposes, using guitars as facilitators of timbres and textures rather than riffs and powerchords' (Reynolds 1994). This working with the body of sound in the music of, for example, Stereolab, Pram, Broadcast and Main again exemplifies the possibilities of the phonographic inscription and its expansion, not reduction.

Dub reggae also demonstrates this inscription mania, or what Kodwo Eshun calls 'bringing the outside into the inside of The Song' (1998: 65). Pioneered by King Tubby in the early-1970s, dub is a process which involves taking a reggae song, 'stripping [the] vocal from its backing track and then manipulating the instrumental arrangement with techniques and effects' (Toop 1995: 116). Working with incredibly primitive equipment in his Black Ark studio, Lee Perry extended the possibilities of dub; a studio innovator on a level with Brian Wilson or Joe Meek, he also 'lifted the studio into virtual space' in his treatments of songs with 'rattling hand drums and scrapers, ghostly voices, distant horn sections, unusual snare and hi-hat treatments, groans and reptilian sibilations, odd perspectives and depth illusions, sound effects, unexpected noises and echoes that repeat to infinity' (Toop 1995: 113, 118).[4] In Perry's hands, the studio is a lo-fi cyborg, an interface between man and machine for the degradation of the song into fragments, multiple 'versions' of itself without an original: as Eshun suggests, the dub version produces copies without original one-off acetates of mixes that have been detached from the 'original' that supposedly produced them (Eshun 1998: 188). Dub detaches sound from reference as it constructs what Eshun terms 'sonic fictions', emphasizing the virtuality of the phonographic inscription. Eshun's book *More Brilliant Than The Sun* develops this idea of sonic fiction in recent black musics, documenting the ways in which a fascination

[4] For more information on Perry, see David Katz (1999). An excellent introduction to Perry's work is the *Arkology* box set (Perry 1997).

with the phonographic inscription is linked to a black science fiction, an Afro- or Black Atlantic Futurism which 'alienates itself from the human', specifically the humanism of Western tradition. The 'real' of the street, so often taken as the referent of black music, is eclipsed by a fascination with the alien in all its forms: 'Techno secedes from the street [...], and from Trad HipHop's compulsory logic of representation and will to realness' (Eshun 1998: 117). This is manifest in the gesture towards the impossible experience of the alien in the music of Sun Ra, or John Coltrane's *Interstellar Space* duets with Rashied Ali, in which the call and response between saxophone and drums dissolves into an almost psychotic incantation of the absolutely other, the alien (Sinker 1992).[5] Similarly, the authenticity and presence of jazz is fragmented in Miles Davis and Teo Macero's use of tape editing on albums such as *Bitches Brew* and *In A Silent Way*, where each track is painstakingly constructed from 10-second phrases, drums loops and vamps spliced together to create a sonic fiction with no 'real' referent of any kind and impossible to replicate live, as can be heard on any of Miles' live albums from this period (Davis 1969, 1970 and 1977). For the Black Atlantic futurist, the recorded sound never will have been a 'natural' phenomenon, and as such takes place beyond all questions of reference and 'keeping it real'.

IV

What all these different musicians exhibit is a fascination with the phenomenality of sound, with the body of sense, the matter of sound that cannot be explicitly grasped, understood, conceptually disciplined. Sound itself becomes an absent referent, a 'black hole' – as Hillis Miller might define it – which is not an ineffable and above all spiritual limit upon interpretation (the ineffable is only truly readable by the beautiful soul, beyond language, beyond inscription), but the return (again and again) of the *aisthetic* (to use Jean-Luc Nancy's term) that never ceases to disturb and surprise, to return to a different place each time. The fascination with the phonographic inscription is a fascination with a materiality that can be moulded, shaped, and yet which always escapes. Whereas a reductive interdisciplinarity reduces this remainder to conceptual structures that will have already determined and grasped the object, a productive interdisciplinarity – which is not interdisciplinarity in its traditional sense – pays attention to the specificity of the musical object. In many ways, this kind of work is already being done in the writing of, for example, Kodwo Eshun, Ian Penman, Simon Reynolds, and the magazine *The Wire*; *outside* the academy and its disciplines a productive interdisciplinarity is at work, finding 'new' objects and new ways of beginning to think those objects, 'new' intersections between disciplines, 'new' ways of reading an object that never ceases to escape. Writing about his unfinished work *Espace*, Edgard Varèse desired:

---

[5] On Sun Ra, see Szwed, (1997); Coltrane (2000).

> [v]oices in the sky, as though magic, invisible hands were turning on and off the knobs of fantastic radios, filling all space, criss-crossing, overlapping, penetrating each other, splitting up, superimposing, repulsing each other, colliding, crashing. (Quoted in Dyson (a))

How do we begin to *do justice* to that?

Bibliography:

Adorno, Theodor, and Horkheimer, Max (1979) *Dialectic of Enlightenment*, trans. John Cumming, London: Verso.

Attridge, Derek, ed. (1992) *Acts of Literature*, London: Routledge.

Baumgarten, Alexander Gottlieb (1954 [1735]) *Reflections on Poetry*, trans. Karl Aschenbrenner and William B. Holther, Berkeley: University of California Press.

The Beach Boys (1996) *The Pet Sounds Sessions*, Capitol.

Caputo, John D. (1997) *Deconstruction in a Nutshell: A Conversation with Jacques Derrida*, New York: Fordham University Press.

Carruthers, Mary (1990) *The Book of Memory: A Study of Memory in Medieval Culture*, Cambridge: Cambridge University Press.

Cassirer, Ernst (1951) *The Philosophy of the Enlightenment*, trans. Fritz C. A. Koelln and James P. Pettegrove, Princeton: Princeton University Press.

Coltrane, John (2000) *Interstellar Space*, reissue, Impulse.

Cormack, Patricia, ed. (1998) *Manifestos and Declarations of the Twentieth Century*, Toronto: Garamond.

Davis, Miles (1969) *In a Silent Way*, CBS.

Davis, Miles (1970) *Bitches Brew*, CBS.

Davis, Miles (1977) *Black Beauty: Miles Davis at Fillmore West*, CBS.

de Man, Paul (1983) *Blindness and Insight: Essays in the Rhetoric of Contemporary Criticism*, second edition, Minneapolis: University of Minnesota Press.

Derrida, Jacques (1995) *Points: Interviews, 1974–1994*, ed. Elisabeth Weber, Stanford: Stanford University Press.

Derrida, Jacques (1995a) "*Khora*", trans. Ian McLeod, in: Dutoit, Thomas, ed. *On The Name*, Stanford: Stanford University Press, 89–127.

Derrida, Jacques (1988) *Limited Inc.*, trans. Samuel Weber, Evanston: Northwerstern University Press.

Derrida, Jacques (1983) "The Time of a Thesis: Punctuations", trans. Kathleen Maclaughlin, in: Montefiore, Alan, ed. *Philosophy in France Today*, Cambridge: Cambridge University Press, 34–50.

Derrida, Jacques (1978) *Writing and Difference*, trans. Alan Bass, London: Routledge.

Dyson, Frances "Circuits of the Voice: From Cosmology to Telephony", http://www.soundculture.org/words/dyson_ circuits.html.

Dyson, Frances (a) "A Philosophonics of Space: Sound, Futurity and the End of the World", http://www.soundculture.org/words/dyson_philosophonics.html.

Easthope, Antony (1991) *Literary into Cultural Studies*, London: Routledge.

Eshun, Kodwo (1998) *More Brilliant Than The Sun: Adventures in Sonic Fiction*, London: Quartet.

Froment-Meurice, Marc (1998) *That Is To Say: Heidegger's Poetics*, trans. Jan Plug, Stanford: Stanford University Press.

Gasché, Rodolphe (1979) "Deconstruction as Criticism", *Glyph* 6, 177–215.

Guralnick, Peter (1995) *Last Train to Memphis: The Rise of Elvis Presley*, London: Abacus.

Hegel, G. W. F. (1993 [1835]) *Introductory Lectures on Aesthetics*, trans. Bernard Bosanquet, London: Penguin.

Heidegger, Martin (1962) *Being and Time*, trans. John Macquarrie and Edward Robinson, Oxford: Blackwell.

Johnson, Christopher (1993) *System and Writing in the Philosophy of Jacques Derrida*, Cambridge: Cambridge University Press.

Kant, Immanuel (1952 [1781]) *The Critique of Judgement*, trans. James Creed Meredith, Oxford: Clarendon.

Katz, David (1999) "Lee Perry: The Primer", *The Wire*, 189 (November), 42–49.

Kittler, Friedrich A. (1999) *Gramophone, Film, Typewriter*, trans. Geoffrey Winthrop-Young and Michael Wutz, Stanford: Stanford University Press.

Lewisohn, Mark (1988) *The Beatles: Recording Sessions, The Official Abbey Road Studio Session Notes, 1962–1970*, London: Hamlyn.

Nancy, Jean-Luc (1993) *The Birth to Presence*, Stanford: Stanford University Press.

Perry, Lee (1997) *Arkology*, Island.

Plato (1929) *Timaeus*, trans. R. G. Bury, London: Heinemann; Cambridge, MA: Harvard University Press.

Pole [Stefan Betke] (1998) *1*, KiffSM.

Pole (1998) *2*, KiffSM.

Pole (2000) *3*, KiffSM.

Reynolds, Simon (1998) *Energy Flash: A Journey Through Rave Music and Dance Culture*, London: Picador.

Reynolds, Simon (1994) "Shaking the Rock Narcotic", *The Wire*, 123 (May), online http://www.thewire.co.uk/articles/ index.htm.

Romney, Jonathan (1999) "Million-Dollar Graffiti: Notes from the Digital Domain", in: Adair, Gilbert, ed. *Movies*, London: Penguin, 186–204.

Sinker, Mark (1992) "Loving the Alien", *The Wire*, 96 (Feb), online http://www.thewire.co.uk/articles/index.htm.

Sokal, Alan, and Bricmont, Jean (1998) *Intellectual Impostures*, London: Profile.

Szwed, John F. (1997) *Space is the Place: The Life and Times of Sun Ra*, Edinburgh: Payback.

Toop, David (1995) *Ocean of Sound: Aether Talk, Ambient Sound and Imaginary Worlds*, London: Serpent's Tail.

Young, Rob (2000) "Worship the Glitch", *The Wire*, 190/191, 52–56.

CULTURAL STUDIES AND AESTHETICS – PLEASURES AND POLITICS

JEN WEBB

Although Cultural Studies writings provide a considerable volume of the academic works on the field of cultural production, they tend to focus on the social, political and economic effects of creative works rather than engage with how artistic texts exist as objects of value and pleasure in their aesthetic identity. This can be understood, given the politics of aesthetics and its history, but it can also be read as a rejection of the private and the affective spheres in favour of the public and the rational. Writing as a hybrid agent – someone who is both a cultural theorist and a creative practitioner – I will offer a brief overview of the connections between cultural studies and aesthetics, discuss the ways in which the deployment of 'scientific' discourse has limited the extent to which we can engage intellectually and affectively with art works, and suggest the value of articulating the politics of Cultural Studies with the pleasures of art.

The existence of the world is justified only as an aesthetic phenomenon.
(Nietzsche 1967: 22)

It is self-evident that nothing concerning art is self-evident anymore, not even its right to exist.
(Adorno 1997: 1)

A considerable proportion of the academic works on the field of art come from cultural studies writings but, for the most part, we seem to be descended from Adorno rather than Nietzsche. Our interest in art seems to lie not so much in considering its part in 'the existence of the world' but in problematising art and, at least implicitly, questioning its 'right to exist'. In this essay I will briefly map out some of the issues that lead cultural studies to diverge from aesthetics, discuss aspects of their problematic relationship, and suggest ways in which a more interdisciplinary attitude could enrich both fields.

The potential benefits of such an approach are raised from time to time in the literature. Pierre Bourdieu, for instance, writes of the need to move beyond conventional ways of appropriating works of art as texts for 'decipherment', and suggests that researchers acknowledge that most people appropriate art below, or beyond, this conceptual framework – at a more visceral level. His suggestion that we develop a 'practical knowledge' in relation to art requires a kind of leaking of thoughts and attitudes between aesthetics and social-cultural theory in order to engage rigorously not just with art works, but also with the way in which people in their everyday lives perceive such works. In making this call he carves out a kind of fork in the road, a point of intersection between these disciplines in which the rigours and reflexivities of each can enrich the other.

Interdisciplinarity is, of course, becoming an increasingly sexy term in the academy. It has a number of practical benefits in the research community: working and publishing across disciplines means, for instance, we have to write for extra-peer audiences, and hence minimise that opacity of style which is a feature of much aesthetic/philosophical and cultural studies writing, in the interests of achieving a greater transparency and accessibility. Further, interdisciplinarity in the academy parallels contemporary practice in the workplace and professions, where it's no longer sufficient (in many cases) to have expertise, however sophisticated, in just one area. Developing an interdisciplinary approach makes it easier to structure courses which will train students for the sorts of environments in which they will be working.

And there are other advantages; working across the disciplines offers a point of entry to the liminal which in turn provides access to synergetic energies and transgressive possibilities, and demonstrates the permeability of the arbitrary boundaries of conventional disciplines. Working across disciplines can also be a way of breaking down particularised interest, and hence extending knowledge and thought in a field. Pierre Bourdieu takes this sort of approach when he writes, in the first lines of *Pascalian Meditations*: "If I have resolved to ask some questions that I would rather have left to philosophy, it is because it seemed to me that philosophy, for all its questioning, did not ask them" (Bourdieu 2000: 1). And, no doubt, philosophy has social-cultural questions which social-cultural researchers are not asking, but which may be worthy of attention. Reading across one another's work can allow such 'dark spots' to become visible, because new points of view – the points of view of outsiders – are brought to bear on the material.

Interdisciplinarity can also be viewed in more negative terms: with the increasing fragmentation of knowledge that is a result of this perspective and structure come the loss of coherent research or knowledge communities and, potentially, of specialised knowledges. On the other hand, the gains attendant on working at the intersections of disciplines and professions may, arguably, outweigh such costs. Certainly, there are considerable areas of shared interests between aesthetics and cultural studies which suggests there are (potentially, at least) considerable benefits available from shared work. The aesthetic sphere, for instance, as noted by Frankfurt scholars and reiterated by practitioners from Hans Haacke to community artists, often has a vital critical role in society, providing a space for creative expression, self-realisation and non-exploitative pleasure and contemplation, and representing an implicit criticism of the mechanical and exploitative character of the wider social world. While it is, like any other professional or practical field, caught up in commodity relations, it maintains an attitude of antagonism towards them, and at its best mobilises resistance to neo-liberal values. All these are matters of concern for cultural studies as much as for aesthetics, and obvious points at which to take up interdisciplinary research. And, given that aesthetics and cultural studies are already interdisciplinary disciplines – with aesthetics encompassing philosophy, political thought and art, while cultural studies appropriates aspects of sociology, literary studies and philosophy, *inter alia* – the material experience of crossing one another's frontiers should not be daunting. Indeed, it can be vitally productive: a blending of the disciplines may mean that we need no longer reject the aesthetic experience *in toto* in order to immerse ourselves in the productive techniques of a work of art, *à la* conventional aesthetics, or in order to immerse ourselves in the reproductive effects of art, *à la* conventional cultural studies. Rather, we can draw on techniques of reading and analysis from each discipline as a way of engaging with artistic practice while rendering problematic the more or less unthinking commitment to the logic, values and capital of the field – what Bourdieu calls *illusio* or "the fact of being caught up in and by the game, of believing … that playing is worth the effort" (Bourdieu 1998: 76).

Having said this, though, there are still major differences in the ways in which the two disciplines address the field of art. Perhaps the most significant is that, in general, cultural studies writings tend not to take into account the identity of art objects and artists *qua* art, or as aesthetic experience. Unlike art historians, literary critics and aestheticists, cultural theorists focus on developing a critique of the field and its practice, rather than engaging directly with the works themselves. So, for instance, we analyse the social and political effects of creative works, describe the conditions of their production, distribution and consumption, discuss socio-political ethics, and point out the role of art as a mechanism of social reproduction. But we rarely look to any great extent at what professional artists actually do and say about their work and themselves, as opposed to what is said about them in the stories that emerge in the public sphere – in films like *Love is the Devil*, *Basquiat* or *Amadeus*, for instance. In short, while cultural studies writings contribute many valuable and interesting perspectives on the field, they typically fail to address what for me is the central point about art: that it is committed to the production of works which "demand to be experienced aesthetically" (Panofsky 1955: 11).

This absence isn't, perhaps, all that surprising. While aesthetics has attracted the interest of a formidable list of thinkers and writers, from Plato and Aristotle, over two millennia ago, to Hume, Kant, Nietzsche, Hegel, Schiller, Adorno, Benjamin, Derrida, Foucault, Lyotard and Bourdieu over the past couple of centuries, its political antecedents are regarded as somewhat suspect. The aim of eighteenth-century aesthetics was precisely to colonise the 'other' world of intuition, sensory experience, emotion and thus make it accessible to (and bring it under the order of) Reason. There's little here to do with art, but a great deal that might engage the interest of a cultural studies writer, particularly because this brand of aesthetics claims an absolute and ahistorical position, and effaces the social practices in and by which meanings are made. In this respect, aesthetics buys into the process of establishing, and universalising, evaluative norms, and thus (potentially) works as a form of social and political control.

This is, though, a limited view even of eighteenth-century aesthetics; aesthetics could equally be read as that which challenges Reason by pointing out that the world can't be derived only from abstract laws, but involves affect and the sensate, and so brings together sensation and reason. This is a point at which aesthetics could be seen as very useful for a cultural studies politics: its role in unsettling the dominance of reason and in offering alternative ways of engaging with the social could offer a productive critique of reason and order, present a resistance to metalanguages by pointing out the interconnections between invention and truth, and thus provide a space for appreciating both the contingency and multiplicity of the social, and the fragility of the hegemony.

Cultural studies also has reservations about aesthetics in general, and art in particular, because it is often posited as a matter of individual taste, which overlooks the extent to which taste is an effect of social and cultural position. This point has been taken up enthusiastically and critically by the post-aestheticists, among whom are many cultural theorists. The approach is perhaps best summed up by Bourdieu's famous line: "Taste classifies, and it classifies the classifier" (Bourdieu 1984: 6). While the art world may indeed be committed to self-expression, social contestation, and the production of works that 'demand to be experienced aesthetically', it is also a prime site for classifying people into groups: the *cognoscenti* – those who 'get' David Lynch's *Eraserhead*, or value modern art – and the 'barbarians' – those who think *Eraserhead* is dead boring, or who can't see the point of a white room filled with white canvases. People may no longer be clearly distinguishable from one another in their external appearance (in terms of their social rank, for instance), but they can still be distinguished in terms of their tastes, and particularly the degree of 'refinement' or 'coarseness' that characterises their sensibility. Bourdieu develops this extensively in *Distinction* and elsewhere, showing on the basis of theoretical and empirical methodologies that aesthetics serves as a crucial marker of social distinction in contemporary society, and arguing that Kant's formalist notion of aesthetic pleasure depends on an unspoken rejection of popular tastes:

> The denial of lower, coarse, vulgar, venal, servile – in a word, natural – enjoyment, which constitutes the sacred sphere of culture, implies an affirmation of the superiority of those who can be satisfied with the sublimated, refined, disinterested, gratuitous, distinguished pleasures forever closed to the profane. That is why art and cultural consumption are predisposed, consciously and deliberately or not, to fulfill a social function of legitimating social differences. (Bourdieu 1984: 7)

And so aesthetics also comes under the critical eye of cultural theorists because of its association with the tastes and interests of the social elite, in which respect it is categorised as capital-A Art, not as a part of everyday life.

This question of art's relation to everyday life is another area in which cultural theorists engage critically with aesthetics, working from Kant's foundational thought. Kant famously posits aesthetic judgment as a form of reason which mediates between abstract and lived experience. But he carefully distinguishes aesthetic pleasure from the ordinary pleasure we take in an object: aesthetic pleasure must be disinterested; 'mere' sensual gratification must be rejected; the aesthetic object is reduced to an image evaluated in terms of its form rather than its status as something to be desired, and is abstracted from the concrete thing to the universal. Where aesthetic theory relies on this Kantian logic, it falls into muddy waters because on the one hand it is attempting to make sense of sensory experience, but on the other hand, it ends up only valuing the formal and universal properties of art objects, rejecting the pleasures of the body.

Bourdieu again, following something of a Nietzschean line, articulates this sort of critique of aesthetics. He writes in *Distinction* (1984: 31, 41) that the aesthetic of disinterest, with its abstract concerns and its distance from social or moral imperatives, addresses only elite tastes and practices, and ignores the workings of a popular aesthetic where art appeals to concrete pleasure and addresses moral concerns. But whether it is concerned with 'high' or 'popular' works, this particular critique demands a curious reversal of the logic in the paragraph above. There aesthetics is criticised because art's pleasures are assumed to be individual and personal. Here aesthetics is criticised because art's pleasures are assumed to be universal. This is because the argument that aesthetics is part of the social elite takes us back into Kant's territory – the territory of refined sensibilities, and of trained (elite) responses to the beautiful or the sublime. This marks a considerable departure from the notion that artistic taste or aesthetic experience can be purely personal because, for Kant, such pleasure would rely purely on sensation and on personal indulgence, rather than being a 'genuinely' disinterested, and hence universal, aesthetic experience.

The Kantian view of aesthetic pleasure and its distance from sensual gratification is surprisingly enduring. In January 2000, for instance, the Australian Office of Film and Literature Classification Board (OFLC) banned the French art-house film *Romance* on the grounds that it exhibits both actual and simulated sex and sexual violence. After massive media and public protest, the OFLC reclassified the movie as 'R' (for restricted adult viewing) partly on the basis that despite its graphic portrayal of sex and sexual violence, it is an Art film. This, we can conclude, classifies it as part of the 'genuinely' aesthetic rather than the 'popular', and therefore only of interest to a small, and elite, segment of the population – those able to engage in sensual appreciation without sexual stimulation; an attitude that would, arguably, raise a snigger from the Nietzsche of *On the Genealogy of Morals*. "If our aestheticians," he wrote there, "never tire of claiming in Kant's favour, that spellbound by beauty one can even view undraped female statues 'without interest', then one can laugh a little at their expense". And as a corollary, this classification of *Romance* as an art film, and hence available for viewing, also works as a social-taxonomical device in its unspoken assumption that it would be unlikely to attract the attention of those without distinction – those who prefer their porn unaestheticised.

These attitudes inscribed within aesthetics – that it is 'pure' and abstract, that it is a matter of personal taste rather than social formation, that it is universal and disinterested rather than specific and interested – position this field as the natural enemy of cultural studies, with its history of engagement with the politics of theory and practice. But if we ignore aesthetics, or engage with it only critically, as the "plaything of a deracinated elite" (Williams, in Hunter 1992: 347) or as something simply self-indulgent, we risk alienating and rejecting the private and the affective spheres in favour of the public and the rational. In other words, we risk doing precisely what we critique, and find flawed, in aesthetics. In the process, we forget the very important and potentially liberatory perspectives that traditional aesthetics offered: its attempts to understand that which seemed to be outside reason (the emotional or sensate realm); its insistence that there is more to life than reason; and its argument that the world of perception and experience can't be derived only from abstract laws, but also involves the sensate.

Cultural studies' tendency to overlook both these features of aesthetics and its own interest in framing up perspectives on art is most clearly demonstrated in a further area in which it takes issue with aesthetics: the matter of evaluating how critics engage with art works. Artists, art historians and aestheticists are often more prepared than are cultural theorists to use as a starting point their personal and emotional response to an art work. For conventional cultural theorists, this attitude demonstrates the 'softness' of artistic sensibility, and shows it to come up short against conceptual and critical rigour – the imperative to reduce an artwork to a specific analysis. But in this, cultural studies is falling into the kind of elitism that it criticises in aesthetics privileging its approaches over the approaches of other disciplines. It also falls into the kind of universalising gesture that it criticises in aesthetics, reducing art to a singular practice and project, focusing on the high art aspects of cultural production, and eliding the extent to which aesthetics is also an everyday practice and an ethics involved in making up the civil society. This cultural studies 'take' on the aesthetic field doesn't necessarily or effectively problematise its elitist features; what it tends to do instead is tip the cultural studies' hat to Reason, and in the process overlook the everyday experience of appreciating art. In this regard, a dialogue between these two disciplines may in fact point out ruptures in the discourses of each. Aesthetics, as we note above, has a bet each way ('it's personal'; 'it's universal'). Cultural studies writings, on the other hand, explicitly distance themselves from master narratives and notions of Truth and yet, when it comes to art, claim the high ground of science, or reason, and demand a careful separation of the affective and the critical selves. The application of a reflexive gaze upon our own positions, and a commitment to view our own position from the point of view of 'the other', can plug such gaps, and help to ensure a perspective on art and society that is at once more rigorous and more engaged.

Cultural studies isn't alone in neglecting aesthetics, rejecting it as a viable reading practice, or treating it as somewhat irrelevant. Artists themselves often reject aesthetic discourses, being suspicious that too much analysis of their art will harm their creativity, or considering that aesthetic analysis is artistically useless – the work of word-smiths rather than creators. Philosophers over the past few decades have also overlooked aesthetics, despite the fact that aesthetics has traditionally been central to philosophy, and that questions of art and beauty were once regarded as among its essential concerns. And social critics and activists likewise often see it as worthless to their interests, positing that because of its claims to disinterest and autonomy it suffers from social functionlessness: that is, it has no social force, or 'teeth', and doesn't necessarily or obviously contribute to social change.

Still, that's not all that can be said about aesthetics – or art more generally, since I'd argue that at this point in history, when the notion of a disinterested aesthetic is being eroded, there is an isomorphism between art and aesthetics. However convincing the arguments of post-aesthetic cultural theorists, art is not only about social representation and reproduction. It's also about making and enjoying art works, practices which have changed significantly over the past century or so, and even more significantly over the past few decades. Taking this line, and bearing in mind the arguments against aesthetics that are mounted from across the disciplines, we can argue that it is no longer relevant to engage with aesthetics in its eighteenth-century concept, as a 'science of beauty'. Rather, we can understand and make use of aesthetics, in Bourdieu's terms, as "a theory of practice *as practice*" (Bourdieu, in Calhoun *et al.* 1993: 266-267) – and address ways of understanding the extent to which the experience of sensual, emotional and 'intuitive' responses is an effect of being produced within, and inhabiting, particular contexts, and not just the effect of 'cultivated literacies', social distinction, or elite sensibilities.

Changes in art and in how we understand art have problematised the conventional approaches of both cultural studies and aesthetics, because what has been emerging in artistic practice over the twentieth century is not the practice of refined distance, or of elevated sensory experience. Rather, there has been a visible rejection of canonical standards and autonomy, and a shift away from traditional evaluative landscapes towards an approach which can be associated with mass culture, commerce, modes of global communication and quotidian practices. And although in many cases art remains identified with alienated, privileged cultural zones – galleries, theatres, colleges of art and music – in all those isolated cultural sites the artists, directors, curators and editors who staff them are commercialising, commodifying, and otherwise finding ways of serving up what people want to see, in a way that they want it; and hence responding to commercial and visceral demand rather than insisting on a discrete aesthetic distance. This change is moving aesthetics out of its traditional elevated, refined atmosphere and into the sphere of communication and commerce. And this is perhaps why, although the criticisms of art and aesthetics are in many ways well grounded, aesthetics keeps coming back, over and over, in various periods and in various guises, as a cultural studies' interest.

One of its recent 'returns' is in the shape of the notion that contemporary aesthetics can provide the grounds for a discussion of democratisation in an increasingly globalised environment. In traditional aesthetics art and life were opposed, with art conceived as that which reflects, and hence is subordinated to, life. More recently, as noted above, art is being conceived as that which captures, rather than just reflects, everyday life. This comes out of post-aesthetic perspectives which are grounded in the notion that aesthetic products are neither intrinsically Beautiful nor emblems of the Sublime, but are *signs*, the meanings of which are field-specific, and open to contestation as part of the struggle to delimit meaning and to formalise the systems of value which constitute the social world. This can provide grounds for theorising the ways in which people, in their everyday lives, consume aesthetic products; which is, typically, not in the mode of an abstract affective response to beauty, but a particular and situated response. So, increasingly, art demonstrably depends on both artist and audience, thus changing its status from a special, priceless 'thing' to simply another commodity. In this change, it carves out a space for everyday life, everyday experiences and everyday responses to be taken seriously. And as a corollary, it demonstrates the possibility of change by moving art away from the distanced and disinterested world of elite aesthetics into a more democratised zone. As Eric Lott wrote, "We have recognized too little … that art and aesthetic activity generally are recognizable human interests" (1994: 545-56); and effectively, the aesthetic is now everywhere, and nowhere. Radio patter and song lyrics play with language in skilful and engaging ways; visual stimuli are everywhere, from billboards to building designs to book jackets; while televisual flows move us from the Beautiful to the Sublime and on to the ridiculous with barely a pause. Everywhere, so the argument goes, we find the aesthetic in the form of an enveloping semiotic, and are touched by it.

Another 'return' is to an area that seems to have remained somewhat under-theorised, though it was arguably the subject of early aesthetics – the art work, and what it does to or in us. In this admittedly murky water, I suggest, lie a couple of very good reasons why, despite all their shortcomings, art and aesthetics remain so resonant for cultural theorists, artists, viewers, governments. Both of these reasons come from Nietzsche – or, rather, use Nietzsche as a springboard. The first is its role in continually calling into question the relationship between truth and representation; and the second is the relationship between aesthetic pleasure and our physical lives.

The issue of truth is, of course, central to aesthetic enquiry, and it is one which Nietzsche apparently takes seriously: "Very early in my life," he writes in the *Nachlass,* "I took the question of the relation of *art* to *truth* very seriously: even now I stand in holy dread in the face of this discordance." Of course Nietzsche's understanding of truth is of something multi-layered and shot through with absences (*There are no facts, only interpretations*). But in relation to art, it can be read as having a more precise meaning, one that begins with the writings of antiquity and follows those 'takes' on the questions of mimesis and reality right through to Kant and his descendants. In this view, Nietzsche's 'dread' can be read as a response to the 'discordance' occasioned by the fact that truth is presented as an absolute, and yet comes to seem less true than art, or at least less true than art's truth-value – which can be more convincing than either reason or empiricism. So, holy dread could most certainly be a response to the realisation that truth is contingent.

But we can also read Nietzsche's dread as a response to the realisation that art is not truth, and not mimesis, but is simply art – just another commodity, just another social practice; one which results in artefacts which draw their value, like other artefacts, from idiosyncratic and socially authorised taste, rather than from absolute standards. This view of 'dread' is made more resonant by the sorts of art work that have been produced over the twentieth century: think, for instance, of the Dadaists and Surrealists, for whom art was a form of madness, a joke, chance, or just the arrangement of found objects. Think of the inclusion in art galleries and literary collections of traditional works and stories, which could equally have been classified as pure ethnography, and which make no claims to Art or Truth. Think too of postmodern works that further attenuate the relation of art to truth, that insist on their status as representation, or even as representation of a representation. Art no longer (if it ever did) simply agrees that it offers a window onto the Real.

If we follow this second reading of the 'holy dread', then the question of the relation of art to truth affords an engagement with the question of ethics. This ethics, of course, is not one which can be situated on an absolute or abstract plain, 'an ideal or subjective domain', but remains firmly in the material realm, constituting an attempt to think through "ways of conducting one's life" (Hunter 1992: 348). At the same time as it questions what is meant by truth, aesthetics can offer a forum for debates over the relations of commodity culture to culture ('culture' in Raymond Williams' sense of 'a whole of life'). In this respect, aesthetics works as ethics because its practices test and expose the limits of the social as well as its own limits. And again, twentieth-century avant-garde art, whether plastic, literary, media or performance, is largely responsible for this because it cannot be read – as is the case with Romantic art – as necessarily beautiful, or as offering a representation of the true-real. Rather, it focuses attention as much on the processes of production and distribution as on how, or why, such work becomes considered Art, problematising the 'truth' of art, and particularly the truth of its disinterest or its universality. So the ethics of the aesthetic can be discussed not as an entry point for truth, but as a site for debate about meanings and value and, perhaps most importantly, debates about who 'we' are, or who and how 'we' should be (see Maffesoli 1991). Aesthetics, seen in this signal question of the relation of art to truth, takes on a role in the constituting and legitimating of a collective conscience and a collective identity. And it does so by authorising the production of works which may be used to undermine the 'natural' authority of the cultural elites (for example, the pianist David Helfgott's immense popularity in the face of the critics' scorn); or by making visible the degree to which artistic distance and autonomy is a fantasy (in the very public distribution of arts grants and cash prizes). In short, aesthetics – or the art world more generally – can be reclaimed as a model in which sociability is foregrounded: not necessarily the violently homogenised Hobbesian view of 'the community', but an agonistic and pluralistic one, in which aesthetic evaluation is connected to pleasure and sociability, where the enjoyment taken in the consumption of cultural products is in part the pleasure of placing oneself in, and competing for position within, a social world.

The notion of pleasure takes us to the second departure point that Nietzsche provides: the status of aesthetics as a part of our physical lives, a part of our being, an 'applied physiology'. Art-as-physiology connects the body and reason, desire and sociality; and, moreover, makes it difficult to appreciate the disinterested possibilities of art. The pleasures of art, from this perspective, are located not in the mind but in the body with all its animality and visceral joy. This means it is difficult, if not impossible, to manage, control or rationalise. Pleasure in art is part of the 'willing' of being, and can threaten to break down the social contract. Here of course Nietzsche's view of art is closer to Plato's, with his rejection of poets from the ideal republic, than to Kant's; but it is worth giving some consideration to the relations between artistic production and 'life processes'. This again brings art away from the cool air of refinement and sensibility and back to the vulgar quotidian. What this suggests too is that aesthetics, and artistic production, make it apparent that everything can be reduced to an artefact, or a commodity. Aesthetics need not make large claims or assert capitalised values, but can investigate the ways in which aesthetics is, in Terry Eagleton's terms, "a discourse of the body" (Eagleton 1990: 13) and a discourse of the social: one which foregrounds desire and physicality, and in so doing can be used to think through justice, ethics, social organisation, power, sex – all those factors that make us human.

In this respect, aesthetics can also offer the sorts of transgressive or contestatory possibilities that are valued by cultural studies. By reflecting on the contingencies of the social, and of the imbrication of the aesthetic with the everyday, and by recalling the body to the world of reason, taste and ethics, it is possible to conceive of a way of appreciating artistic works that might further the political ends of cultural studies – to break down taxonomies, destabilise privileged practices, and disturb the boundaries between disciplines, so that there are no claims made for universal aesthetic or ethical truth, but only useful and equitable ways of accommodating the social and its exigencies, and of making us what we are. And finally, an attitude of interdisciplinary curiosity between cultural studies and aesthetics may allow us to take up the strengths offered by post-aesthetic thought, without reducing art objects to simple commodities or texts for analysis; and without, on the other hand, restoring art to its former place as capital-A Art. Cultural theorists can make use of aspects of aesthetics, especially the notion of sensate experience and, without insisting on a Kantian infinite deferral of pleasure or the redirection of pleasure into social performativity, view the aesthetic experience as offering a site for multiple, and potentially playful, but always contestatory subjectivities. Drawing on both cultural studies and aesthetics, with their shared antecedents, we can critique and defamiliarise the art world while restoring the notion of pleasure and the sensate to the experience of art.

Bibliography:

Adorno, Theodor (1997) *Aesthetic Theory*, trans. Robert Hullot-Kentor, ed. Gretel Adorno and Rolf Tiedemann, London: Athlone Press.

Bourdieu, Pierre (2000) *Pascalian Meditations*, trans. Richard Nice, Cambridge: Polity.

Bourdieu, Pierre (1998) *Practical Reason: on the theory of action*, Cambridge: Polity.

Bourdieu, Pierre (1993) "Concluding remarks: for a sociogenetic understanding of intellectual works", in: Calhoun, Craig; LiPuma, Edward; and Postone, Moishe, eds. *Bourdieu: critical perspectives,* Cambridge: Polity Press, 263–75.

Bourdieu, Pierre (1984) *Distinction: a social critique of the judgement of taste,* trans. Richard Nice, London: Routledge.

Eagleton, Terry (1990) *The Ideology of the Aesthetic*, Oxford: Basil Blackwell, Oxford.

Hunter, Ian (1992) "Aesthetics and Cultural Studies", in: Grossberg, Lawrence; Nelson, Cary; and Treichler, Paula, eds. *Cultural Studies*, London and New York: Routledge, 347–72.

Lott, Eric (1994) "The aesthetic ante: pleasure, pop culture, and the middle passage", *Calloloo* 17: 2 (Spring), 545–56.

Maffesoli, Michel (1991) "The ethic of aesthetics", *Theory, Culture and Society* 8, 7–20.

Nietzsche, Friedrich (1967) *The Birth of Tragedy*, trans. Walter Kaufmann, New York: Vintage.

Panofsky, Erwin (1955) *Meaning in the Visual Arts: papers in and on art history,* Woodstock, NY: Overlook Press.

Section C:

The Translation of Cultural Studies – Translation Studies

TEACHING NOMADISM: INTER/CULTURAL STUDIES IN THE CONTEXT OF TRANSLATION STUDIES

RUSSELL WEST

This essay places Anglo-American Cultural Studies in an international context, specifically, that of translation studies degrees in contemporary Europe. It explores the conditions under which cultural studies can be relevant to professionally oriented translation studies. The discussion goes on to interrogate the ways in which cultural studies and translation studies intersect, with the help of a reading of the recent novel by the Australian translator, academic, critic and novelist Robert Dessaix, *Night Letters* (1996), and its German translation, *Breife aus der Nacht* (1997). The cultural conflicts and tensions typically examined by cultural studies, and exemplified in Dessaix' novel and its translation provide the basis for the concluding discussion on the models of subjective agency which a novel inter/cultural studies can offer students of translation studies today.

'Translation' has been at the heart of some of the most momentous interdisciplinary innovations in the social sciences in the twentieth century. Lacan's 'translation' of Freud using the instruments of structuralist linguistics produced a novel theory of subjectivity; Lévi-Strauss, similarly wielding Saussurian linguistics, undertook a 'translation' of traditional ethnography; and Marx found himself 'translated' by Althusser in a further application of the notion of 'structure'. Translation figures in all these cases as a metaphor for transgressive hybridisation across disciplinary boundaries which produces radically new possibilities of knowledge and critique in the social sciences. Translation in the broadest sense is an operation which establishes continuity across a space of discontinuity, making heterogeneity productive for intellectual pursuit.

Anglo-American cultural studies is itself a case in point, as it has grown out of a fruitful dialogue between literary studies and studies of popular culture, with linguistics, psychoanalysis and ethnology being co-opted as powerful analytical instruments. The 'translative', interdisciplinary operations at work in the genesis of cultural studies as a new disciplinary area are perhaps symptomatic, in a sense, of what Homi Bhabha discerns as the operations of translation in the very object of cultural studies' enquiries, suggesting that: "all forms of culture are in some way related to each other because culture is a signifying or symbolic activity. The articulation of cultures is possible not because of familiarity or similarity of *contents*, but because all cultures are symbol-forming and subject-constituting, interpellative practices." Bhabha goes on to specify that by "translation" he primarily means "a process by which, in order to objectify cultural meaning, there always has to be a process of alienation and of secondariness *in relation to itself*. In that sense there is no 'in itself' and 'for itself' within cultures because they are always subject to intrinsic forms of translation" (Bhabha 1990: 209-10). In this essay, I wish to give this 'translative' turn in cultural studies a further interdisciplinary revolution by confronting Anglo-American cultural studies with a double translation – on the one hand into the specific pedagogic context of teaching translation studies, and on the other, beyond its own English-language/cultural sphere into the European context.

This project involves a number of 'translative' steps. The first is that of explicitly situating cultural studies in a concrete pedagogic context, an increasingly prominent issue of discussion among cultural studies theorists, as the success of the Internet discussion group 'cspedagogy' indicates. This first translation implies an ethical task which can be helpfully elucidated with reference to some of the underlying principles of Levinas' philosophy of alterity. Three aspects of Levinas' philosophy of the Other are pertinent in the context of teaching in institutes of higher education. First, the notion that Selfhood does not contain its own origin, but is preceded and founded by an an-archic the Other (Levinas 1990: 125). Secondly, that the Other questions my existence, that the face of the Other person casts into question the self-sufficiency of my existence, and imposes upon me a responsibility which is not of my choosing (Levinas 1990: 203-77, Levinas 1987a: 50 ff.). And thirdly, that the duo of self and Other, with the potential dilemma of moral responsibility for an Other whose action is immoral, needs to be complemented by responsibility for a "Third Party" [*tiers*] (Levinas 1987: 97, 101). Translated – in a manner perhaps too cavalier and inadequate to do justice to the complexity of Levinas' philosophy, but in a way which, I hope, nonetheless remains faithful to the spirit of his ethical undertaking – into the context of tertiary teaching, it is the students who found our teaching practice and in the last analysis provide its *raison d'être*. The faces which confront me in the classroom impose upon me a responsibility to address their immediate present as learners and their future as prospective graduates. What increasingly intrudes upon the teacher-student duo is the employment market and the demands of the subsequent profession. This situation has led academics such as Ansgar Nünning and Andreas Jucker, in a recent paper on the teaching of English studies in Germany, to suggest that the content of tertiary teaching should be dictated more by the needs of students than by the teachers' own research (Nünning and Jucker 1999: 169-92). Here I would like to suggest that the teacher-student relationship functions as a sort of transfer relation in which the reciprocal translation of apparently quite heterogeneous discourses into hitherto autonomous domains transpires to be highly fruitful. Where some teachers have written of generic conflicts arising from the translation of the imperative of professional orientation into the classroom space with its pedagogical imperative, I would like to stress the "complementarity" of the two genres (see Plotnitsky 1994), suggesting that the needs of students for a later entry onto the employment market can fruitfully guide our teaching practice (Cowley and Hanna 1997: 119-34).[1] This does not mean slavishly subordinating our teaching to a set of narrowly pragmatic criteria, but rather, responding to the ethical imperative to find out market uses for the skills imparted by a critical and even oppositional pedagogy.

The reason why this apparent clash of genres in reality manifests complementarity is that operations of 'translation' in fact form a common denominator which establishes a continuum linking the classroom, professional contexts towards which the classroom can constantly refer, and the culture in which teaching practices are inserted. Taking translation seriously as a unifying figure across a range of pedagogic, professional and cultural practices means responding to the ethical imperative to abandon what Appadurai calls "the kind of illusion of order that we can no longer afford to impose on a world that is so transparently volatile" (Appadurai 1996: 47). In other words, the corrosive and creative confrontation with Alterity pervades the form, content and function of what I shall call an inter/cultural studies informed by translative processes at every level. This essay argues that the notion of "nomadic thought" proposed by Rosi Braidotti as an adaptation of Deleuze's concepts of nomadism and the nomadic war-machine is an apposite one to take account of the transformations wrought by pedagogical responses to encounters with a foreign culture (Braidotti 1994: 1-40). Translation can be understood here as a broad process, the key to which is the learning of nomadic thought.

The suggestions in this essay arise out of my own experience of taking up a teaching position in a German University of Applied Sciences ostensibly to provide technical translation students with cultural competencies corresponding to their technical translation skills. This aspect of their training is clearly seen within the department as subordinate to the technical skills imparted, as the area-studies positions, reserved for English, Spanish, French and Russian native speakers respectively, are pegged lower down the seniority scale than the technical translation professorships. Such an attitude is also shared by the students themselves, who, understandably, are vigorously resistant to theoretical or non-technical teaching (Nünning and Jucker 1999a: 138). Two challenges are contained in this situation: to allow the intrusion of the professional world into the academic space of cultural studies to produce new stimuli for that discipline; and to offer students a range of critical perspectives which simultaneously break apart a relatively narrow insistence upon instrumental technical skills and equip them for the genuinely ubiquitous cultural processes at work in the translation profession.

The underlying dynamic of the translation act itself, however, can offer the basic model for a form of cultural studies which both responds to the clearly

[1] Many thanks to Barbara Hanna for giving me access to her work, some of it not yet published.

expressed needs of students and asks them to confront a series of questions about the location, constitution, and relevance of cultural practices within their profession. Indeed, I would suggest that cultural studies, with its claim for the interlocking of cultural process, cultural practice and the construction of subjectivity, provides the theoretical basis for a personal interpellation of the translation student in her or his very identity as a translator.

In order to unfold the full pedagogic potential inherent in cultural studies when interrogated in an intercultural context, however, a degree of transgression of disciplinary boundaries is necessary. Though schematic, the gestures of disciplinary iconoclasm which follow are intended as ways of responding to the translation of the teaching context into that of intercultural professions and vice versa. The first gesture consists of radicalising area studies (or *Landeskunde* as it as known within the German-speaking university system). This discipline is generally seen as a supplement to language teaching as such, and consists of the transmission of a body of knowledge regarding the politics, geography and institutions of the culture being studied, as well as ostensibly typical quotidian cultural practices. Three questions can be asked about this approach to the teaching of culture. A first question is that of the utility of such knowledge. How is such knowledge to be implemented, what is its place in an increasingly practical thrust of language teaching, in my case, the training of technical translators? (See Liedke, Redder and Scheiter 1999: 155). A second question is that of the definition of cultural configurations underlying such an approach, one in which culture is generally regarded as static, homogenous, and restricted to institutional or political traditions or some reified aspects of 'high culture' or 'typically English/German/French/Spanish characteristics'. This questioning comes from the direction of cultural studies, which problematises assumptions of the homogenous and static character of culture, as well as highlighting the complex interactions of high culture, popular culture and political structures. Thus Annalie Knapp-Potthoff vigorously criticises the (diachronically) static and (synchronically) speciously representative character of cultural knowledge for students of a foreign culture (Knapp-Pothoff 1997: 181-205). The third question is that of the relationship between cultures which is constitutive of the act of acquiring knowledge of another culture. This question is of course particularly present in the context of a translation degree, where it is impossible to avoid drawing attention to the processes of transmission linking cultural activities of various national or language areas. How then do students situate themselves in relation to the other culture? Is the other culture seen as a homogenous entity held at a critical distance and regarded by a homogeneous group in the classroom? (Cowley and Hanna 1999: 6). Or is the process of observation itself reflected as a practice carried out within a cultural space no less heterogeneous than the culture being studied?

My second gesture against disciplinary boundaries is that of the radicalisation of cultural studies, following a lead suggested by Paul Gilroy in the opening sections of *The Black Atlantic* (Gilroy 1993). There, he claims that cultural studies has been dogged in its emergence as a radically critical interdisciplinary pursuit by its clinging to a national (English) paradigm. This maintenance of national boundaries as the defining framework for cultural studies constitutes a blind spot which elides the inherently syncretic and hybrid influences contributing to the construction of modern British society, in particular that of Black slaves transported across the Atlantic. It suppresses the cross-cultural origins of radical politics in Britain, and the on-going syncretism of much compound cultural production in contemporary British society. Closer to the activity of cultural studies itself, it also forgets the role of English-speaking outsiders in contributing to the development of conceptions of Englishness (Carlyle, Swift, Scott, Eliot) – to which one would have to add contemporary names such as Williams, Hall, Bhabha and Gilroy himself. "I want to develop the suggestion", writes Gilroy, "that cultural historians could take the Atlantic as one single, complex unit of analysis in their discussion of the modern world and use it to produce an explicitly transnational and intercultural perspective" (Gilroy 2000: 449). We need to couch the parameters of our programmes for learning and research increasingly in inter/cultural terms, partly in response to the mounting recognition of the significance of translation processes in the reciprocal constitution of cultural identities, as Susan Bassnett's recent work stresses (Bassnett 1993: 138-61) and partly in response to the increasing intensity of cross-cultural contacts in the contemporary world.

Out of these two radicalising moves, I wish to propose a hybrid pedagogical area which I term inter/cultural studies – one which interrogates cultural identities across a dialectical reflection upon foreign cultures and the students' own culture, working on the assumption that national cultures, in a postmodern and global era, increasingly constitute each other in processes of reciprocal if not symmetrical translation (Nünning and Jucker 1999a: 139-40). The diagonal bar within inter/cultural studies points towards the difference, heterogeneity and articulation at the heart of such a discipline, and its inherently composite character as a '*bricolage*' of several already available models. Not so much the didactic content of the material studied, as the very form of this reflexive dialectic (the 'inter' of inter/cultural studies) embody a translative operation. Culture itself is always a hybrid entity, always constituted in a process of border-crossings. Furthermore, individual identities are also caught in processes on ongoing translation and reciprocal modification; in the context of my own teaching practice, an awareness of identity-as-translation is crucial for the professional identity of intercultural communicators such as translators. In the realm of translation, the capacity to deal with differences between languages is predicated upon a subjective configuration which sits easily with ambiguity and multiple realities: "The polyglot", suggests Braidotti, "also knows intimately what de Saussure teaches explicitly: that the connection between linguistic signs is arbitrary. […] Thus the polyglot becomes the prototype of the postmodernist speaking subject; struck by the maddening, fulminating insight about the arbitrariness of linguistic meanings and yet resisting the free fall into cynicism" (Braidotti 1994: 14).

To offer a rough idea of what teaching inter/cultural studies in the context of translation studies might look like, I'd like to take a detour by way of a text used in a recent seminar in Magdeburg, in order to propose a reading of Robert Dessaix's 1996 novel *Night Letters* (Dessaix 1996), translated into German as *Briefe aus der Nacht* (Dessaix 1997, and Dessaix 1999). It contains nightly letters written to a friend in Melbourne by an Australian traveller suffering from an incurable disease. Alongside the several translators who figure in the narrative, the novel as a whole offers an image of 'translation' in the spatial sense as it is ostensibly a collection of letters, and in the literary and cultural sense as it constantly has recourse to much transmitted and translated texts (the Gospels, Dante, Mann, as well as Lermontov and Tolstoy [see Vladiv-Glover]) to weave the fabric of its own symbolic work.

One intertextual element which embodies transmission and translation is the recurrent narrative of the Annunciation, which is parodied early on to describe the Chinese-Australian doctor's informing the narrator of his disease. This parodic version of the Annunciation – the narrator wryly observes that there was "no point in my murmuring '*virum non cognosco*', of course" (*Night Letters*, 6) – is one element in a thematic strand concerned with death and disease, contamination, sexuality as a threat to hegemonic order, and homophobia. A later translation of the Annunciation is the narrator's account of a visit to Giotto's chapel in Padua, containing the painter's representation of the event, on the Feast of the Annunciation (*Night Letters*, 209). Padua, significantly, is also the place where the narrator celebrates heresy as a form of productive translation, opening up dogma, always centrifugal, leading beyond ready-formed answers to persistent questions – a rogue genetic mutation that makes the species multiply (*Night Letters*, 231). Thus this second perspective on the Annunciation figures an iconoclastic mode of translation of news, itself translated into many different versions, not the last of which is Dessaix's own irreverent version of it. The Venetian St Mark's lion also figures a similarly double figure of translation. The narrator is plagued by recurring dreams of being pursued by a lion and faced with the choice of running away from it, or being torn to pieces by it. Towards the end of the novel, the dream changes, with the narrator springing onto the lion, and riding through the jungle on the creature's back (*Night Letters*, 272). Once again, the evangelist's feline mascot embodies the narrator's nemesis, until, by appropriating prior textual models as a mode of transmission, it is transformed into a resolution of the problem of mortality. The writer is no less mortal than before, but is able to ride irreverently on the back of the literary works of the past. This positive appropriation of the lion is never definitive, but needs to be constantly reasserted: in the last chapter, the view of the Venetian lions motivates the narrator to move on (*Night Letters*, 271).

What is at stake for Dessaix's terminally ill narrator is the transformation of selfhood through a mode of story-telling based upon translation and transmission both as textual and spatial principles. He comments, "I needed a story, probably because the story of my own life is in danger of petering out in a series of incomplete sentences, the main thread well and truly frayed" (*Night Letters*, 153). Against this image of phrasal disintegration as an expression of the incipient extinction of the self, Dessaix's novel offers images of forms of travel that cannot end because they have no end, and of a selfhood that cannot be obliterated because it is always already in flux. Thus the narrator fantasises about an aimless, unpredictable journey lacking telos and terminus, based upon "the desire to be, of course, not to have" (*Night letters*, 13-14). The narrator yearns for "*travel* in the old sense [...] travelling to whet your appetite, to pique your hunger, not to satisfy it" (*Night Letters*, 213). Here, travel challenges and thus reworks selfhood. Here the transmission of the self through time and space is to be understood as a constant process of interrogation, just as translation can be construed not as reconstituing, but rather questioning an original, opening up novel aspects of the original instead of closing them down. In this view of travel, the famed Marco Polo is a failed traveller: "There's no sign at all that his thinking changed about anything – he left Italy as an Italian teenager and returned to Italy twenty years later as Italian as he'd left it. Nothing he saw seems to have had the slightest effect on is medieval Italian view of the world. [...] he just started at the beginning and ended at the end – all very linear. [...] Essentially, [...] what I'm saying is that Messer Marco Polo had not *been* anywhere" (*Night Letters*, 246-7).

This impoverished stability of the self in conjunction with the absence of a true voyage and a true narrative reverses the principle set down earlier in the novel by the rather fanciful story of an amulet which is sent from place to place, successively surviving its various possessors and senders who one after another die in a colourful variety of ways (*Night Letters*, 47-54). Selfhood is ephemeral, a mere vehicle for the amulet and the narrative it generates. The amulet passes via its respective owners just as a text passes from translator to translator, the whole translation history thereby making up a global picture of what the translation has meant for various generations. The self merely articulates one of the translative fragments whose mystical sum total Benjamin saw as making up true speech. A similar example of translation as a governing metaphor for subjective global existences would be Eva Hoffman's autobiography, *Lost in Translation*, which employs the writer's profession as a metaphor for the entire pattern of her life, ceaselessly characterised by nomadic, cross-border movements (Hoffman 1998). This mode of selfhood, I would argue, is one of the underlying principles of education for work in an intercultural context today.

But lest this all sound too idealist, it is worth underlining that Dessaix' novel is entirely aware of the material aspects, and in particular the costs of translation. If the novel is concerned on the diachronic axis with the subject's fight against death, predicated upon a questioning of a stable selfhood, it is equally concerned on the synchronic axis with translation as a dangerously transgressive activity. One of the metaphors of translation which structures the novel is that of contamination or infiltration. Dessaix writes: "The streets around the Roman ghetto were gated shut as well, but in Rome Jewishness could quite easily leak out into the city – without canals defilement of the Christian body could not be completely prevented. In Venice at night the ghetto was a sealed-off island. Christians were safe from the polluting sensuality of the Jew. [...] All foreigners, in fact – the Armenians, the Turks, the Albanians – were segregated like lepers. At night" (*Night Letters*, 131-2). Venice is a contradictory city, both protected by its island status, and made vulnerable by its canals. Venice embodies this paradoxical mixture of water as vehicle for traffic, the basis of the city's wealth, and of the body criss-crossed with canals which make of it an open body vulnerable to infection. According to this simile, translation is both a means of material gain and a transgressive threat to be strictly policed. Translation as a form of transgression is brutally punished in two episodes of the novel. In one story told to the narrator by a German professor staying in the same hotel in Venice, the Renaissance courtesan Camilla gains such power to seduce her lovers, members of a noble Venetian family, that they eventually orchestrate a gang rape to punish Camilla's symbolic infiltration of the Venetian establishment and the affective if not effective power she wields (*Night Letters*, 167-8). The same movement of brutal ejection of a foreign body is rehearsed when the professor himself is beaten up by the staff of the Venetian hotel he stays in every year, late one night upon returning from a gay club (*Night Letters*, 198-201). It is precisely this event which motivates the narrator to move on from Venice, tempering his new found optimism with a sober appraisal of his own prospects in the city.

These novelistic images of retribution levelled against translation as a contamination of infiltration point to a real history of political consequences of translation. Lawrence Venuti documents the potential disruptive force of translations with the example of Jerome's translation of the Bible from the Hebrew; Christopher Hill describes the caution evinced by seventeenth-century translators into English and the real threat to absolutist authority posed by their work (see Hill 1997: 27ff; Venuti 1995: 19-20). More recently, Anthony Pym has listed the names of twelve literary translators whose work has earned them political persecution, imprisonment or death, while journalists investigating the activities of Serbian militia in Kosovo have reported threats against the Serbian interpreters charged with betraying too much information to outsiders (Pym 1997: 11-12; see also Schirra 1999: 19). All intercultural transaction takes place within a configuration of power relations, with the result that communication between cultures and its individual representatives is seldom symmetrical or equally balanced; such asymmetry will be vigorously defended by those bound to profit from it.

This omnipresence of attempts to control translation is enacted in Dessaix's novel by the framing introduction and notes written by the letters' editor, a certain Igor Miasmov. His intervention within the text, in his own account, is one of radical censorship: "references to matters of no conceivable interest to anybody apart from close acquaintances (details of menus and railway timetables, complaints about [...] rates of exchange, amorous encounters and the like) have been omitted from this edited version." What Miasmov claims to have cut are, precisely, the everyday aspects of translation or transaction – digestion, transport, monetary exchange, love. More radically, Miasmov claims to have standardised the defective English of the narrator's foreign interlocutors in the letters' reported speech: "As a non-native speaker myself, I considered I was ideally equipped to make the necessary sensitive adjustments" (*Night Letters*, ix). Once again, tangible evidence of the process of intercultural translation is suppressed, in a gesture which I take to be symptomatic of some form of projection of an immigrant's own impulse to elide his own intolerable foreignness (Miasmov's deep implication with the semantic and moral contamination he attempts to extirpate is revealed in his own name, etymologically a mix of Russian and the Greek for 'pollution' [see Vladiv-Glover]).

But let us return from the text-immanent level of Dessaix's novel to the real processes by which a translation is produced and distributed – in other words, the material and professional context to which inter/cultural studies should always be oriented. In Wolf Koehler's German translation of 1997, which was studied in the recent seminar in Magdeburg, the process of editorial intervention is radicalised even further. Miasmov's end-notes are both censorious and censoring, where, to cite only one of many examples, Miasmov signals the excision of passages of bad taste (*Night Letters*, 202), but they are at least gathered discretely at the conclusion of the three parts of Dessaix's text. In the German translation, however, the end-notes become marginal notes which actually bite into the substantial sections of the text. (Their position in the margins of the German text also works to elongate them, with the result that the notes intrude into proportionally more text.) In this way, the control instance is made immanent to the text flow, in contrast to the distance and thus relatively weak action of the end-notes of Dessaix's original. This typographical aggression is a tangible analogy of the translation strategy undertaken by Koehler throughout the text, which is to weaken the parts of the text where the English directly refers to the disruptive force of translation. Thus when the narrator disputes the agency of a naked sexual drive motivating cultural activity, suggesting rather that culture is simply driven by layers upon layers of cultural encoding reminiscent of the endless productivity of the translation process, Köhler replaces Dessaix' "the desire to fuck" (*Night Letters*, 188) with the trivialised and harmless "*pimpern*" (*Briefe aus der Nacht*, 216). Likewise, the narrator's visceral reaction to the discovery of the professor being beaten up by his own hotel staff ("I felt quite shaken" – *Night Letters*, 269) is watered down by the German into the mildly surprised "*Ich war ziemlich platt*" (*Briefe aus der Nacht*, 300). Even more disconcerting is the translator's decision to cut the most brutal sections of the description of the retributive pack rape of the courtesan Camilla (*Night Letters*, 167-8/*Briefe aus der Nacht*, 194-5). Thus Koehler consistently intervenes at the points where the English text insists upon underlining the transgressive force of translation by couching that activity or its punishment in explicitly sexualised terms.

Despite a plethora of other translation howlers of an elementary kind, and a generally stilted style, the translation appears to be selling quite well in Germany, having progressed from the hard-cover version published by the Krüger Verlag to a paperback put out by the prestigious Fischer Verlag in Frankfurt. I suspect the reason for this is that the book foregrounds two exotic sites of European escapist fantasy, Venice and Australia. In a Germany in the midst of a slow but steady economic downturn, political disorientation, with neither Left nor Right offering any genuine political programme, and hovering uncertainly between a clearly exhausted Welfare State and a plunge into truly Neo-Liberal deregulation, such sites of enshrined collective fantasy offer a welcome alternative for imaginary investment. For a nation reluctant to deal with issues from the Nazi era such as massive damages to be paid to former forced-labour workers, or the current necessity of adapting unwieldy immigration policies to the urgent needs of the high-tech industry, Koehler's translation offers two convenient sites of projection which he is careful not to let Dessaix's original subvert. Amusingly, Dessaix appears to have anticipated this, remarking that as an Australian, "you are a kind of blank to other people, I usually find, and so of little interest to them until they have written on you" (*Night Letters*, 46). Contemporary Australia, however, has much more in common with the ambivalences of the Venice of the novel than would appear to fit the innocuous tourist images that the German translation proffers. The novel vigorously resists such nostalgic images of Australia: "Quite untypically for me, images started to cross my mind of bushland outside Melbourne – thickly wooded hills scarcely stepped on in millennia, escarpments gazed at but never climbed, views out across valleys with no house or road in sight, cockatoos squawking somewhere up behind you in the trees. [...] I was getting irrational and maudlin" (*Night Letters*, 122).

Rather, Venice, in Dessaix's narrative, functions as a decidedly unflattering mirror for today's Australia: an island nation, a paradise, an open-ended multicultural society – but one whose government actively maintained a policy of destruction of the fabric of indigenous society and culture by removing children from their parents through to the 1970s; a country which is is reluctant to follow through the full consequences of the 1992 Supreme Court ruling rejecting the *terra nullis* doctrine and thereby establishing a legal basis for Aboriginal land claims and still refuses to make a representative gesture of apology and reconciliation for almost two centuries of genocide directed at the indigenous population; and which is constantly tightening immigration legislation and culpabilising asylum seekers. Dessaix remarks: "on the one hand, Venice sent Marco Polo to Cathay and Sumatra, inspiring Columbus to sail west and discover the Americas; traded with India, Egypt and England; was home to multitudes of Germans, Dalmatians, Armenians, Turks and Persians; yet on the other hand it was a closed society, riddled with spies and double-agents, which locked up its foreigners at night for fear of contagion" (*Night Letters*, 129-30). Venice is both open and closed, welcoming to outsiders, yet controlling and sanctioning them, thus offering a parable of modern Australia. It is also a parable of Koehler's translation strategy, simultaneously ushering in this symbolic bearer of foreign places, and yet concerned to moderate their foreignness.

This attempt on the part of the translator to purify the foreignness of the text is subverted, however, by the form in which the translator presents himself in the dedication. Koehler docilely translates Dessaix's enumeration of his debts, inexplicably deleting the acknowledgement of the study used as the source of information of courtesans in Renaissance Venice, and rather oddly transplanting Dessaix' dedication to Peter Timms into the acknowledgments. Furthermore, Koehler replaces the Dante version cited by Dessaix with the corresponding German translation – at which point it abruptly becomes difficult to know who precisely is speaking in the acknowledgements. For Koehler was most certainly not funded by the Australia Arts Council, and Dessaix did not cite Dante from the translation by Herman Gmelin. Yet the same textual voice records this debt to prior sources, whether financial or textual (*Letters from the Night*, vi/*Briefe aus der Nacht*, 5). It is precisely in the recording of a translative, intertextual debt to the foreign (text) that Koehler betrays his project of purifying and controlling the foreign bodies with which he comes in contact. If the notes, alongside other paratextual elements, are one of the privileged sites of the pragmatic aspect of textuality, its action upon the reader, in the Dessaix/Koehler acknowledgements, another aspect of paratextuality comes to the fore: that of the closure of the text, its self-sufficiency or conversely, its lack of hermetic boundaries, and with that, the issue of the status of subjectivity and subjective identity within intercultural transactions (Genette 1992: 10-11).

What Dessaix's novel makes clear is that the synchronic contact between cultures and translation, and the diachronic process of translation and transmission presume a certain degree of contamination, permeability, perversion, distortion, which inevitably encounter resistance, rejection, ejection and retribution. This is the wider political context in which translation as an individual or subjective undertaking needs to be understood. Thus Dessaix's text sets both individual and collective parameters for translation as a practice of the postmodern world. Dessaix's novel suggests that our world is one where boundaries continue to exist, but are increasingly frequently crossed; and that a new subjective hybridity is not only the inevitable result of border-crossing, but more radically, its prerequisite.

Inter/cultural studies, then, to return to the larger context of this essay, must work at two levels at once. On the one hand, this pedagogic undertaking must offer students an understanding of the strategies of translation which structure the globalised postmodern world in which we live. Whence the relevance of Appadurai's concept of "Cultural studies conceived [as] the basis for a cosmopolitan (global? macro? translocal?) ethnography". Such a discipline would help students to appreciate the complex interactions of texts and cultural forms across the world and the places in which they are produced and consumed: "To translate the tension between the word and the world into a productive ethnographic strategy requires a new understanding of the deterritorialized world that many persons inhabit and the possible lives that many persons are today able to envision" (Appadurai 1996: 51-2).

On the other hand, cultural phenomena of contamination and permeability at the collective level carry with them similar experiences at the individual level, much written about in recent years under the heading of experiences of cultural hybridity anchored in the individual migratory subject. Inter/cultural studies in the context of translation studies has the task of better equipping translation students for work in the area of cross-cultural relations, and this means addressing not just collective cultural structures and their instability, but also crucial issues of subjectivity. Dessaix's novel suggests that the sort of decentering of subjectivity integral to the poststructuralist thought upon which cultural studies depends does not signal the death of selfhood, but far more, a flexibilised and radicalised mode of individual agency freed of what Lacan called the alienation and servitude of the Imaginary. For students of a foreign culture, this means confrontation with a certain degree of questioning of their own culture-bound subjectivity: thus Jürgen Kramer states that our "appropriation of a foreign means of signification (like the English language) does not leave [...] us 'untouched'... [it] is a hermeneutic process in which we expose our own cultural identity to the contrasting influence of the foreign language and culture" (Kramer 1993: 28-9). In a rather different context, Bhabha has suggested that "the possibility of producing a culture which both articulates difference and lives with it could only be established on the basis of a non-sovereign notion of self. [...] It is only by losing the sovereignty of self that you can gain the freedom of a politics that is open to the non-assimilationist claims of cultural difference" (Bhabha 1990: 212-3). For politics, read here: the translator's professional work on the borders between cultures. But what does this mean in pragmatic terms? If the structuralist and poststructuralist decentering of subjectivity implies that cultural structures transcend individual subjectivities, providing the very conditions of existence within which individual subjectivities are constituted, at the same time, however, such cultural structures cannot exist outside of subjective bearers of structures, whose agency maintains and perpetuates structures within time (see Liepietz 1997: 250-84). The subject is like Lévi-Strauss's *bricoleur*, obliged to construct an existence from the materials at hand; yet the subject can also work as an second-order *bricoleur*, reworking the structures within which it comes to being. As Peter Cowley and Barbara Hanna comment, "Part of our job as we see it is to teach our students to cut and paste, to engage with a complex system in evolution, rather than perceiving culture as a finished masterpiece, to be at best forged, at worst admired from afar. Effective language and culture teaching is not just about teaching generic rules, but showing how and where rules can usefully be broken" (Cowley and Hanna 1997: 120). Recognition of the heterogeneity, open-endedness, the process-determined character of cultures, all standard topoi of cultural studies, needs to be matched by a similar acceptance on the part of students of their own power to act provisionally, to take risks, to engage in an open-ended manner with open-ended intercultural space, to see their *own action as process* interlocking with *culture as a process*. Thus opening up collective and individual cultural entities to contaminating translation is not merely a risk, but the very qualification for a translator's optimal performance and exercise of her or his professional skills.

Foucault's notion of "technologies of the self", or Keupp and his colleagues' projects of "Identity-work" or "Identity-construction" helpfully describe the meeting point of the creative appropriation of new social forces to remodel the shape of subjective experience and action in a risk-bound postmodern age – not to make the self infinitely flexible in Sennett's sense, but to capture the possibilities inherent in working on the borders of, the overlaps and spaces between cultures (see Foucault 1994: 783-813; Keupp and Höfer 1998; Keupp *et. al.* 1999; and Beck 1986). If, as Wolfgang Welsch suggests, postmodern identities are made up of fragmented and disparate elements whose coherence is assured by processes of 'transition' and 'translation', then teaching cultural processes as cross-border processes would appear to take on a broader significance in the field of cultural studies. The "plurality competencies" which Welsch sees as a necessary element of postmodern processes of identity construction are equally central to the translator's professional skills (Welsch 1995: 845-7). This means that postmodern projects of identity are not merely philosophical speculations but rather, entirely apposite responses to changing social conditions, and one of the necessary qualifications for successful performance on today's local-global market.

It should be stressed, in order to avoid misunderstanding, that the task of inter/cultural studies is not to provide some sort of a therapy, or to mould personalities. Quite rightly, Knapp-Potthoff notes that some students possess a set of personal qualities – flexibility, tolerance, curiosity about other cultures – which make them excellent intercultural communicators, but that an academic discipline cannot and should not aim to inculcate such personal qualities (Knapp-Potthoff 1987: 425-7). Rather, the role of inter/cultural studies, via the study of texts, cultures and their borders and boundaries with neighbouring cultures, and the insertion of collective and individual agents in those inter/cultural spaces, is merely to offer strategies for learning and action. Likewise, *which* strategies are appropriated by students, and *how* subjective configurations are modified, however, is not the teacher's prerogative to determine (see Gnutzmann 1998: 135).

In the teaching of the profession of translation today, inter/cultural studies becomes instrumental in offering not only strategies, both linguistic and textual, for dealing with alterity, but also, in the very form of its pedagogical project, making available models of subjective configurations which students can appropriate for themselves, and which the successful acquisition of instrumental translation skills in fact implicitly presupposes. In Levinas' *Totalité et infini*, to return to the meditations of the opening lines of this essay, the author states that "*La différence absolue, inconcevable en termes de logique formelle, ne s'instaure que par le langage*" (Levinas 1990a: 212). Translation would thus appear to be a privileged site of the confrontation with and the negotiation of difference, both in the form and content of operations whose dimensions are both individual and collective, linguistic and social. In this general context, the notion of translation possesses a paradigmatic significance for the modes of existence of subjects acting and working within increasingly hybridised cultures in our late-modern times. Translation, as an operation which is always already at work in the constitutional hybridity of culture as process, and thus inherently a dynamic force in the disciplinary identity of cultural studies itself, continues, in the contemporary moment, to demand interdisciplinary re-configurations of our ways of knowing, and of wielding knowledge both within the university and beyond its walls.

Bibliography:

Appadurai, Arjun (1996) *Modernity at Large: Cultural Dimensions of Globalization,* Minneapolis: University of Minnesota Press.

Bassnett, Susan (1993) *Comparative Literature: A Critical Introduction,* Oxford: Blackwell.

Beck, Ulrich (1986) *Risikogesellschaft: Auf dem Weg in eine andere Moderne,* Frankfurt/Main: Suhrkamp.

Bhabha, Homi (1990) "The Third Space", Interview by Jonathan Rutherford, in Jonathan Rutherford, ed. (1990) *Identity: Community, Culture, Difference*, London: Lawrence and Wishart, 207-21.

Braidotti, Rosi (1994) *Nomadic Subjects: Embodiment and Sexual Difference in Contemporary Feminist Theory,* New York: Columbia University Press.

Cowley, Peter, and Barbara Hanna (1997) "Is There a Class in this Classroom?", *Australian Review of Applied Linguistics* [Special Issue: "Teaching Language, Teaching Culture"] Series S, 14, 119-34.

Cowley, Peter, and Barbara Hanna (1999) "Teaching Cultural Skills", Unpublished Paper.

Dessaix, Robert (1996) *Night Letters,* Sydney: Pan/New York: Picador.

Dessaix, Robert (1997) *Briefe aus der Nacht*, trans. Wolf Koehler, Frankfurt/Main: Krüger.

Dessaix, Robert (1999) *Briefe aus der Nacht*, trans. Wolf Koehler, Frankfurt/Main: Fischer.

Foucault, Michel (1994) *Dits et écrits 1954-1988*, ed. Daniel Defert and François Ewald, Paris: Gallimard, Vol. 4: 1980-1988.

Genette, Gérard (1992) *Palimpsestes: La littérature au second degré* Paris: Seuil/Points Essais.

Gilroy, Paul (2000) "The Black Atlantic as a Counterculture of Modernity", in Kwesi Owusu, ed. (2000) *Black British Culture and Society: A Text Reader*, London: Routledge, 439-52.

Gnuztmann, Claus (1998) "English as a Global Language: What does it Mean?", *Neusprachliche Mitteilungen* 51:3, 130-37.

Hanna, Barbara (1996) "Spies Like Us: Thoughts on Cultural Conformity and Language Teaching", *Australian Journal of French Studies* 33: 2, 262-77.

Hill, Christopher (1997) *Intellectual Origins of the English Revolution – Revisited,* Oxford: Clarendon Press.

Hoffman, Eva (1998) *Lost in Translation: A Life in a New Language,* London: Vintage.

Keupp, Heiner, and Renate Höfer, eds. (1998) *Identitätsarbeit heute: Klassische und aktuelle Perspektiven der Identitätsforschung*, Frankfurt/Main: Suhrkamp.

Keupp, Heiner, *et. al.* (1999) *Identitätskonstruktionen: Das Patchwork der Identitäten in der Spätmoderne*, Reinbek: Rowohlt.

Knapp-Pothoff, Annalie (1997) "Interkulturelle Kommunikationsfähigkeit als Lernziel", in Annalie Knapp Potthoff and Martina Liedke, eds. (1997) *Aspekte interkultureller Kommunikationsfähigkeit*, München: Iudicum, 181-205.

Knapp-Potthoff, Annalie (1987) "Strategien interkultureller Kommunikation", in J. Albrecht, H. W. Drescher, H. Göhring and N. Salnikow, eds. (1987) *Translation und interkulturelle Kommunikation,* Frankfurt/Main: Lang, 422-37.

Kramer, Jürgen (1993) "Cultural Studies in English Studies: A German Perspective", in Michael Byram, ed. (1993) *Culture and Language Learning in Higher Education*, Special Issue of *Language, Culture and Curriculum* 6:1, 27-45.

Levinas, Emmanuel (1987) *Humanisme de l'autre homme,* Paris: Livre de poche.

Levinas, Emmanuel (1987a) "Interviews", in François Poirié (1987) *Emmanuel Lévinas – Qui êtes-vous?* Lyon: La Manufacture, 61-136.

Levinas, Emmanuel (1990) *Autrement qu'être ou au-delà de l'essence,* Paris: Livre de poche.

Levinas, Emmanuel (1990a) *Totalité et Infini: Essai sur l'extériorité,* Paris: Livr de poche.

Liedke, Martina, Angelika Redder and Susanne Scheiter (1999) "Interkulturelles Handeln lehren – ein diskursanalytischer Trainingsansatz", in Gisela Brünner, Reinhard Fiehler and Walther Kindt, eds. (1999) *Angewandter Diskursforschung*, Opladen: Westdeutscher Verlag, Vol. 2: *Methoden und Anwendungsbereiche*, 148-79.

Lipietz, Alain, "Warp, Woof and Regulation" (1997) in Georges Benko and Ulf Strohmeyer, eds. (1997) *Space and Social Theory: Interpreting Modernity and Postmodernity*, Oxford: Blackwell, 250-84.

Nünning, Ansgar, and Andreas H. Jucker (1999) "Anglistik/Amerikanistik 2000: Plädoyer für einen studentenorientierten Kurswechsel", *Anglistik: Mitteilungen des deutschen Anglistenverbandes* 10:2, 169-92.

Nünning, Ansgar, and Andreas H. Jucker (1999a) *OrientierungAnglistik/ Amerikanistik: Was sie kann, was sie will,* Reinbek: Rowohlt.

Plotnitsky, Arkady (1994) *Complementarity: Anti-Epistemology after Bohr and Derrida*, Durham: Duke University Press.

Pym, Anthony (1997) *Pour une éthique du traducteur,* Arras: Artois Presses Université/Presses Universitaires d'Ottawa.

Schirra, Bruno (1999) "Die Gräuel der Frenkie Boys", *Die Zeit*, 2 December 1999, 17-20.

Venuti, Lawrence (1995) "Translation and the Formation of Cultural Identities", in C. Schäffner and H. Kelly-Holmes, eds. (1995) *Cultural Functions of Translation*, Clevedon, PA: Multilingual Matters, 9-25.

Vladiv-Glover, Slobodanka "Aids as the Ultimate 'Real' of the Writer: Robert Dessaix's *Night Letters*", http://www.arts.monash.edu.au/gsandss/slavic/ aids.html.

Welsch, Wolfgang (1995) *Vernunft: Die zeitgenössische Vernuftskritik und das Konzept der transversalen Vernunft,* Frankfurt/Main: Suhrkamp.

MEDIATING THE POINT OF REFRACTION AND PLAYING WITH THE PERLOCUTIONARY EFFECT: A TRANSLATOR'S CHOICE?

DAVID KATAN

Translators have an extremely important responsibility in communicating ideas to society. Much of what we read, from Aesop and the Bible to Voltaire and Weil is (re-)created by an invisible and little respected writer, the translator. This paper explores two fundamental areas: the possible refractions and perlocutionary effects that can be engendered by a translator; and secondly, what possibilities a translator has given the traditional subservience to a habitus which values translator invisibility and fidelity to the source text. A proposal is made for the translator to take more responsibility for the potential perlocutionary effect through taking a third, disassociated perceptual cognitive position. From this position the various forces acting on the translator and the translation can be controlled through mediation focussed on the benefit to the reader.

Introduction

Cultural studies and translation studies have traditionally trodden separate paths, though both have been fundamentally concerned with the processes of communication and meaning. To a large extent the former has viewed translation as a necessary but unimportant vehicle (and necessary only because many cultural studies scholars are foreign), while those involved in translation have tended to assume that culture, and the study of it, has little to do with the art of translating a text. As we shall see, though, times are changing.

This essay takes as its starting point that language is one of four filters affecting perception of reality, the other three being physiological, individual and socio-cultural (Katan 1999a: 88-90). It is, as Hanks notes (1993: 139) "one of the central vehicles of habitus". I will refer to habitus as Simeoni (1998: 17) does, as a "convenient stenograph for different default functions applying at different levels and in different domains", a global catch-all for context of situation, map of the world and context of culture (see Katan 1999a: 71-74). It is, according to Bourdieu (1990: 53- 60): "a system of durable, transposable dispositions", of "internalised structures, common schemes of perception, conception and action", the result of inculcation and habituation, simultaneously structured and structuring, and directed towards practice.

Language re-presents a person's particular vision of reality for the benefit of others. Barthes (1993: 109) calls this socially constructed representation a "myth", suggesting that "everything can be a myth provided it is conveyed by a discourse". This is a useful metaphor to bear in mind. Myths do not exist in the objective reality, but are parables or allegories with an array of possible significations. The reader, in interpreting the succession of words as coherent discourse (locutions or signifiers) will give the words meaning, and experience a certain effect, known in speech act theory as the perlocutionary effect.

Speech act theory deals principally with three levels of language and meaning, each of which anyone interested in communication should be aware of. The locution and the locutionary meaning, according to J. L. Austin (1962), is the dictionary or referential meaning. However, what is important in communication, both for culture studies and for translation studies is the force of the locution (the illocutionary force), which will be related to the interlocutor's intention, and the way in which the locution affects the hearer or reader (perlocutionary effect).

The Importance of Translation

For centuries translation in Britain has been a Cinderella profession with little theory behind it, little prestige, and little idea about how monumentous its role in influencing what people do, what people know and what people believe in. The stories that moulded our childhood are written by the translators of Collodi, and his Italian Pinocchio; the German Grimm's brothers; the Danish Hans Andersen, and the Greek Aesop. As we grow up so we may be influenced, for example, by "the word of God" or rather the words of various translators, the results of painstaking attempts to render original words into 21st century English (Katan 1996). Most of the world's greatest thinkers, from Aristotle to Voltaire and Weil are read in translation.

It is also true that the vast amount of translation has been out of rather than towards English (Venuti 1995: 12-14). Some language-cultures get the vast amount of their literature through translation. Slovene, for example, has only recently become the official language of Slovenia. As a result, translators are working round the clock to supply schools and bookshops with translations of everything, from computer manuals to histories of the world. Hence, the bookshops in Ljubliana are lined with translations; and thus the cognitive environment of Slovenia, and many other countries, is being formed by the choice of words made by translators.

On Italian TV, the world news is interpreted not only by journalists and news editors but by little known (or respected) groups of translators and interpreters, translating texts from CNN, internet and from world leaders speaking mainly in English. The same is true not only for documentaries (bought from the BBC), but for soap operas (bought from America) and chat shows, which thrive on the live interpretation of famous foreigners.

So, translators have an extremely important responsibility in communicating ideas to society. In many cases, it is only through a translator that groups of people can have access to another individual's or culture's view of the world, and whatever it is that they intend to mean through their writings. The translator is pivotal not only in re-producing a writer's words, but also in directing the reader to much more. First, in writing, as in any other system of signs, the writer has only a limited control over understanding. Unconscious choices of words will be noted or absorbed by the reader who will give meaning to them regardless of intention. Second, the reader will experience a wider variety of feelings and meanings, due to the intertextuality of texts. The specific choice of words themselves cue a series of other words and associations in the reader's own mental lexicon. How the reader interprets will, to a large extent, be determined by decisions made by the translator, both as critical reader and as writer.

The Art of Translation

There is, contrary to what might be thought, no "correct translation", though there are various levels of appropriate translations related to specific contexts – and this is true even for purely technical texts (Katan 1999a: 8-11). Benjamin ([1923] 2000: 18) famously pointed out that even lexical equivalents, such as *bread, brot* and *pain*, do not relate to the same thing. "Brot" is German bread, with a significantly different taste, texture and colour to French "pain" or English *Mother's Pride* or *Allison's Stoneground*. The same is true of language. So, translators, at the lexico-grammatical level have no choice but to choose from a social semiotic (Halliday: 1978) of approximate possibilities. Halliday has also pointed out that the act of choosing one element also means not choosing another paradigm, which marks the beginning of how meaning is made of a text (see also Hermans, 1999: 12-13). Each meaningfully linguistic expression, or locutionary act, chosen entails an array of potential reader responses or perlocutionary effects. The organisation of the array of effects becomes more complex as the locutions begin to weave discourse patterns. These locutionary acts, paradigms, and patterns can clearly have no exact equivalents across languages. As Sapir (1929: 214) pointed out: "no two languages are ever sufficiently similar to be considered as representing the same reality". Yet, and oddly perhaps, a literary great such as Milan Kundera, "assumes that the meaning of the foreign text can avoid change in translation, that the foreign writer's intention can travel unadulterated across a linguistic and cultural divide" (Venuti 1998: 5). As the author of *The Art of Translating Poetry*, Raffel (1988: 51), notes: "Alas, translation is nothing like that easy."

There is a second problem for translators, which we will investigate in more depth. It concerns the fact that not only do the language signifiers point to different significations across languages, but also that the reader has an extremely limited capacity to respond to "the Other" (see Barthes 1993: 151) except by distorting the reality of Other-ness till it either fits his or her own reality or is denigrated (Katan: forthcoming).

The Task of the Translator

Walter Benjamin summed up the task of the translator in terms of the illocutionary force of language:

> The task of the translator consists in finding that intended effect [*Intention*] upon the language into which he is translating which produces in it the echo of the original" ([1923] 2000:19-20)

Concern for intention and the echo (equivalent effect) has been a carrot and stick in the history of Translation Studies (Katan 1999a: 126, 140). On the one hand, scholars have taken the related concepts as the holy yardsticks of translation quality (such as Newmark 1982: 132), while on the other, it has been forcefully argued that the former is undecipherable and that the latter is not only unmeasurable, but "a chimera" (Bell, 1991: 6). Nevertheless, the "basic issues in twentieth century translation theory", according to Venuti (2000: 34) are (or were) "equivalence and shifts, audience and function, identity and ideology". Hence, the perlocutionary effect remains a key element in discussing the task of the translator.

Refraction

In Lefevre's seminal paper, "Mother Courage's Cucumbers" ([1982] 2000: 234), he introduces the idea of 'refraction':

> Writers and their work are always understood and conceived against a certain background, or if you will, are refracted through a certain spectrum, just as their work itself can refract previous works through a certain spectrum".

Cultural Studies' readers are not, by the way, immune to refraction (Postone *et al* 1993: 7):

> One effect of translation, as simply of the passage of time, is to tear works from their original intellectual contexts and insert them in new ones. The negative effects of this process are particularly evident in the case of Bourdieu.

This is something he is well aware of himself: "the meaning of a work (artistic, literary, philosophical, etc.) changes automatically with each change in the field within which it us situated for the spectator or reader" (1983: 313). The idea of refraction is closely related to recurrent themes in cognitive psychology and to habitus: reality is filtered and then modelled or downsized to become a mental map of the world. An individual reader's interpretation of a text (the reality in this case) will be governed by the type of map or mental model s/he has of the world. This cognitive map will tend to filter or refract the meaning gleaned until it fits the way things *should* be (Bandler and Grinder 1975; see also Katan 1999a: 87-92; 1999b: 413-417).

As with the cultural arbitrary in the habitus, through enculturation individuals grow up with strong beliefs attached to the value of signs; and then learn to react according to *a priori* categorisation. This categorisation is quite simply not pan-cultural, but is bound to the map groups of people share. And, like topographical maps, these maps are simplifications of reality. Each culture will tend to focus on and expect certain phenomena of the text, while ignoring, or refracting those aspects foreign to their shared map.

Hence, according to many translation scholars today texts will need to be "manipulated" if they are to be translated for reading in a target culture. This means, for example, "adding remarks if the translator feels motivated, and adding entire passages to make the text relevant to the contemporary reader" (Gentzler 1993: 100). Gentzler, however, is not the only scholar unhappy with this approach. He believes that the translator's loyalty should be to the source text.

However, loyalty to source content only, focussing on the literal translation of locutions, can often be as devious as any conscious manipulation of the text. Nixon's trade discussions with Japanese prime minister Sato are a case in point. The interpreter translated faithfully the locutionary act "Zensho shimasu" into "I will deal with the matter in a forward looking matter". However, Nixon's uptake was totally different to the intention. The intention was to send a strong but diplomatic refusal to look into the matter of import quotas. Nixon, on the other hand, unused to this type of normal Japanese "off the record" face saving utterance, took the locution to be a statement of intent. The final perlocutionary effect, when Nixon realised that the Japanese had no intention to negotiate the quotas was that: "Nixon felt betrayed and thought all Japanese politicians liars and utterly untrustworthy" (Kondo 1990: 59). So, even when a translator does not refract (the form) refraction will take place.

Refraction also takes place over time. New translations are constantly being commissioned, creating new readings. Take, for example, the following book catalogue description:

FRENCH LITERATURE
[...] recent stage adaptations of *Liaisons Dangereuses* and Hugo's *Les Misérables* show that there is much to rediscover in one of the world's richest cultures, through a continuing process of translation and re-evaluation, vital to our understanding of our nearest neighbours and of ourselves.
Penguin Classics Catalogue (1995: 35)

I mentioned at the beginning how important the invisible translators have been in shaping beliefs about "the word of God". Recently, the word of God has been further manipulated to take account of the increased sensitivity to the lexical signifiers of gender (Katan 1996). For example, "Let us make man in our image" (Genesis 1:26) has been retranslated to "Let us make human beings in our image", and: "If anyone says, 'I love God', and hates his brother, he is a liar" (John's first letter 4:20), has recently become "But if someone says 'I love God', while at the same time hating his fellow-Christian, he is a liar".

These prime example of the translators' conscious manipulation of a text are an attempt to rebalance the refracted readers' perlocutionary response. However, in many of these cases the translators were commissioned to make these alterations, which points to the translator's subservience to the dominant norms practised by scholars (religious and non) today.

The Translator's Perceptual Positions

The translator's various positions and roles can be usefully analysed in terms of perceptual positions, a concept developed in Neurolinguistic Programming. First position is that of total association with self. The translator immersed in a syntactic or semantic view of meaning does not go beyond the confines of the signifier. Uptake in the real world of a target reader is irrelevant: "There is no other: you […] look at the world completely from your own [textual] point of view, your own reality within yourself, in a completely associated way" (O'Connor and Seymour 1990: 87). In terms of speech act theory, the locutionary act is paramount here. This is the position that Benjamin is referring to when discussing the *intention* inherent in the text. He felt that the force or the intention lay in the text language itself. In fact, one of his solutions to retain the *intention* was "above all, by a literal rendering of the syntax…" ([1923] 2000: 21).

In theory, according to this perceptual position, meaning can be obtained simply from the signifier in the text. One can analyse the potential illocutionary force, as Levinson says, "by virtue of *the conventional force* associated with it" (1983: 236, emphasis added). The conventional force may well be a source of conflict and struggle between those with the authority to determine the convention and those who are only in the position to follow or submit to the convention. Gender in language would be a case in point.

Here, I am not so concerned with the ethics of the translator in transferring power/subservience across languages as much as a more ontological consideration. What is necessary for transference to take place; to what extent is the convention universal, or at least cross-cultural – and to what extent can the translator reveal the source habitus to the target reader? If we return to gender again, for example, the conventional force of politically incorrect language and its perlocutionary effect is not universal. The effect is habitus specific (Katan, 1999a: 75-79). As we shall see, it will be very difficult to subscribe to the structural view that there is an objective social reality. Actors in reality interpret and make sense of the symbolic system of meanings through the habitus they are part of.

In fact, translation scholars today (cf. Hermans, 1999, Katan 1999a) accept that text readers interpret and make sense of reality through a set of filters which distort the potential perlocutionary effect according to their own habitus. Each habitus will encourage a different uptake, through a different set of arbitrary significations. What Barthes (1993: 151), in translation, says about one class of readers should really be made much more universal: "The petit-bourgeois is a man unable to imagine the Other. If he comes face to face with him, he blinds himself, ignores and denies him, or else transforms him into himself".

Hence, a translator must also take the second perceptual position: the vantage point from which the difference can be entertained, where "you can consider how it would look, feel and sound from another person's point of view. It is obvious that the same situation or behaviour can mean different things to different people" (O'Connor and Seymour, 1990: 87). Clearly *conventional* acts have consequences, and these depend on "the uptake including the *understanding* of both the force and the content of the utterance by its addressee(s)" (Levinson 1983: 237, original emphasis). And gender-sensitive readers here, for example, may be affected by the force they have attached to Annette Lavers' use of "man" and "he" in her translation of Barthes above.

So, a translator, whose task it is to at least gauge intention and effect will need to take a further, third position, if he or she is to choose between one set of target-language signifiers and another. This third position has rarely been discussed, with most discussion in Translation Studies focussing on the faithful/free debate, the first or second position. In the third, meta, position, s/he disassociates from the dynamic moment-to-moment creation of meaning between source text and reader, but watches the interaction with keen interest. S/he will be equally interested in the potential interaction between the virtual target text (Katan 1999a: 125) and the imagined reader.

The Translator's Habitus

This third position, essentially is the mediator's habitus. The translator is neither bound to the text nor to the norms of the domestic culture. However, this habitus is just as norm and value governed as any other habitus is: relativity is valued, and mediation is the norm; the structure, the inculcation, though will either be a- or multi-cultural (see Katan: 1999b, forthcoming). Fundamentally, the translator is now no longer confined to dictionary style equivalence, but is a mediator; and thus is free to choose - and all options are open. There is understanding of both source and target text values, norms and practices, rather than submission to one or other dominant type. Not only should the translator-mediator be free from the constraints of the source and target cultures, but s/he should also have the ability to choose, and the desire to play with, the potential perlocutionary effect in each particular translation circumstance; knowing full well that reader response will be guided not only by the conventional force of the words but by the procedural contexts (of situation and of culture) brought about through the interplay of text, implicature and reader cognitive environment.

Reaching this position is easier said than done, for two reasons. First, this requires a form of bi-, if not multi-, culturality which few are able to attain at an individual level (Katan forthcoming); and second the norms inculcated in any system tend to be asserted as universal and absolute, and therefore tend to restrict relativisation or contextualisation, which is a pre-requisite for bi-, or multi-, culturality.

Structural Limitations

A number of scholars have mentioned the knotty problem of the translator's habitus (Hermans 1999: 82-85; Simione 1998). Successful translators, it is argued, are necessarily subservient to their own native norms: success equals subservience. Toury's (1995) conclusion neatly summed up in Simione (1998: 6) is clear: "the horizon of the successful translator heralds near-complete submission to the norms effective in the subsector(s) of society in which s/he is professionally active". Logically then, according to Simione, translators are encouraged to carry out their task within another's specialised field (such as cookery or cultural studies), following the respective norms, and within the domestic habitus. The structuring nature of the habitus leads to what Simione calls "*servitude volontaire*", the translators' active role in maintaining the norms. This effectively prevents most from moving freely into a third system of mediation. This is the real problem Kondo alludes to in his paper on Nixon. The interpreter was "right" not to interfere, because the first perceptual position is the overriding norm: the translator should be faithful to the source text words.

It is also true, in other fields such as literature, that the 2nd position has been the dominant norm, what the translator and scholar Venuti, has called "domestication". He cogently makes the point that "[t]ranslation can never simply be communication between equals because it is fundamentally ethnocentric" (1998: 11). His point is that the more seamless and flawless a translation (the translator's benchmark of quality) the less the reader will "see" the translation; and therefore will be less likely to perceive the foreign. The text becomes subservient to the tastes of the target reader habitus. So, foreign texts, potentially cueing other realities, come into Britain and America through a process of colonisation, losing their otherness on the way.

However, Venuti's struggle against the translator's subservience to the domestic norm does not take the translator to the third perceptual position, which respects both source and target culture habitus. Instead, his first aim is based very much on the non-acceptance of one habitus: "it is this evocation of the foreign that attracts me [...] This preference stems partly from a political agenda that is broadly democratic: an opposition to the global hegemony of English" (1998: 10). Clearly, this strategy reduces the translator's ability to choose in much the same way as conformity to domestication, and results in subservience to the foreign.

The Translator's Status

In reality, whatever the scholars might say, a translator's symbolic capital is, in reality, extremely low; a factor which also severely reduces the ability to make choices. Choices are often made by other agents instead (see Venuti, 1998). And here, in total agreement with Venuti, it is clear that the translator will need to become visible if s/he is to earn any respect (Venuti, 1995, 1998). One of the scandals of translation, as Venuti (1998) notes is that the translator is often not acknowledged in print or through royalties. After all, "Translation and Interpretation" is nothing but part and parcel of the EU job class "74.83 Secretarial and translation activities".

In a corpus of 27 best-selling published versions of *Little Red Riding Hood* available in Italian bookshops, only 7 (25%) clearly state who was responsible for the translation. The other 20 do not even point to the fact that the text is a translation. Of these 20, 6 (22%) give absolutely no indication of who might be responsible for any of the changes from the original French (Perrault) or German (Grimm). In the other cases there is a mixture of "edited by", "adapted by" and "revised by" (Dobrowolny 1998), giving no indication if this is the translator or a second, "more important" person.

Regarding "more important" people, Imre Barna (1993: 31) talked about his translation into Hungarian of "Il nome della rosa" in the presence of the (original) author, Umberto Eco. As he took the podium he said: "[...] ho scritto qualcosa di bello.... Ho scritto un romanzo di successo mondiale, e ne sono fiero/I wrote something beautiful ... I wrote a world bestseller, and I'm proud of it". He actually also added at the conference, though not included in the published article: "Il nome della rosa è mia"/The Name of the Rose is mine". The royalties, of course, speak otherwise.

Very rarely does a translator stand up to be counted. Most are too busy keeping up with increasingly tight deadlines, made even tighter through increasing use of semi-automatic translation software and commissioning on the internet. So, even more rarely today does the translator have the opportunity to discuss the text with his/her often distant client. Translators, in general, are not in a position to choose the final version of a text, nor can they choose whether or how they themselves will be presented to the target reader.

Until Barna's cry is replicated by other translators, and they are in a position to take ownership of what they produce, the profession will not begin to be given responsibility or credit for the work done. So, where can translators choose? They still retain their hidden, and largely unused, power to influence reader perception and uptake at a micro-level. Working on the edges of their restrictive and restricting norms, translators as mediators can pro-actively decide *where* to make the refractions, rather than simply transposing words subserviently to one or another norm.

Refraction Strategies

There are basically 3 refractive strategies open to the translator, which can be conveniently subsumed in the following diagram:

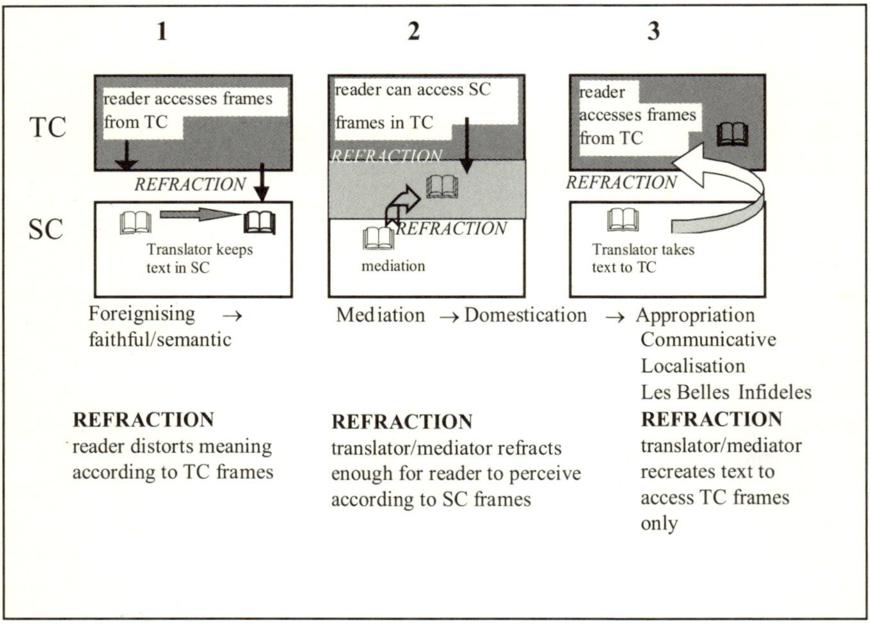

There are 4 main factors here: habitus, text, translator and reader. In each case there are two aspects: source, or original, and target. Refraction will occur where there is a significant gap between cognitive environments. At one extreme (3) the translator can refract the foreignness of the ST (i.e. make it domestic) on the reader's behalf; or, at the other extreme (1), allow the reader to perform the refraction for themselves, which means that the reader will filter the language of the text and refract according to the norms and values of his/her habitus. We will now look at this idea in a little more detail.

Foreignising Translation (1)

With this term, Venuti and others wish to make the foreignness of the text explicit and the translator visible. He believes that "its most decisive occurrence depends on introducing variations that alienate the domestic language…" (1999: 11). His aim, as we have already noted, is to allow the reader to appreciate the foreign. There is, however, a big difference between appreciating the foreign looking locution and appreciating the foreign illocutionary force – as Nixon discovered. At this point we need to investigate further the idea of uptake and perlocutionary affect across cultures.

We can be fairly sure that the illocutionary force may well be taken up as intended by the author in the source language as a result of our understanding of conventions. However, from a purely pragmatic point of view, we have already mentioned that uptake depends on the ability to share a similar map of the world or habitus. The reader, following the Theory of Relevance (Sperber and Wilson 1986) will apply the minimum cognitive reading effort while looking for the maximum cognitive effect. If the cognitive distance between the two habitus is too large, the perlocutionary effect will simply be to leave the text unread due to too much cognitive effort for too little cognitive effect.

Domestication/Localisation (3)

As the names suggest, the translator manipulates (refracts) the target text until it can be read without refraction by the target reader. It becomes a source culture text, to be read once again by insiders. The reader will not notice that the text is a translation, will have the resources to process the implicatures to the full, and will be guaranteed a rich cognitive effect. The disadvantage is that the foreign text author becomes domesticated according to the canons of the domestic readership. Pinocchio, for example, is appropriated by Disney (Katan, 1999a: 28); Guglielmo in the English version of "The Name of the Rose", becomes William, and, according to *The New York Times*, "*our* learned and ironic monk-detective" (in Katan 1993: 158, emphasis added). Not only that, but with regard to the book:

> getting out the American edition required a bit of additional work mainly reducing the Latin content by about 10 per cent so as not to scare off the less-erudite reader. The 200,000 hardcover copies sold so far in the U.S. indicate that this was probably a wise move.

Sari Gilbert in *The Washington Post 9.10.93*

One field that has developed domestication to its limits is information technology. Localization is the term used by the computer industry for the production of seamless software manuals, translated to provide the user with 100% clear, explicit guidance – with no distraction. Hence, typically American communication styles designed to please the user have been deleted in the Italian versions because the perlocutionary effect would be the opposite. The changes range from icons of the American school bus, baseball and other references to encyclopaedic knowledge through to the "*poco serio*" informality of the first and second person singular in the text. Entire paragraphs, deemed too childish have been deleted. Referring to the proposed Italian translation of Encarta, an internal Microsoft document states: "70% of the product requires editorial changes. It is of paramount importance to hire a reference material editor and a proof-reader". The task of editor is clearly not yet within the remit of the translator.

Mediation (2)

The mediator is in third position (which would encompass the role of editor) and is able to see the consequences of both domestication and foreignisation. The task of the mediator will always be to empower the reader enriching his or her cognitive environment, whether through accessing what is foreign or what is new. The key concept is access, and the question to be asked is "what minimum changes are necessary to ensure the maximum level of uptake and cognitive effect?" The type of effect desired will depend on what the translator wants or is required to produce. Manipulation will be necessary to push the text out of the source culture and refract it so that either the text can be accessed by the target culture reader or, paradoxically, the source culture itself.

The example below will give an idea of how the three strategies will create different reader perlocutionary effects.

Perlocutionary Effect

As mentioned earlier, through enculturation individuals grow up with strong beliefs attached to the value of signs. Individuals learn what proper social conduct means, and the signs used to demonstrate it. The perlocutionary effect will depend on the situation, and more importantly, the extent to which the language used follows or flouts listener expectancy.

The following text, from Italo Calvino's (1970) *Gli amori difficili*, clearly shows us an example of day to day social conduct: that of a customer requesting a drink. This is potentially a face threatening act (Brown and Levinson 1987) which we would expect to be countered with an adequate face saving act.

Stefania finds herself outside a coffee bar in the early hours of the morning after her unexpected and secret "*avventura*". The translation is already domesticised to some extent through the localisation of Italian "bar" into "coffee bar". However, what I wish to focus on is the perlocutionary effect on both the barman and the reader of Stefania's as yet untranslated words in bold.

L'avventura di una moglie

Nel bar c'erano le sedie accattate, la segatura in terra.	In the coffee bar, the chairs were stacked, the sawdust on the floor
C'era solo un barista, al banco.	There was only a barman, at the counter.
Stefania venne avanti; non provava nessun disagio a esser lì a quell'ora insolita.	Stafania went in; she didn't feel at all uneasy being there at that unusual time.
Chi aveva da sapere nulla?	Who could have known anything, anyway?
Poteva essersi alzata allora, poteva essere diretta alla stazione, oppure arrivata in quel momento	She might have got up at that time, she could have been on her way to the station, or else just arrived.
Poi, lì non aveva da render conto a nessuno. Sentì che le piaceva sentirsi così.	Anyway, she didn't have to explain herself to anyone. She sensed she was enjoying the way she felt
- **Un ristretto, doppio, caldissimo**, - disse al cameriere.	"-**Un ristretto, doppio, caldissimo**" she said to the waiter.
Le era venuto un tono di confidenza sicura di sé, come se ci fosse una consuetudine tra lei e l'uomo di quel bar, dove invece non entrava mai.	A relaxed and self-assured tone came to her as if it were a perfectly normal exchange between her and the man at this bar, though she had never been there before.
- Sì, signora, un momento che scaldiamo la machina ed è pronto, - disse il barista.	"Yes, madam. One moment while we warm the machine up and it'll be ready," said the barman.
E aggiunse: - Ci metto di più a scaldarmi io che a scaldare la macchina al mattino;	And he added: "It takes longer to warm me up than to warm the machine up in the morning.
Stefania sorrise, si rannicchiò nel bavero e fece: - Brrr... [...]	Stefania smiled and drew tight inside her collar: "Brrr... [...]

The illocutionary force of the locution is clearly described by Calvino. The tone is relaxed and self-assured; the force is that of "*consuetudine*": a perfectly normal, and hence we can assume, perfectly appropriate social conduct. This is confirmed by the barman's affirmative and friendly reply, further confirmed by Stefania's smile. Literally her words are as follows:

Un ristretto (a small)
doppio (double)
caldissimo (very hot)

Clearly, there can be little uptake here. This is where the translator has the power to choose. S/he can choose, as I have said, between 3 types of translation possibilities, though, in reality each blends into the other, depending on the exact point of refraction:

Foreignised target text	**Mediated Target text**	**Domesticated Target text**
REFRACTED by reader	**REFRACTED by translator and reader**	**REFRACTED by translator**

The most foreignised target text possibility would be to keep the actual words spoken: "*Un ristretto, doppio, caldissimo*", which would have no significant uptake for the vast majority of readers. The next most foreign would be: "a strong double and very hot", domesticising "*ristretto*" into "strong". The reader here will be left to look for the coherence in what is a particularly elided sentence; i.e. that this is a request, the request is polite, and that the request is for a coffee.

However the uptake will be as intended only for the privileged few insiders, those who will have full access to the beliefs, values, norms and practices of Italy – and in particular, morning counter exchange talk. If the translator decides to make explicit what is shared *conceptually* by the insiders, we have: "a strong double and very hot coffee". An outsider reader can now, from knowledge of his or her *own* culture expectancy schemas infer that the locution has the force of a request. However, the main problem lies with the reader's use of his or her own expectancy frames to understand the intention of the request, which will be cued through the choice of words in the target language. As Hanks (1993: 139) points out: "To speak is inevitably to situate oneself in the world … In its structure and in its use language is one of the central vehicles of habitus". In fact, with regard to language, it is the speaking rather than anything else that the reader will tune into. Questionnaire research on translation and reader uptake came to the following conclusions: "the words uttered […] condition reader perception more than the visual description" (Katan 1992: 114, my translation). So, the reader will tend to focus on the lack of verbal politeness more than the clear description of the normality of the encounter.

Hence the reader response is likely to attribute a misplaced level of rudeness on Stefania. A foreignised translation requires that the readers have the resources themselves to translate the foreign locutionary act into the appropriate perlocutionary effect. The only readers who will be empowered to do this will be those who probably do not need a translation.

The English reader, who needs a translation to have access to the foreign, will only have access to his/her own prototypical script for morning counter exchanges on the lines of "Morning, a large cup of strong coffee please – and could you make it really hot?" A translator may well decide to localise the script, and choose similar words to those above, to fit the target culture. As a result, the perlocutionary effect will be as intended both for the barman and for the reader – as far as politeness is concerned.

However, the domestication of the sight, taste, rituals and meanings of a small, thick, black "*ristretto, doppio, caldissimo*" *caffè* into a large (paper) cup, or mug of watery instant milky coffee or *cappuccino* means no uptake of the foreign. The directive remains an illocution with little or no perlocutionary effect; there is no improved accesss, no learning, and the target reader is poorer as a result.

The culture of "*il caffè*" in Italy is ubiquitous. A tourist brochure for Trieste (translated into an imperfect English) states:

> No longer called 'thinkers milk' as it was in 16th Century Constantinople, coffee's popularity is practically unlimited. Is there anyone who does not set aside at least 5 minutes of their day to savour a cup of coffee?

Coffee, in Italy, transcends class and all other social groupings. The price is a political, state-controlled 0.77 Euros; and though each coffee bar will have its selected *clientele*, the ritual is the same for all - as is the attention to the aesthetics and social ritual pleasure taken in satisfying the national addiction. The ritual is so ingrained in the national way of life, that it is, by and large, the only drink drunk until around 11 am. Also, the default "normal" coffee, is just that: black coffee with extremely little water (the quantity is crucial) - though numerous other permutations are possible. The morning coffee is drunk standing up, away from the work place, usually in a coffee bar. When coffee is available in vending machines, the machine will tend to have an eternally smiling neon barman beaming down from the front of the machine; the most popular button to be pressed will have but one word "*normale*"; and the coffee will never be taken away. Instead it will be enjoyed (or not) next to the eternally smiling barman, in the company of other coffee drinkers.

If we compare this with the domestic, watery large cup or mug of (usually) white, possibly frothy, coffee, the difference in perlocutionary effects are manifold. There is no national ritual or complicity with the barman. Coffee is also different in Britain not only in terms of quantity, quality – but also in terms of its symbolic capital today.

Times, as we noted at the beginning, change how texts are translated. When Calvino's book was first published, coffee, and in particular Italian coffee, meant very little to most readers. In the year 2002, the drink is either exotic, foreign, sophisticated or a mundane, simple "refreshment". In the first case the nation is being taught what to drink and how. The pronunciation of "*cappuccino*" is highlighted in Italian coffee bar windows. Italian coffee is "in". Adrian Mole has his "*Cappuccino* Years", and comedians regularly make fun of the trend. This new myth has penetrated the *petite bourgeoisie*, yet the drink is being diluted and consumed according to domestic patterns which has made Italian coffee, as Barthes (1993: 152) would have noted: "a pure object, a spectacle, a clown". In an article entitled "Desperately Seeking Cappucino" (Sunday Times 25/8/01) Morris states: "Iy you are lucky you might get a half-decent cup. But sadly, it seems that in coffee-chain land, coffee and its production … are little more than a convenient façade for a lot of pricey posing." The *bourgeoisie*, on the other hand, have been quietly drinking it and "can at least imagine the place where [it] fits in".

The words "instant" and "real" may now be leaving the language to make way for "freeze dried", "*cappuccino*" and "*espresso*", but whatever the word or the concoction, a decision is being made, which will have a class distinction. There is no such thing as a "normal coffee". Normality, with regard to this particular myth, does not depend on your national culture habitus but on your particular field within it.

Mediating the Point of Refraction

It is at this point that the translator should take the third position, and begin to play with the words uttered and the immediate co-text. Though, as I have underlined, the translator is very much subservient to many other forces, and as yet has little control over his or her production at a macro-level, the translator should begin exercising control over the translation at a micro-level. This means being aware of, and extending the strategies of manipulation to allow the target reader to have access, and experience at least some of the source culture. This means, first, considering the perlocutionary effect. The translator will realise that the default reaction to the foreign may well misattribute impoliteness to Stefania, or domesticate the ritual; and in both cases distort the intention of Calvino.

We can, in fact keep the directive exactly as she made the order, but change the co-text so that the reader no longer reads it as *an* order. Hence the locution is not judged according to a reader's internal value system, but simply as an illocution. Next, we can guide the reader to Italian coffee in the text by adding "*espresso*" to contextualize the request. By leaving the projecting directive as direct as before, this leaves the politeness to the context, so there is no distortion of the target text within the projection; and leaves the readers (and, in reality, the barman too) to add the politeness from their own expectancy frame:

She asked the waiter for an *espresso*, "thick, double and really hot".

This solution allows the readers to glimpse, from the safety of their own maps, something of the Italian directness in projected requests - without distorting the illocutionary intent. The choice of the foreignising "thick, double", rather than the domestic "large, strong", takes the reader away from the domestic towards the look, feel, taste and aroma of an *espresso*. In so doing the reader is likely to experience a richer perlocutionary effect, and will have begun to learn something new.

Clearly, refraction still exists, but the translator has taken control of choosing from between the potential perlocutionary effects – which marks the beginning of the structuring of a new translatorial habitus.

Bibliography

Austin, J.L. (1962) *How to Do Things with Words*, Oxford: OUP.

Bandler, R. and Grindler, J. (1975) *The Structure of Magic*, Palo Alto California: Science and Behaviour Books Inc.

Barna, I. (1993) "Monologo del copista con commento di G.L. Beccaria", in L. Avirovic' and J. Dodds, eds., *Umberto Eco, Claudio Magris: Autori e Traduttori a Confronto*, Udine: Camponotto, 31-36.

Barthes, R. (1993) *Mythologies*, London: Vintage.

Bell, R. T. (1991) *Translation and Translating*, Harlow, Essex: Longman,

Benjamin, W. ([1923] 2000) "The Task of the Translator", in L. Venuti, (ed.) *The Translation Studies Reader*, London: Routledge, 15-25.

Bourdieu, P. (1983) "The Field of Cultural Production, or the Economic World Reversed", in *Poetics*, 12 (Nov): 311-356.

Bourdieu, P. (1990) *The Logic of Practice*, Cambridge: Polity Press.

Brown P. and Levinson S. (1987) *Politeness: Some Universals in Language Usage*, Studies in Interactional Sociolinguistics 4, Cambridge: Cambridge University Press.

Calvino I. (1970) "L'avventura di una moglie", *Gli amori difficili,* Turin: Einaudi.

Dobrowlney, K. (1998) *Che fine ha fatto "Capuccetto rosso"?: Orientament culturali e traduzione delle trasformazione italiane della fiaba di Perrault*, Undergraduate thesis deposited at SSLMIT, University of Trieste.

Gentzler, E. (1993) *Contemporary Translation Theories*, London: Routledge.

Halliday, M. A. K. (1978) *Language as Social Semiotic: the Social Interpretation of Language and Meaning*, London: Arnold.

Hanks, W: F. (1993) "Notes on Semantics in Linguistic Practice", in Calhoun, C., LiPuma E., and M. Postone, eds., *Bourdieu: Critical Perspectives*, Cambridge: Polity Press.

Hermans, T. (1999) *Translation in Systems: Descriptive and Systemic Approaches Explained*, Manchester: St. Jerome.

Katan D. (1992) "Traduzione e significato Pragmatico ne I Morti', in *Rivista Internazionale di tecnica di Traduzione*, 0: 111-119.

Katan, D. (1993) "The English Translation of 'Il Nome della Rosa' and the Cultural Filter", L. Avirovic and J. Dodds, eds., *Umberto Eco, Claudio Magris: Autori e Traduttori a Confronto*, Udine: Campanotto, 149-165.

Katan, D. (1996) "Signs of the Times: Religious, Secular and Pragmatic English for the Year 2000", in C. J. Taylor (ed.) *Aspects of English II*, Udine: Campanotto, 11-26.

Katan, D. (1999a) *Translating Cultures: An Introduction for Translators, Interpreters and Mediators*, Manchester: St. Jerome.

Katan, D. (1999b) "'What is it that's going on here?': Mediating Cultural Frames in Translation", in S. Bassnett, R. M Bolletteri, Bosinelli, M. Ulrych, eds., *Textus: Translation Studies Revisited*, XII, No. 2, 409-426.

Katan, D. (forthcoming) "Mind the Gap: Modelling the Translator's Response to Outsider Reading", Paper presented at the International conference on Social and Ideological Contexts of Translation and Translation Research, 28-30 April 2000, Leeds.

Kondo, M. (1990) "What Conference Interpreters Should Not Be Expected To Do", in *The Interpreters' Newsletter*, 3: 59-65.

Lefevre, A. ([1982] 2000) "Mother Courages's Cucumbers: Text, System and Refraction in a Theory of Literature", in L. Venuti, ed., *The Translation Studies Reader*, London: Routledge, 233-249.

Levinson, S. C. (1983) *Pragmatics*, Cambridge: Cambridge University Press.

Newmark, P. (1982) *Approaches to Translation*, Oxford: Pergamon Press.

O'Connor, J. and J. Seymour (1990) *An Introduction to Neurolinguistic* Programming, London: Mandela.

Postone, M., LiPuma, E. and Calhoun, C. (1993) "Introduction: Bourdieu and Social Theory", in Calhoun, C., LiPuma E., and M. Postone, eds., *Bourdieu: Critical Perspectives,* Cambridge: Polity Press, 1-13.

Raffel, B. (1988) *The Art of Translating Poetry*, University Park and London: Pennsylvania State University Press.

Sapir, E. (1929) "The Status of Linguistics as a Science", *Language* 5: 207-214.

Simione, D. (1998) "The Pivotal Status of the Translator's Habitus', *Target* 10, 1-39.

Sperber D. and Wilson, D. (1986) *Relevance*, Oxford: Blackwell.

Toury, Gideon (1995) *Descriptive Translation Studies and Beyond*, Amsterdam/Philadelphia: John Benjamins.

Venuti, L. (1995) *The Translator's Invisibility – A History of Translation*, London and New York: Routledge.

Venuti, L. (1998) *The Scandals of Translation*, London and New York: Routledge.
Venuti L., ed. (2000) *The Translation Studies Reader*, London: Routledge.

VISIONS OF THE AMERICAS AND POLICIES OF TRANSLATION

EDUARDO J. VIOR

Many Latin-American authors and intellectuals in the last 100 years have tried to define "Our America", i.e. Latin-American identity, against the growing political and economical pressure of the "Other America", the USA. At the same time the USA have projected their own ethno-cultural conflicts onto their relation with Latin America. In this way the image of Latin America played also an indirect role for the construction of US American identity. Each phase in the history of the US / Latin-American relations links up with a re-definition of both identities. This essay follows the history of these (self-)reflections, with specific reference to policies of translation between the USA and Latin America (mainly of technical and economical texts, from English into Spanish).

Emphasising the Difference.

In 1891 José Martí, the father of Cuba's independence, published an essay entitled "Our America" in the Argentinian newspaper *La Nación.* In this essay, circulated in the same year throughout Latin America, he attempted to characterize Latin American identity as the result of the mixture of European, indigenous and African elements. The latter two contributed as much to the construction of subcontinental culture as classical and modern European culture. Following Bolivar he asserted the unique *mestizo* character of Latin American culture. He concluded:

> We came resolutely to the world of nations with our feet in the rosary, a white head and a body with the colours of the Indians and Creoles. (quoted in Zea 1993: 123).

He did not define Latin American culture, but he designated it as the opposite of the *"Other America's"* culture, i.e. of "Anglo-Saxon" American culture.[1]

This opposition has been constitutive of Latin American culture throughout the Twentieth Century. The perception of the United States, held by Latin American intellectuals and decision-makers over the last hundred years, has been

---

[1] For some reference works on José Martí and his significance for the building of Latin American identity see Ette and Heydenreich 1994; Fernández Retamar 1995; and Zea 1993.

dominated by the USA's desire to exercise its power over the continent. The reaction to this perceived desire was either to vigorously oppose it or to adapt to it. This uncertainty has been a determining factor in the definition of Latin America's cultural identity and, as a consequence, in the formulation of values, norms and symbolic images that were intended to orientate Latin American societies. The perceptions Latin Americans have of the external world and of themselves constitute two complementary "visions" in the sense that they contain both interiorised projections of themselves and desires projected onto others.

Nevertheless it would be wrong to paint an unchanging picture of the history of the relations between the two Americas in the Twentieth Century. The changing view includes the "naïve" attitudes of the young Latin American states towards the US-American Intervention in the war of Cuban independence, the bargaining policies of the nationalist regimes between the 1930s and the 1970s, continuing with the radical hatred of the revolutionary youth against the USA in the sixties and seventies, to the disenchanted and sometimes cynical attitudes of the present intellectual life. Each confrontation with the USA deepened the separation between the two parts of the continent and, as a consequence, led to their "individualization". One simply cannot understand Latin America's contemporary identity without taking into account its repeated confrontations with its Northern neighbour.

On the North-American side the stereotypes of lazy and boasting Mexicans, of sleepy villages and Latin lovers runs through the history of literature and cinema, from the Cuban War to the end of the1980s. The image of bearded revolutionaries and bloodthirsty dictators, since the fifties, has been associated with a Latin America that, on the one hand, is unable to democratize its political life and to achieve and safeguard continuous economic grow, while on the other hand, it continues to be represented as sensual and happy, and above all distinct from the white protestant "ethic".

But the image of Latin America that the American elite fostered already includes, at least since the Ibero-American independence at the beginning of the Nineteenth Century, a perception of the threats these attributed features could constitute for US national security. These "weaknesses" ascribed to the new Southern nations might call for extra-continental interventions which, in turn, might put American security at risk.[2] Since the proclamation of the Monroe Doctrine, in 1823, one of the pillars of Washington's continental policies consisted in reducing this Latin American "weakness" to a minimum. Thus, since the early Nineteenth Century, the differences with Latin America also play a very important part in the constituting process of national identity of the United States. But as well as the construction of the Latin American Other, the continental policies of the United States have also sought to preserve Latin America as an

---

[2] For reference works to the Monroe Doctrine and its background see in Aguilar 1968; May 1975; and Whitaker 1954.

ideal field of projection for non-resolved internal conflicts, especially in terms of racism (see Campbell and Kean 1997: 248-49).[3]

Since the beginning of the Nineteenth Century American elites have been interpreting the subjection of Latin America either as an opportunity for advancing America's mission to propagate and safeguard their own idea of freedom throughout the world, or simply as a good opportunity for doing business, or last but not least, as an opportunity for exercising and ensuring national defence policies. The "puritan" spirit helped to justify American presence in Latin America as an "evangelization of the innocents", which sometimes even sanctioned violence. Therefore, the usual reaction by American administrations to attempts by the peoples of the American continent to take the principles of freedom and democracy in their own hands, have been rather hostile. Indeed, the combination of peaceful "constructive engagement"[4] and violent subjection has informed American policies for the continent for most of the past two hundred years. Teddy Roosevelt's "Big Stick" and Franklin Roosevelt's "Good Neighbourhood" policies are not really two successive strategies, but two sides of the same coin (see Gellman 1979; Tulchin 1971).

This essay attempts to illustrate the power that this confrontation has had for processes of identity construction. I will consider three phases within the relations between the Americas between 1900 until the 1970s and I will conclude by invoking a fourth, namely the current phase of the mutual perceptions between both Americas in the context of globalisation.[5]

In this context the essay focuses on some characteristics of the translation practices in both Americas. If the translator is "the invisible third" (cf. Derrida 1997 [1985]), who, by relating to two cultures, modifies them both, then the institutionally guaranteed continuity revealed in "policies of translation"[6] must have implications on both sides of the border. The essay will consider some of

---

[3] For further references to internal conflicts and world-perception as reflected in American foreign policies see Hunt 1988; Rosenberg 1982; and Takaki 1979.

[4] "Constructive engagement" is the phrase employed by the Reagan administration, after 1983, in order to refer to its policy of democratization in South American countries (mainly Argentina, Chile, Bolivia, Brazil and Uruguay) after their military dictatorships (Smith 1995:286-87)

[5] I have been developing this view concerning the search for identity in both Americas for the past seven years while teaching *"Latin American Culture and Society"*, first at the Institute for Translation and Interpretation at the University of Heidelberg and later at the Department for Technical Communication at the University of Applied Sciences of Magdeburg, in Germany. In this essay (which is part of a larger project), I am bringing together all the aspects of that pedagogical experience and a systematic reflection on Pan-American development.

[6] In the broad sense, I am here following Michel Foucault's understanding of "politics" (see Foucault 1984; Minson 1987; and Wickham 1987).

these "policies" of translation with special reference to technical and economical texts circulated between the United States and Latin America.[7]

Theoretical Background

My argument is based on a modified evolutionary view of the history of Latin America.[8] Human evolution depends on the ability of individuals and human

---

[7] This is motivated by my own experience as professor for the Translation of Technical Special Languages from German to Spanish at the University of Applied Sciences of Magdeburg (1999-2000), which has given me some opportunity to study the reactions of the receivers of a text that was translated from a "superior" culture (see also Gémar 1997).

[8] Taking into account the significance evolutionism has achieved in the international scientific debate in the 1990s, it is impossible to give a succinct account of the diversity and range of its positions and its ground covered. However, I would stress the following:

- The term "evolution" refers to a systematization of the continuities and changes within natural and human organisms introduced and perfected since the Nineteenth Century under the conditions of scientific practice mainly carried out in the Anglo-Saxon world. Evolutionism is thus neither independent from the interrelationship between natural and human organisms and their interaction with the environment, nor can it be thought in its application to human societies as independent from its conscious use by social actors. This term implies, then, a non-explicit discourse about continuity and change in nature and humanity. It therefore means, that this scientific term is also an instrument for social action.
- Evolution has no *a priori* stipulated purpose, but it begins with a repetition of significant breakdowns within the information structure of organisms and develops further until the degree of complexity radically contradicts the ability of organisms to adapt themselves to their environment.
- This lack of "purpose" within evolution makes it impossible to constitute a hierarchy of various evolutionary "strategies", especially not in human societies. Evolutionary changes merely represent specific answers to special environments; they have different development times and, therefore, have to be judged according to their ability to satisfy their own necessities without damaging external developments.
- The three points mentioned above also make it impossible to induce from evolution an immanent ethic. "Evolution" therefore does not refer to the process itself but to the prevailing discourse about human development. However, as a scientifically founded discourse, it allows various inferences which do have theoretical and practical consequences.

Based on these four provisions I propose three reasons for applying evolutionism:

- the highly systematic character of evolutionism's categorizations;
- these categorizations allow for conclusions to be drawn across various fields of knowledge. They may also be transferred from an ontogenetic to a phylogenetic approach. The current predominance of evolutionism in scientific discourse can be explained mainly through the development of certain information

groups to adapt themselves to changing environments, to select between different alternatives, to vary these solutions under changing conditions and thus to ensure their continuity. Through this ability social beings and societies increase their knowledge of the world and of themselves, i.e. they learn "together".

Since evolution depends on collective learning, it has to be understood as a social process that also brings about social stratification, inequality and violence. In order to overcome resulting counter-productive consequences, human societies are able to reverse these relations, in their "world views", through psychological mechanisms of negation, projection, displacement and suppression.[9] These mechanisms lead to consensus-building affirmation of the dominant elites.[10] Following Gramsci (1975, [1932]) I would like to call this combination of

---

technologies within the "historical natural sciences" (to differentiate them from other "non-historical" sciences, such as chemistry and physics) within the last thirty years. These sciences include palaeontology, biology, epidemiology, geology, climatology, oceanography, hydrology, astronomy, etc. They can provide numerous insights into the working of society. Provided we accept the fundamentally historical character of the social sciences, there seems no reason why there should not be more translations of theoretical knowledge from other historically oriented sciences;

- evolutionism also provides numerous opportunities to relate the materiality of phenomena to categories of causality and necessity (see Diamond 1997: chapters 1 and 2).

[9] These form the constitutive aspects of a theory of ideology K. Lenk (Lenk 1986) formulated fifteen years ago, incorporating aspects taken from psychoanalytical theory. In his model ideology occupies the place of the "I" in Freud's theory. If we start from the two fundamental Lacanian statements ("the subject is an illusion" and "the unconscious is structured like a language"), the analyst of public discourse, referring to the four categories mentioned above, should be able to restore "the truth" of the (individual or collective) unconscious. Although postmodernism teaches us to disbelieve in truth, human beings and societies continue to search for some "truth" to believe in. "Unconscious" only exists in its homologic relationship with "conscious" and manifests itself historically. We can then suppose that – similar to the world wide web – the collective unconscious organises itself today round changing "truth-nuclei".

[10] Following Foucault (1984 and 1994) power can be understood as a strategic system to restore the control over the unconscious and thus ensure the possibility of producing, disseminating and reproducing life forms. This system concentrates on certain nodal points which are selected contingently but which allow for establishing and using the kind of coercion and persuasion apparatuses that are needed to impose power strategies. Therefore one can neither speak of "power" (but rather "power centres"), nor is it possible to "seize power" (but rather to achieve control over power centres, or indeed, create them). Power constitutes a strategic and tactic play with forces that are designed to restore equilibrium through externalizing violence. If the restoration of equilibrium is an evolutionary question, it is also one that concerns culture. This means that the constitution of the Nietzschean "will to power", which is required to restore this equilibrium, can only be achieved in a specific historical and cultural framework, which has to be analysed in terms of its performances.

domination and consensus "hegemony". Since hegemony combines both elements and also "hides" violence, it is fundamental to collective identity-construction. For my analysis of identity-construction on the American continent, in Twentieth Century, I shall here concentrate on the projection of Latin America's own conflicts onto the United States, as a specific process of identity-construction.

These considerations have nevertheless a provisional character, because only by dealing with the "monological exchange" between both cultural spaces can the role of mutual perceptions be understood for the work of identity-construction.[11]

Collective identity-construction in Western societies occurs through two recurrent differentiating processes: the first distinguishes "I" or "we" from the "Other" and the second "before" from "now". The differentiation regarding the Other is carried out through two contradictory and complementary projections: a) the permanent reference to an external subject, which may be perceived as threatening (see below) and b) the segregation (suppression or negation) of minorities in order to restore the lost symbolic unity.

The mere constitution of differences is not enough for the process of identity-construction: one or more symbolic "cuts" are necessary to construct the Other as "alien". Without this transformation there is no "marking out" of the subject. As violence is almost always a constitutive factor for political communities, who have to be ideologically maintained, most identity-construction work is achieved through the projection of internal violence onto the image of a threatening externalised Other. On the other hand, the differentiation between "before" and "now" is historically necessary to turn the contingent character of dominant ideas into a "timeless" absolute "essence". These identity-construction processes also take place in the relation between languages and are thus relevant for translation practices.

Hierarchy of Languages and Translation

Differences between languages are not "neutral": they are implicated in relations of power and domination which help to establish hierarchies between languages. These relations determine the differences between and, therefore, also the structures within languages. Since every language in its history has been interacting with other languages, each language shows signs of the effects of these power relations. Translating is thus not merely a carrying across of information and meaning from one language to another, but interferes with an "Other" equilibrium of power relations.

[11] For a first step into this direction see Vior 2001.

My objective here will be to provide some introductory reflections on the character of the translation flow between the United States and Latin America and its implications for the identity-construction processes on both sides of this cultural border. The following reflections are based on impressions of prevailing mentalities in the business world and the universities, with specific relevance to the flow of texts related to technology and economy from North to South.

The next research stage will have to be to collect more historical and empirical evidence in order to establish regularities and changes within the translation practices between the Americas. Despite great variation throughout the Twentieth Century it is possible, by analysing translations of specialised technical and economic texts, from the United States to Latin America, to establish the following general points:

- What is striking in almost all areas of translation is the predominant direction of translations, namely from English to Spanish and Portuguese (around 90 per cent).

- Before the 1980s, morphological and syntactic levels of expression in the translated texts across all fields and purposes are of very poor quality.

- Throughout the period considered there is an evident lack of concern on behalf of the (North-American) emitters for adapting the translations to the great lexical, dialectal and communicative varieties prevailing in different parts of Latin America. This negligence is explained by the general choice of a hybrid Cuban-Puertorican-Mexican register in the translated texts, which in turn of course can be explained by the relative availability of translators from these specific countries in the USA.

- One can also confirm a general lack of concern of American companies to adapt their texts to Latin American mentalities. Most translations are still starting from the (more or less tacit) assumption, that the American way of life is evidently desirable for all people and universally valid and therefore does not need to be adapted to any local circumstances.

- The effect of these translations on the Latin American public is an enduring inferiority complex, a feeling of powerlessness (there often is no alternative to products or services from the North) and a repeated necessity of *"secondary translation"*, i.e. to make up for the lack of information provided and the fragmentation of cultural meaning in the texts.

- The translated texts thus contribute to American culture being seen in Latin America as a myth – a process that accentuates the heterogeneity of the cultures in question. Elitism, ethnocentrism and sexism are some of the consequences of these policies of translation.

- The ambivalence the South displays in its reaction to the unilateral attitude embraced by the North also has consequences for the identity-construction process of the latter. The inability or unwillingness of American politicians and managers to make their intentions and goals more understandable to the Latin American peoples, throughout "the short twentieth century" (1898-1989), and the resulting "surprise" over averse reactions by Latin Americans, have considerably increased America's disenchantment with the Southern cultures and, as a reaction, the tendency to impose the US will through force. However, since the early Seventies, these differences have begun to find their often brilliant expression in many literary and artistic translation practices. This gradual change is still waiting to reach the business world and the translation of technical and economical texts.

In the following I will consider some of the "visions of the Americas" occurring throughout the Twentieth Century, before I will eventually return to some reflections on translation at the end of this essay.

In considering evolution as a collective learning process, it is important to view the efficiency of rules of behaviour (which are derived from a confrontation with external circumstances) as dependent on a collective's ability to restore an internal equilibrium and to adapt to the changing environment. Nevertheless, an environment can change so dramatically, that adaptation along the lines of the learned rules becomes impossible and thus threatens the restoration of internal equilibrium. In this case new rules have to be introduced and their application leads to a new understanding of the world, i.e. to entirely new meanings.

Establishing the meaning of an historical process implies the possibility to identify its significant breakdowns.[12] I have therefore structured the history of the mutual perceptions of the United States and Latin America in three stages which are distinguished by four significant breakdowns.

The Visions of the Americas in the Twentieth Century

"The short twentieth century", as E. Hobsbawn (1994) called it, was not as short in Latin America as in Europe. It began in 1898 with the US-American Intervention in the Cuban Independence War against Spain and ended at Christmas 1989, when the US-Army killed 4,000 civilians in Panama in the search for their ex-ally General Noriega. This act demonstrated to the whole continent who was the dominant power behind the conservative restoration,

[12] On the concept "significant breakdowns" see Chiaramonte 1982.

beginning 1982 (Mexican debt crisis and Falkland War), and after the end of the Cold War.

First Breakdown: The Rise of a Great Continent

When the United States intervened in the Cuban War in April 1898, they did so with the conviction, that, having suppressed the last indigenous upheaval in 1890, and having established control over their internal affairs, their mission to disseminate their idea of freedom all over the world required the US to end colonialism in the Western hemisphere and to create order within the administrations and economies within the Caribbean. In the geopolitical understanding of that time the reigning "disorder" in the region threatened the giant's "belly" (Koenig 1992: 409-18; Rosenberg 1982; Zuleta 1998).

The reactions by intellectuals to this intervention all over the continent started with the famous speech by Paul Groussac (the French founding director of the National Library in Buenos Aires) in May 1898 entitled *"Caliban's spirit"*; followed shortly afterwards by the Nicaraguan poet Ruben Darío's *"Caliban's victory"* (first published in New York); and two years later, young Uruguayan journalist José E. Rodó with *"Ariel"* (a continental best-seller with a lasting impact). All three used the Shakesperean motive of *The Tempest* in the version popularized by Ernest Renan in 1878. The struggle between Ariel and Caliban, linked to the spiritualism-materialism debate, allowed Latin American intellectuals to incorporate French discourse about "Latinity" and to turn the continent's material backwardness into a virtue, without having to worry too much about the necessary social reforms.[13] "Arielism" constitutes the first "Latin-Americanism" in opposition to "Yankee" spirit. Latin American intellectuals had to look for literary and mythical motives to express their desire for political activism, because they could not rely on anything within the history or the social reality of their peoples (Fernández Retamar 1995 [1971]; Vior 2001a).

American intellectuals of the period, like John Dewey and William James, however, did not look towards the past. Their pragmatism pushed them to the kind of vision of America as the "liberated Jerusalem" that promised the United States to "be" the future. However, it is important to stress the humanist character of James' universalism for he had already voiced his protest against the imperialist motives of American intervention during the Cuban War (Zuleta 1998;

[13] In his essay "Caliban's victory" (1878) Ernest Renan had proposed the antinomy Ariel-Caliban as a metaphor for the opposition between elites and the democratic masses. Renan's conservative connotations were modified by Rodó's ethical attitude, who saw in "the government of the elite with their intelligence and education" the necessary corrective for the massification already taking place in the USA. Rodó's work had great influence on Latin American identity-construction. Recent appreciations have seen him as founding figure of Latin American philosophy (see Acosta 2000; Fernández Retamar 1995 [1971]; and Vior 2001a).

Koenig 1990: 414-15). This contradiction between expansionist universalism and liberal humanism dominated the internal discussions on American continental policies throughout the Twentieth Century (Hunt 1988).

The Mexican Revolution (1910 – 1920), the first successful agrarian and social revolution worldwide in the Twentieth Century, modified the confrontational message proposed by Rodó ten years earlier. Instead of a contradiction between spiritualism and materialism it refocused the intellectual and political attention on the contradiction between the attempt to build a Mexican nation state and US expansionism in Central America and the Caribbean. The continental university reform movement after 1918, on the other hand, emphasized Marti's claims for an education for all people grounded in regional traditions, justice and freedom. This "trinity" of building a nation state, egalitarian education and distributive justice by the reformers and revolutionaries all over the continent was regarded, from 1920 to 1980 as the main instrument for political progress. It was the reformatory state and not individuals who had the responsibility to promote social development. The continent regarded this new view of itself, based on an ethic of justice, as opposed to US-American pragmatism and thus consolidated the first autonomous view of Latin American culture and politics. The perception of "imperial America" produced the vision of a "free Latin America".

Second Breakdown: Developing Nationalism and Bargaining

The world-wide economic crisis in 1930, the need to satisfy the consumption requirements of a growing urban population, the influence of anti-liberal movements in Europe as alternative ideologies to dominant Anglo-Saxon liberalism and the will to build an independent bargaining power in world politics during and after the Second World War influenced the rise of "popular nationalism" in the major Latin American countries, Brazil, Mexico and Argentina (Anderle 1992). From 1930 to 1982 popular nationalism determined the political and cultural life throughout the continent. It was an integrative, modernizing nationalism, which included the search for Latin American unity and sought a balanced relation with the United States, who were seen as too ambitious, business-oriented, but also as rational and willing to negotiate (Carmagnani 1992; Vior 1984).

This nationalism (cf. Vior 1985) represented a peculiar way to achieve modernization, internal integration and differentiation. It expanded the urban market, accelerated industrialization and promoted social policies. But it excluded the rural population (except in Argentina, who did not have such a significant number of peasants) and was strongly authoritarian. In its attempt to construct "national unity" it polarized political and cultural life and tried to subsume all social contradictions by putting forward a few leading figures. Vargas, Cárdenas and Perón were its main representatives. Although being successful as far as economic growth, and social and educational affairs were concerned, it proved in the end unable to provide an alternative to the growing international influence of the United States in the post-war era. Nationalist action does not rely on external conceptual frameworks for its legitimation, but derives its justification from the actions and discourses of their leaders.[14] Thus the popular nationalist leaders and intellectuals explained their defeat in the Fifties and Sixties exclusively by reference to US-interventions. It was the period of the Cold War and US diplomats and agents *did* intervene frequently, however, as indicated below, the fall of nationalist regimes in Latin America had more complex causes.

Third Breakdown: Revolution and Total Negation

The frustration about the unachieved nationalist reforms and the faltering of development strategies in the Fifties in general, the ideological confrontation during the Cold War, US intervention in Guatemala in 1954 and the Cuban Revolution in 1959 led to a radical turn within nationalism and to the dramatic expansion of anti-imperialism. The growing popular demands for structural reforms and the rise of a rebellious intellectual youth facilitated the emergence of revolutionary movements (Aguilar 1968; Hunt 1988; Koenig 1992: 454-73; Whitaker 1954).

The United States reacted to the Cuban Revolution with an exaggerated militarization of all Inter-American relations. The radical turn of the confrontation with Castro in 1959-61 and his alliance with the Soviet Union sharpened the American perception of being threatened from overseas. Protest and popular upheavals on the continent were no longer perceived by US public opinion and decision-makers as internal problems, but as part of a communist global plan for the take-over of the Western hemisphere. In this way US administrations, from Kennedy to Reagan, submitted all Latin America policies to the strategic necessities of the Cold War. For many Latin American countries this contributed to the replacement of civilian with military governments; for some it brought dictatorial regimes; for others, civilian administrations adopted strongly repressive measures with regard to public protests in order to prevent military and/or US-interventions (Collier 1979; Linz and Stephan 1978; Loveman and Davies, 1978; Malloy 1977; O'Donnell 1972; Petras and La Porte 1973, Tapia V. 1980).

In the face of this polarization of the Inter-American relations old nationalist leaders and elites were unable to react efficiently, while, at the same time they tried to satisfy popular demands, to control revolutionary upheavals, to confront American pressure and to continue economic growth. Therefore, between the end

---

[14] For an analysis of the structure and functions of popular nationalist discourses see Vior 1984: chapters 4, 6 and 12.

of the 1960s and the beginning of the 1970s the break between the reformist and revolutionary elites throughout the continent arose.

The bloody repression of the student movement at the "Tlatelolco Place" in Mexico City in October 1968 and the public Montoneros' break with Peron in May 1974 in Buenos Aires were events which marked the separation of the revolutionary generation from their political parents. The young embraced the old nationalist views of the internal and external fractures in Latin America's societies, but blamed the earlier generation for making compromises with the elites and the USA.

As regards these anti-imperialist, nationalist and socialist movements, the USA was unwilling to accept reforms in Latin America and only their defeat could open the way for freedom and equality. The history of the Algerian War against France and the Vietnam War seemed to confirm this demand (Vior 1991: chapter 13). The negation between the US administrations and the revolutionary youth modified the split character of the continent. From the beginning of the 1960s the Second Declaration of Havana (1962) and the National Security Doctrine replaced the earlier combination of negotiation and conflict by a war-climate.

There is no simple nor single causal relationship between the gradual setting up of a link between "economic development and national security" in the US policies for Latin America from 1947 to 1961 and the radical turn towards anti-imperialism in Latin America. However, there were factors, which contributed to the rise of a critical attitude towards anti-imperialistic reformism in Latin America. These factors included the modernization of the most important Latin American towns, which in turn brought about the growth of the middle classes (however, without giving them a proper place within the power structures), the radicalization of the Cold War, the increasing international influence of the Soviet Union, the Cuban revolution, the crisis within the Catholic Church and the radical critique of modernity in the industrialised countries.

The revolutionary anti-imperialism movement never developed its political and social programmes into governmental strategies, because to that effect, elites would have had to formulate global orientations, i.e. decide on symbolic and normative frameworks. Heroic mythology and frequent affirmations of their will to power took the place of constructive explanatory discourses. Their underlying desire for continental unity can be seen as "cesarist" and close to "bolivarism" (following the ideas and actions of Simon Bolivar). The anti-imperialists expected liberating military action to immediately create a revolutionary consciousness and produce their own legitimation as leading elite. Their mythification of the revolutionary ethics and their hope for a "new human being" (both aspects also deeply rooted in Christianity) are reminiscent of Latin American traditions from the time of the independence and civil wars in the Nineteenth Century, but also of the missionary spirit of the Sixteenth century.

While condemning the arrogance of the revolutionary elite, one cannot deny the intellectual boom brought about by the new movements, at least until the revolutionary *élan* came down to mere terrorism. Throughout Latin America this period constitutes the renaissance of utopia. The continent's "South" has a long utopian tradition, but in these years it showed in a particularly productive way. Thus many innovative creators attempted to articulate originality in the fields of literature, music, the arts, advertising and design.

In both Americas the cultural apparatuses were paralysed in their legitimate functions by the counter-cultural movements and (especially in the USA) by the Anti-Vietnam-War movement. The alliance between the middle-class revolutionary youths and the popular protest undid the dominant cultural and national images and created the basis for new popular-national identities. But these new crystallizations either had insufficient time to achieve systematic formulation, because of the military coups after 1973, or were stopped short by the leading elites.

The Latin American revolutionary movements between the 1960s and the 1980s remained in the end dependent on the worldview of the old nationalist movements. After the first oil-crisis in 1973 and the American defeat in Vietnam in 1975, revolutionary elites in Latin America were unable to understand the new trends of capitalist recovery and scientific-technological development. While their criticism of capitalism remained uni-directional and moralist, the conservative revival in Great Britain and the United States in the second half of the seventies that led to the empowerment of Margaret Thatcher 1979 and Ronald Reagan 1981 was equally "fundamentalist".

The End of the Dichotomy and the Building of Post-National Identities

It was Ronald Reagan who, in the 1980s, advanced the conservative restoration throughout the continent. The so-called "globalisation", the dominant discourse about the new expansionist phase of capitalism, weakened the nation states across the continent and submitted them to the decision-making processes in Washington or Wall Street. Nationalism collapsed and the majority of Latin American governments hastened into the adoption of neoliberal policies. The continent was reorganized by big international corporations through their investments in export-oriented agriculture based on bio-technologies, giant infrastructural works, mining and finances. After the debt-crisis, the fall of the Berlin Wall and the replacement of military dictatorships in South America by weak democracies, a sense of fragility and lack of orientation has been dominating Latin American thought. US dominance has never looked more assured. The penetration of "turbo-capitalism" (Ramonet 2000: 1) into Latin America's last corners coincides with the extension of surveillance throughout the social networks. The new American regime over the continent shows strong totalitarian traits.

But, ironically, whoever pushes integration too far, lives in constant danger of breaking up. The end of nationalism and neoimperialist discourse in Latin America have been creating a widespread feeling of disempowerment and confusion. The dissolution of the nation states caused the disappearance or de-legitimating of its referential settings. In the face of this crisis the elites and Latin American intellectuals have again been divided along the old lines, namely whether either to submit themselves to American influence or to withdraw from the debate.

While the Latin American economies grew at high rates during the first half of the 1990s, the neo-conservative governments seemed to be "in the right". But the "Americanization" of Latin American societies has also multiplied forms of segregation and fragmentation of groups who are organizing themselves within non-national, ethnic, regional, religious, mafia-looking and/or revolutionary identities. These signs of social dissolution also involve a search for new, post- or non-national meanings that will redraw Latin America's internal borders.

However, the dissolution of nation states, and the crisis of continental identity that used to be based on them, is being accompanied by the rapid expansion of Latin American cultural space deep inside the United States. The "dollarization" of Latin American economies, and the recognition that these economies are winning for the American companies, are leading, for one part, to an internalization of Latin American economic "problems" by the USA. For the other part, the unstoppable migration from the South and the accelerated growth of the Spanish-speaking minority in the United States are introducing to US society the typical problems existing within the Latin American cultural space itself. In this way, the borders of the Latin American cultural space have extended 3.000 miles towards the North.

Since 1823 the United States has repeatedly asserted its right to make the continent its backyard, justifying itself through universal mission, requirements of national security and interests of US corporations. But this triple justification worked on the assumption that Latin America was external to the space of American cultural and political practice. Only thus could the "export" of US internal conflicts be assured and the "filtering" process by US cultural apparatuses of the violence exercised abroad be guarded from the repercussions "at home" (see Campbell and Kean 1997). However, what has actually occurred is that US borders have extended to such a degree that Latin America's conflicts are now part of its own.

The US / Latin America dichotomy, which, for ninety years, served to guarantee both cultural identities, has disappeared to be replaced by *new borders*. One can no longer conceive of these borders in the traditional sense in terms of customs and rangers. They constitute a process which has neither yet crystallized nor found its limits. It is only now starting to reach a more "fixed" condition.

The dissolution of the nation state may pave the way for a new Latin America. A new continentalism can give meaning to the multiple searches for identity. This also presupposes a new, more detached Latin American approach to the United States. The Latin American governments and the media, in the 1990s, created the assumption that nothing can be done against the only remaining superpower. Obedience seemed to be the only possibility. Nevertheless multiple expressions of rebellion are signs of the need for internal differentiation and individualization. Instead of experiencing fear or the urge for confrontation, many people in Latin America are beginning to feel the need to understand the United States in order to compete successfully with it, and thus to prevent unnecessary conflicts and to plan their own development.

In the last century, Latin Americans have tended to swing between a search for recognition by and hatred of the USA. Concerned with the marking out of a Latin American cultural identity, the actual analysis of American society was neglected. The double "slide" of borders outlined above now makes it impossible to go on as before. At the same time, Latin America realizes that it has been too preoccupied with the recovery of its language, history, archaeology and arts. Sight of the scientific and technical revolution has been lost ever since the Seventies. But US-American politics and culture also need to realign themselves with reality. The US cannot resolve its minorities issues without a new, more differentiated approach to Latin America. It has to understand that if it does not want to reduplicate the old dichotomies within its borders it must now appreciate that Latin American problems are also its own.

The same applies to translation theory, didactic and practice. Latin American theoreticians should not wait for help from their American and European colleagues to achieve a critical "rewriting" of their own texts that would adapt them to the receiver's necessities in the Southern countries. Neither can American text producers expect that their texts will remain unchallenged in the South by inter- and re-contextualizations. Especially in technical and economical translations it is necessary to move towards a translation-practice guided by the receiver's necessities. Translations that fulfill these criteria will have to be informed by:

- an Ibero-American pragmatism: i.e. the purposes of the texts ought to be clear from their beginning;
- attention to the polysemy of Romance languages;[15]
- a restoration of con- and inter-textual references in order to allow for a critical reading of the source-texts;

[15] Taking also into account the growing significance of interferences with Amerindian languages and, in selected regions, translations also into these languages.

- a complementation of the source-texts through oral discourses, which often are constitutive elements of Latin American identity (Berg 2000);

- a relativization of the European and American space-time-notions, in order to be able to set them side by side with Latin American patterns: space and time are in the Latin American white and *mestizo* cultures subjective, and in the indigenous and Afro-Latin-American cultures part of the relationship between humans, the mythical and religious world and nature.

The whole American continent currently seems to be moving towards new mixed forms. The breakdown of the borders between both Americas is opening the doors for the re-definition of both. The differences between them will not disappear, because they have phylo- and ontogenetical causes, but on their redefinition will depend the future relationship between both cultural spaces: ie. mutual recognition or negation.

If social evolution is a matter of learning, we have perhaps now to begin to study the continent as a whole. Maybe, we have to overcome the division between "American" and "Latin American studies" and begin to analyse both parts in their inter-connection, and in their interrelatedness with indigenous- and Afro-American cultures. The same is valid for linguistic and translation studies. Only when American and Latin American intellectuals (in the broadest sense of the term) begin to recognize themselves as equal, different and inter-dependent, will the continent definitively have overcome its North-South divide.

Bibliography

Acosta, Y. (2000) "Ariel de Rodó, un comienzo de la filosofía latinoamericana y la identidad democrática de un sujeto en construcción", Lecture at the Instituto Superior del Profesorado Artigas, Montevideo, 7th. September.

Aguilar, A. (1968) *Pan-Americanism. From Monroe to the Present*, New York and London.

Anderle, A. (1992) "El Populismo (1929-48)", in: Lucena Salmoral, M. *Historia de Iberoamérica*, Tomo III, Madrid.

Berg, Walter B. (1995) *Lateinamerika: Literatur-Geschichte-Kultur*, Darmstadt: Wissenschaftliche Buchgesellschaft.

Berg, Walter B. (1999) "Apuntes para una historia de la oralidad en la literatura argentina", in: Berg, and Schaeffauer, Markus, eds. *Discursos de oralidad en la literatura rioplatense del siglo XIX al XX*, Tübingen: G. Narr Verlag, 10-37.

Brockman, John (1995) *The Third Culture*, New York: Simon & Schuster.

Campbell, Neil, and Kean, Alasdair (1997) *American Cultural Studies*, London: Routledge.

Carmagnani, M. (1992) "El Nacionalismo", in: Lucena Salmoral, M. *Historia de Iberoamérica*, Tomo III, Madrid.

Chiaramonte, J.C. (1982) "Coyunturas de ruptura y crisis de sistema", *Revista Mexicana de Sociología*, Año XXXIX, Nro. 152.

Collier, D., ed. (1979) *The New Authoritarianism in Latin America*, Princeton.

Derrida, J. (1997 [1985]) "Theologie der Übersetzung", in: Hirsch, A., ed. *Übersetzung und Dekonstruktion*, Frankfurt a.M.: Suhrkamp.

Diamond, Jared (1997) *Guns, Germs and Steel*, New York: W.W. Norton Co.

Ette, O. and Heydenreich, T., eds. (1994) *José Martí 1895/1995, Literatura Política-Filosofía-Estética*, Frankfurt a. M.: Vervuert Verlag.

Fernández Retamar, R. (1995) *Calibán / Contra la leyenda negra*, Lleida: Universitat de Lleida.

Foucault, M. (1984) *The Foucault Reader*, ed. P. Rabinow, New York: Pantheon Books.

Foucault, Michel (1994): *Dits et écrits 1954-1988*, vol. III: 1976-1979, Paris.

Gellman, I.F. (1979) *Good Neighbour Diplomacy 1933-1945*, Baltimore.

Gémar, J.C. (1997) "Traduction et civilisation: fonctions de la traduction et «degrés» de civilisation", in: Morillas, E. and Arias, J.P., eds. *El papel del traductor*, Salamanca: Colegio de España.

Gramsci, A. (1975 [1932])"Americanismo e fordismo", in: Gramsci, *Quaderni del Carcere*, Vol. II, Torino: Einaudi.

Hobsbawn, Eric (1994) *Age of Extremes*, London: Abacus.

Hunt, M. (1988) *Ideology and U.S. Foreign Policy*, New Haven, Conn.: Yale Univ. Press.

Koenig, Hans-Joachim (1992) "El intervencionismo norteamericano en Iberoamérica", in: Lucena Salmoral, Manuel, ed. *Historia de Iberoamérica*, Vol. III, Madird: Ed. Cátedra.

Linz, J.J. and Stephan, A. (1978) *The Breakdown of Democratic Regimes: Latin America,* Baltimore.

Loveman, B. and Davies, T.M. (1978) *The Politics of Antipolitics the Military in Latin America*, Lincoln, Nebr.

Malloy, J. (1977) *Authoritarianism and Corporatism in Latin America*, Pittsburgh.

May, E. R. (1975) *The Making of the Monroe Doctrine*, Cambridge, Mass.

Minson, J. (1987) "Strategies for Socialists? Foucault's conception of power", in: Gane, M., ed., *Towards a Critique of Foucault*, London and New York.

Morales Padrón, Francisco (1988) *Atlas histórico-cultural de América, Tomo II*, Las Palmas de Gran Canaria : Gobierno de Canarias.

O'Donnel, G. (1972) *Modernización y autoritarismo*, Buenos Aires.

Petras, J. and La Porte, R. (1973) *Cultivating revolutions*, New York.

Ramonet, Ignacio (2000) "Un délicieux despotisme", *Le Monde Diplomatique*, 5 May.

Ramonet, Ignacio (2000a) "L'aurore", *Le Monde Diplomatique*, 1 January.

Rosenberg, E. (1982) *Spreading the American Dream: American Economic and Cultural Expansion, 1890-1945*, New York: Hill and Wang.

Smith, Tony (1994) *America's mission*, Princeton: Princeton University Press.

Takaki, R. (1979) *Iron Cages: Race and Culture in Nineteenth-Century America*, London: Athlone.

Tapia Valdez, J. (1980) *El terrorismo de Estado: la Doctrina de la Seguridad Nacional en el cono sur*, Mexico.

Tattersall, Ian (1996) *The Fossil Trail. How We Know What We Think We Know About Human Evolution*, New York and Oxford: Oxford University Press.

Tulchin, J.S. (1971) *The Aftermath of War. World War I and U.S. Policy Toward Latin America*, New York.

Vior, E.J. (2001) "Las visiones de Nuestra América, las de la Otra y las nuevas fronteras", in: Fornet Betancourt, R. and Wojcieszak, J., eds. *Filosofía e interculturalidad: una Perspectiva universalizable desde las Américas*, Aachen and Warszawa.

Vior, E.J. (2001a) "Visiones de Calibán – Visiones de América", in: El Hermes criollo, Montevideo, año 1, nro. 1, November, 24-45.

Vior, E.J. (1991) "Bilder und Projekte der Nation in Brasilien und Argentinien", Doctoral thesis, University of Giessen.

Vior, E.J. (1985) "Nación y nacionalismo en América Latina", *Concordia*, 8.

Vior, E.J. (1984) "Der Peronismus, populärer Nationalismus in Argentinien", M.A. thesis, University of Heidelberg.

Whitaker, A. P. (1954) *The Western Hemisphere Idea. Its Rise and Decline*, Ithaca and London.

Wickham, Gary (1987) "Power and Power Analysis: Beyond Foucault?" in: Gane, M., ed., *Towards a Critique of Foucault*, London and New York.

Wright, Robert (1994) *The Moral Animal*, New York: Pantheon Books.

Zea, Leopoldo (1993) *Fuentes de la cultura latinoamericana*, Vol. I, México D.F.: FCE.

Zuleta Alvarez, Enrique (1998) "Los Estados Unidos y la Guerra del 98", *Cuadernos Hispanoamericanos*, Nros. 577-78, 111-57.

Section D:

Translating Cultural Studies

BUILDING CULTURAL STUDIES FOR POSTCOLONIAL HONG KONG: ASPECTS OF THE POSTMODERN RUINS IN BETWEEN DISCIPLINES

STEPHEN C K CHAN

Under the impact of post-Fordist globalism, scholars who consider themselves part of "a community of thinkers" would realize today that they dwell in none other than a "ruined institution", where Culture no longer matters for the education they deliver. Without a guiding idea of human culture *inside* the university, understanding the multiplying perspectives and wide-ranging voices of dissent *outside of it* has become impossible. By outlining the institution of Cultural Studies in postcolonial Hong Kong, I discuss the educational project of the *BA Cultural Studies* launched by Lingnan University in 1999. The first such programme found in the Chinese-language world, the Lingnan case of critical Cultural Studies emerged in the context of the HKSAR where intellectual efforts are being driven to the matrix of sociohistorical factors shaping the reproduction of "thinking subjects" in universities. The problem is that postmodern institutional structures have not been adapting as much as they can to the processes of cross-fertilization and trans-disciplinary interaction of the new knowledge formations that affect them.

University and Culture in Ruins

> *To speak of the university and the state is to tell a story about the emergence of the notion of culture.* (Readings 1995: 466)

The modern university has been growing to monstrous size, and in monstrous ways. Those of us who still want to consider ourselves belonging to a community of thinkers would no doubt realize that we dwell in none other than a sort of monumental ruin, otherwise known as "the University of Excellence", in which, students "are not *like* customers, they *are* customers" (Readings 1996: 22). Here I borrow the use of the terms 'ruin' and 'excellence' in describing the critical condition of our university institution from the late Bill Readings. In a provocative article entitled "The University without Culture?", published posthumously in a special issue on Higher Education in *New Literary History*, Readings (1995) reminds us forcefully that the university is as much a workplace as a community – that whatever we do there, between consumer service and cultural manicure (where Excellence presumably lies), we do so in our role as educators. In *The University in Ruins,* after an account of the general decline of the nation-state in the contemporary age (Readings 1996: 44-53), he asks educators to "recognize that the University is a *ruined* institution, while thinking what it means to dwell in those ruins without recourse to romantic nostalgia" (1996: 169). Struck by the power of Readings' ruin metaphor, I have been trying hard lately to think of myself as part of a community who, at a time when a decolonized Hong Kong returns to the cultural and historical homeland of China, need to come to grips with the meaning of the teaching and learning of culture.

According to Readings (1995: 466-7), the university and the state have essentially been *modern* institutions; he points out that the strong idea of culture has arisen with the nation-state, and we now face its disintegration as the site for establishing meaningful values at a collective level. As national identity loses its relevance, the original notion of culture becomes effectively unthinkable, not least for the university community. For coupled with the commodification of culture as such is also the decline in the function of the university as an institution in the public sphere, alongside the disappearance of the intellectual as a public figure. Today, in Hong Kong, we have more or less come to accept that there is nothing authentic to be said, much less to be done, in our tertiary institutions about culture or the immanent intellectual mission the latter is supposed to carry. Despite our move into a new political era after the 1997 handover of sovereignty to China, the available postcolonial rundown of social reforms, nationalist movements or managerial discourses nowadays appear to be pathetically degenerate, if not unconvincing or downright hypocritical within the local educational context.

Hence, the changing role of culture Readings is concerned with reflects aptly our collective reaction and indifference to the changing partnership between the two grand institutions of modernity, namely, the university and the state, which have indeed always been closely aligned. The result has long been known: decolonized or not, culture is impossible; or, in Readings' words, "Culture ceases to mean anything *as such*; it is dereferentialized" (1996: 99).

Culture as Impossibility

The undeniable reality is that the collapse of the guiding, liberal idea of human culture *inside* the increasingly homogeneous and bureaucratic university has made it extremely difficult for teachers and students alike to appreciate the multiplying perspectives and wide-ranging voices of dissent *outside of it*, let alone to try to grasp the form and meaning of education as a liberating cultural experience. In order to be able to re-invent a story about the business as well as the *art* of university education, let us digress for a while from the dominant ideology of managing culture in our modern institution, to move around, even beyond, the existing institutional boundaries and disciplinary territories available therein. Adopting Homi Bhabha's view that culture as a strategy of survival is "translational" in nature (1994: 172), I hope that such strategic displacement of culture as an institutional space would make it possible to reach those texts and contexts that have since the recent crisis of modernity been changing our views of others, and that of others of ourselves. I would like to believe that there is still room for us to translate and re-articulate culture within the university *after the ruin*.

In what follows, we shall therefore take a serious look at the educational possibility of such a culturally impossible programme, i.e., to engage with reality despite the ruin. Our attempt is *to translate the significance of culture (or the lack of such) in pragmatic pedagogic terms through strategic border re-alignment of our institutional realities*. Locally, such a focus will present Hong Kong as a case of critical cultural studies. This would put the demand on our universities to open up new space for the engaged study of various problems on identity politics and the new global cultural economy, but also allow intellectual efforts of the university community as a whole to be channeled pragmatically to fruitful re-development, indeed re-invention, of "thinking subjects" in the postcolony.

On this paradox of cultural possibility Readings has spoken ironically of "a strange contemporary coincidence" which marks the simultaneous decline and rise in the state of our art. Together with the erasure of a certain kind of speaking position tied to the role of the teacher-intellectuals occupying key posts of culture-building throughout the history of modernity, he argues that there is a recent rise within the university of this "quasi discipline" of cultural studies, which "promises to install a new paradigm for the humanities that will either unite the traditional disciplines… or replace them… as the living center of intellectual inquiry, [thus] restoring the social mission of the university" (1995: 467). In short, "Cultural Studies… arise when cultures ceases to be the immanent principle in terms on which knowledge within the University is organized, and instead becomes one object among others" (1996: 87). In this uncertain crossroad we shall seek to see how cultural studies can be a project to break away from the given positions of subjectivity made possible within the existing institutional borders. Specifically we want to suggest that contemporary studies of culture have to involve disciplinary re-alignment in concrete strategic terms. Any curricular plan to re-articulate subject matters within a viable set of disciplinary parameters (of the new Cultural Studies) ought to address the need to situate new subject positions (of cultures thus articulated) under the condition of that ruined institution we still call university.

Interdisciplinarity has always been recognized as part of what constitutes Cultural Studies as an intellectual project. Lloyd and Thomas recently pointed to the historical shift in its own trajectory as an interdisciplinary practice: "Cultural Studies increasingly takes as its objects the highly differentiated forms of cultural production *and* reception that have emerged in time with the increasing intervention of capitalism in civil society, in the domain of 'values' and recreation, through the intensification of a commodification of culture that is indifferent to aesthetic distinction except in the instrumental form of audience and consumer stratification" (1998: 160-1). Realizing that interdisciplinarity itself is a marker of culture's very *un-translatability* under the postcolonial perspective (Bhabha 1994: 224), we shall discuss how a contemporary transdisciplinary space of Cultural Studies may now generate a base for nurturing the open perspectives needed to understand the current changes, and to change the current understanding, of our disintegrating social world, known to have been affected significantly by the global cultural economy today. It is quite true that some of the more recent tendencies in the institutionalization of Cultural Studies have been worrying, as they seem to have revealed that the very dissenting voices (and their un-translatability, as it were) which gave rise to the kind of (inter-)disciplinary transformation we find in the early history of its development are no longer there. They are now distorted, contained, if not silenced, by a new guise of professionalism, housed respectfully within newly drawn authoritative (often also disciplinary) borders of knowledge. In developing cultural studies for our current needs, we have cautioned ourselves to address this institutional paradox or pragmatism involved through what I refer to as the re-alignment of the borders of culture in the state of the contemporary ruin.

Given the absurdity of this modern ruin, I propose to diverge from the norm of our institutional practices, not in order to lament the loss of the idea of culture, but to find ways of re-emerging from the ruin and to dwell *radically* (if we can) upon the paradigm shift of culture-building as an educational project. In the process, we would also try to negotiate our future work with the ideal *conservative* notion of liberal education as the institutional home base for a community of thinkers *cum* educator-scholars who constitute still the `university` albeit in a state of ruin.

Re-imagining a Community of Thinkers

> Toni Morrison refers specifically to "the violence of representation" in the 1993 Nobel Lecture in Literature. "Oppressive language," she writes, "does more than represent violence; it is violence." ... "We die. That may be the meaning of life. But we do language. That may be the measure of our lives." She does not state: "language is agency," for that kind of assertion would deprive language of the agency she meant to convey. (Butler 1997: 6-7)

> The language of my education was no longer the language of my culture. (Ngugi 1986: 11)

For sure, what is required of us now is *not* the building of a better institution, nor the setting up of another model of efficiency, another project of grand integration. The university, rather, has to find a new *language* in which to make a claim for its role as a locus of higher education. If we acknowledge that the university today has been "busily transforming itself from an ideological arm of the state into a bureaucratically organized and relatively autonomous consumer-oriented corporation" (Readings 1995: 467), then we must indeed begin to identify this more pragmatic, mundane role within the context of humanist education it might still want to deliver today. Now that the agency of liberal education has been abstracted from the organizing matrix of culture as meaning, we would need to ask how, and indeed whether, the measure of the sort of education we continue to provide in the university relates to the kind of culture we live in, live with and live for. As Terry Eagleton's recent analysis shows, "Culture is not only what we live by. It is also, in great measure, what we live for. Affection, relationship, memory, kinship, place, community, emotional fulfilment, intellectual enjoyment, a sense of ultimate meaning: these are closer to most of us than charters of human rights or trade treatises" (2000: 131). Hence, while culture as the object of the humanities may no longer be assumed these days, as educators still engaged with the subject of culture we do need to identify and reflect on the disciplinary and pedagogical framework we are left with, or left to live for within the ruined institution of excellence. Even more so, we need to ask with what guiding educational orientations we would lead our students through the virtual elimination of our "common culture" (Raymond Williams' term, as discussed in Eagleton 2000: 112-31), understood as the array of grand narratives and experiences of humanity which have shaped the various individual and social practices in the institutions of modernity?

Instead of making any further redemptive claims about the university as a locus of culture, what we want most in this new age of postmodern contingency, incoherence and ambivalence,[1] is paradoxically, *a turbulent, cruel, indeed what must be called "hypermoral" attitude* toward the progressive, enlightening and communicating function of the humanities.[2] This requires rigorous communication indeed, through which the new subjects of humanistic education may be made aware of "the complexity and historically marked status of the spaces in which we are situated, while recognizing that these are spaces that we cannot *inhabit*, from which we are alienated" (Readings 1995: 480). Readings calls this attitude "institutional pragmatism," with which we tend to accept that the modern university, as "a ruined institution," is no longer charged with the responsibility of making transcendental claims as part of its cultural function (1995: 485, 480; 1996: 168). Dwelling in the ruins means, therefore, to confront

---

[1] Cf. Mike Featherstone in "Localism, Globalism and Cultural Identity": "postmodernism entails a loss of confidence in the master-narratives of progress and enlightenment which have been central to Western modernity. The confidence in the universality of this project is replaced by an emphasis upon contingency, incoherence, and ambivalence" (Wilson and Dissanayake 1996: 59).

[2] The notion of "hypermorality" is borrowed from Georges Bataille; see his *Literature and Evil*: "Literature is either the essential or nothing. I believe that the Evil – an acute form of Evil – which it expresses, has a sovereign value for us. But this concept does not exclude morality: on the contrary, it demands a "hypermorality"... Communication requires loyalty. A rigorous morality results from complicity in the knowledge of Evil, which is the basis of intense communication" (Bataille 1973: "Preface").

persistently the complexity of the space the university now occupies, functions within and makes real. Having become more and more specialized and professionalized, this modern institution can no longer guarantee the revelation of a unifying idea under any of its universal claims. In fact, at the cost of full-range bureaucratization, the university has been expanding rapidly nowadays with perhaps only one clear ambition, that of disciplinary specialization in particular and academic professionalization in general, a direction which has already come under strong criticism.[3]

Accepting the ruin is hence not in itself any reason to abandon culture and education; far from it, it demands that we not take for granted the significance of our professional circuits and the kind of academic bureaucracy they in turn support, that we do not in short, "satisfy ourselves with rebuilding a ghost town" (Readings 1995: 485). As a matter of fact, having been trained and re-trained by the institutions we work in, we are now all thoroughly equipped with one brand or another of institutional pragmatism, not only in the sense that we see clearly the need to render ourselves "professionally" according to prevailing rules, but also in the way we allow ourselves to sit through the range of teaching and research routines in a discipline without a single thought for education as a liberating experience.[4]

Can we still hope to imagine a notion of community in the ruined institution such as ours today? *That* is indeed the question. Our challenge is to test our imagination against the pragmatic limits of our teaching and research activities. In the midst of ruins, what can we do, to protect our institution from the violence of representation Toni Morrison alludes to? How can we re-build the university as a locus of dissensus (Readings 1995: 478) and yet retain the *unplannable* nature (Williams, quoted in Eagleton 2000: 119) and *untranslatable* character (Bhabha 1994: 163, 172-3, 224-9) of culture? Can the university in general and humanistic education in particular acquire new meanings and new forms as an institution of culture in the 21st century?

---

[3] Readings, for one, has written: "Professionalization deals with the loss of this subject-referent of the educational experience by integrating teaching and research as aspects of the general administration of a close system: teaching is the administration of students by professors, research is the administration of professors by their peers, administration is the name given to the stratum of bureaucrats who administer the whole" (1995: 477). See also Damrosch (1995), and Said (1994).

[4] In the attempt to re-imagine the university as a community, we might want to be reminded that, "recognizing the university as ruined means abandoning teleologies and attempting to make things happen within a system without claiming that such events are the true, real meaning of the system. … [Thus, it] liberates new spaces and breaks down existing structures of defense against thought" (Readings 1995: 489).

Cultural Studies as an Educational Project

> The question of our relation to regimes of value is not a personal but an institutional question. (Frow 1995: 16)

> Thus, the emergence of the University of Excellence in place of the University of Culture can only be understood against the backdrop of the decline of the nation-state. (Readings 1995: 476)

There has been a clear tendency of the institutionalization of cultural studies. More and more degrees in cultural studies are being offered by institutions of higher education in many parts of the world, and a growing number of academic journals and conferences have come out of cultural studies worldwide. Since the 1960s, when a group of loosely related projects in media studies and cultural history broke off from traditional borders of knowledge and research to form the famous Birmingham Centre for Contemporary Cultural Studies, cultural studies has had tremendous impact on such academic disciplines as English studies, sociology, anthropology, media and communication studies, comparative literature, linguistics and history. In British cultural studies, the key moment has been the development of studies in post-war social history with a strong focus on "popular culture," the culture of "the people", or "the culture in common". These forms of what Raymond Williams calls "ordinary culture" have often been represented and re-invented in clear political terms. Instances of popular struggle and traditions of ideological dissent have since been associated with the critical project of cultural studies.

The question two decades after the initial Birmingham projects on cultural studies was the issue of institutionalization. In "What is Cultural Studies Anyway?" Richard Johnson wrote, "To put the question most sharply: should cultural studies aspire to be an academic discipline?" (Johnson 1986: 38). The issue before us here, fifteen years after it had been brought up, is rather culture's specific relevance to university education in Hong Kong. How meaningful is the intellectual cause of dissent to the form of pedagogic discourse we are familiar with? To what extent is the disciplinary formation of cultural studies a matter of concern for liberal education under the post-colonial condition of Hong Kong? My discussion below will focus on the consideration of cultural studies education in relation to the institutional borders and disciplinary territories it has been engaged with. Questions pertaining to the institutional management of knowledge and subjectivity in the local context will also be considered.

The first question of pedagogy and curriculum to concern us is, if dissent is the *content* of cultural studies, what *form* – of knowledge, of subjectivity – would it take in the process we call education? Here Bhabha's point on the *translational* character of culture may again be helpful. Along the line of his suggestion, what might be called the acts of "translation" in cultural studies would serve to highlight "the performative nature of cultural communication" (Bhabha 1994: 228). In more positive terms, Johnson (1986) suggests that "critique" be considered the key component in the development of cultural studies as an educational project. He analyzes cogently how the codification of method or knowledge runs in principle against some main features of cultural studies as a critical tradition: its openness and theoretical versatility, its reflective even self-conscious mood. Defining critique as the identification of "procedures by which other traditions are approached both for what they may yield and for what they inhibit," Johnson (1986: 38) argues that making it a basic strategy of cultural studies allows the latter to "steal away" from disciplines in the humanities and social sciences certain useful elements and "reject the rest." From this point of view cultural studies is a process of appropriation that involves constant re-negotiation and dialogue: "codify it and you might halt its reactions". Attempt to institutionalise it, and of course you would get into trouble with what Bhabha calls the untranslatablity of culture, and you are bound to confront an array of disciplinary problems: Should there be a formal set of methodology for cultural studies? Need there be a canon in the tradition of cultural studies writings? Refusal to specify all these in formal disciplinary codes would not allow you to translate at all in your educational project – to be able to claim any role at all in the process of institutionalization which captures all our educational resources today. Define any of these and you risk the reification of its function of critique, and losing hold of the powerful untranslatability of culture itself. But perhaps such a paradox is at the root of our education.

Not without a touch of black humour does Readings point to the swift degeneration of culture as such in the rapid rise of cultural studies as a half discipline. "The idea of cultural studies," he remarks, "arises at the point when the notion of culture ceases to mean anything vital for the university as a whole. The human sciences can do what they like with culture, can do cultural studies, because culture no longer matters as an Idea for the institution" (1995: 466-7). The university, meanwhile, cannot be bothered; everywhere, it has been busy setting up what have come to be known as "centres of excellence."[5] Under the

---

[5] In Hong Kong, the idea of "excellence" was first raised with regard to tertiary education in the 1993 Universities and Polytechnic Grants Committee (UPGC, later UGC, or Universities Grants Committee) by the interim report on Higher Education 1991-2001. The most relevant paragraphs read: "The [UPGC] institutions should incorporate centres of excellence having local, regional and international functions. They should provide very high quality bilingual manpower for both Hong Kong and the hinterland and should act as points of reference, particularly in Business and Social Studies and in innovative science and technology for developments in Southern China and more widely (paragraph 25. iii)"; also: "There is no such thing as an excellent university. Indeed it is only rarely that every part of an academic department can be said to be of excellent quality. What we hope to foster within our institutions is a number of excellent groups, recognised internationally as of equal status to their peers in the same subject area, and justifying the investment in state-of-the-art facilities and activity which will maintain them among the world leaders. We hope that a significant proportion of these "centres of excellence" will be working in areas of direct interest to Hong Kong industry, commerce and culture and that their existence will precipitate curriculum development which is also locally and regionally

current system, "excellence" cannot serve as a carrier of content, for it seems capable of drawing one single boundary, that of "the unrestricted power of the bureaucracy" (Readings 1995: 469, 473, 491; 1996: 21-43). Worse, it permits exhaustive accounting, often taken to mean the same thing as accountability. In short, it would appear that the quest for "excellence" work only to tie the university into an "excellent" net of bureaucratic institutions. Needless to say, this work of institutionalization runs against the very liberating cause that distinguishes the initial moments of cultural studies. With the representation of dissent placed at the core of its intellectual programme, cultural studies holds a firm belief in the language of culture, even though the latter must now be articulated with a certain notion of power. It is now truly difficult to fix the content of culture. In that particular sense, culture no longer matters, thus opening up the gate for everyone to plough its common, ordinary field, with divergent and sometimes rather isolated concerns for its formal constitution, ideological ramification, policy implementation, and the rest.

For us the relevant question has therefore to do with attempting to re-invest meaning into a label such as "cultural studies" within an institution which is no longer being developed on the groundwork of Culture, but led to dwindle under the banner of Excellence.[6] My own inclination is towards the impossible, towards counter-disciplinarity if you want, holding on to the cruel, hypermoral stance to dwell in the ruins without nostalgia or hope. Granted that it is no longer possible to re-gain the guiding idea of culture for the university, there may still be chance for an alternative view or a dissenting voice to capture culture in its secular, public forms for us. Given the extreme difficulty to reach the values or regimes of values made accessible in our educational process, perhaps the option left for educators is to imagine the return of culture as a programme that matters, in minor ways, for the university as a now dislocated community of scholars. And if cultural studies has still a role to play there, we might as well try to see if that would be one of (counter-) discipline, catalyst, interlocutor or clown.

---

orientated" (paragraph 27a); "The existence of internationally recognised "centres of excellence" has a catalytic effect in an institution far beyond the subjects directly concerned. It produces a liveliness and confidence in teaching and research and in overseas contacts which will help in the production of the high quality bilingual manpower..." (paragraph 27b).

[6] "Under the rubric of excellence, interdisciplinary programs can be created, allowing the application of university-wide standards of straightforward and objective evaluation, so that we will all become more excellent. Is it surprising that corporations resemble universities, healthcare facilities, international organizations, which all resemble corporations?" (Readings 1995: 472).

Global Development in the Contemporary Critiques of Public Culture

Invoking the all-time question *What is cultural studies*? Johnson suggests that, ultimately, its object of study are the historical forms of consciousness or subjectivity, or what he calls "the subjective side of social relations" (1986: 43). I think this formulation has strong implications not only for understanding the meaning of education cultural studies provides, but also for re-thinking the liberating function of culture as a form of experience, one that is strongly rooted in pedagogy as a process of open negotiation. We need to add that this form of experience becomes fundamentally historical when situated in the knowledge formation of cultural studies. It becomes historical at the same time as it remains subjective; it regains subjectivity, that is, through a pedagogical process of historicization. Culture, and especially contemporary culture, become liberating as they return to us from history. And as subjectivity becomes historicized, history also takes root in subjective, cultural forms.

Roughly approximating the work of a "historian-of-the-contemporary," the cultural studies scholar does not limit the field of research to specialized practices, genres or texts. Hence all social practices can indeed be viewed from a *cultural* point of view, for the role they play and the work they do in the *historical* constitution of subjectivity (Johnson 1986: 42, 45). Within this basic intellectual perspective, Johnson identifies three main models of cultural studies research: namely, production-based studies, text-based studies, and studies of lived cultures, and urges that we see the vigorous but multiplying field of cultural studies, not as a *unity*, but as a *whole* (1986: 41). In what follows, I shall adopt this division in my attempt to outline an account of a cultural studies programme for Hong Kong.

Production-based cultural critiques – are studies which deal with the means of cultural production. While they often involve the making public of private forms of experience or representation, public texts are regularly consumed or received in private (Johnson 1986: 52), thus fostering an active process of cultural interflows between the private and the public, between the local and the global. As we know, the cutting edge for contemporary changes are those *public cultures* being brought into contact by a global media industry and cultural economy; these worldwide "contact points" have for the past two decades become the catalysts for change at all levels of society across the globe. As the global development of democracy movements since the 1980s has shown, economic proposals, foreign policy statements, journalism, human rights reports, resistance literature, non-mainstream screenplays, avant-garde multi-media installations, as well as pop music concerts can become potent forms of sociopolitical criticism when they are enacted in mass-mediated public contexts. The trajectories of this new range of social movements are linked to a variety of cultural sites, including the media, internet, performing arts, academic institutions, and popular culture, all of which are being pulled into international networks of global cultural communication. Cultural studies thus treats in fundamental ways the interplay between global commodity culture and the localized patterns of everyday life with perspectives both culturalist and structuralist.[7] All in all, it is clear that the condition of production cannot be limited to the material means of production and the capitalist organization of labour. These need to be examined in relation to the analysis of textual forms and the modes of their reception, as part of the cultural circulation process in which a particular act of consumption is implicated.

Text-based cultural critiques – the second major kind of research commonly found in cultural studies – deals with the various forms and flows of cultural products through well-developed strategies of formal description. With the demise of the Cold War with its bilateral model of nation-state relations, traditional area- or discipline-based models of global process seem to be out of touch with the hybrid and multilateral nature of the current sociocultural changes worldwide. The prototypes of such textual organization of cultural forms, now considered indispensable in global cultural analysis, are drawn from disciplines conventionally grouped under the arts or the humanities. Traditional academic programmes (e.g., international relations) that do engage in global thinking tend to lack a rich, "thick" understanding of local forms of culture, especially in the most dynamic area of sociocultural changes, not to mention that of textual mediations and their ties to crucial contextual redefinitions. On the other hand, area programmes (e.g., Chinese studies, Asian studies, Oriental studies, African studies, Afro-American studies, English studies, even Hong Kong Studies) and conventional disciplines (e.g., literature, anthropology, sociology, communication, philosophy, fine arts, film studies) sometimes encourage work on local culture, but tend to overlook the global processes which are changing them. In any case, they allow themselves readily to be consolidated and contained within a single-disciplinary knowledge formation.

Our present forms of education, not least in the field of culture, are therefore rather slow in addressing the complications that the local, national, and transnational are creating – and this seems especially the case with academia in Hong Kong making its way through phases of late- and post-colonial change. At their best, the disciplinary boundaries conform to the main circuits of cultural flows, but restrict the agency of knowledge and understanding in significant ways. Recent global developments of cultural flows and identity politics (Appadurai 1996, Gole 1996, Hardt and Negri 2000, Jameson 1998, King 1990,

---

[7] "On the one side there are those who insist that 'cultures' must be studied as a whole, and *in situ*, located, in their material context… [culturalist]. On the other side, there are those who stress the relative independence or effective autonomy of subjective forms and means of signification. The practical theory here is usually structuralist, but in a form which privileges the discursive construction of situations and subjects... If the first set of methods are usually dervied from sociological, anthropological or socio-historcial roots, the second set owe most to literary criticism, and especially the traditions of literary modernism and linguisitic formalism" (Johnson 1986: 50).

Ray and Sayer 1999, Sassen 1994, Taylor 1994, Tomlinson 1999) can in no way correspond to the compartmentalization of academic knowledge. They provide strong support to the cultural studies position that no single academic discipline can grasp the full complexity of the phenomena of culture. In view of such changes in the field, cultural studies must not only take seriously its commitment to develop interdisciplinary perspectives, it needs also to think of itself as rigorously counter-disciplinary in its basic orientation. While it often holds a deep, imaginative perspective on various kinds of representation, textual analysis tends to *translate*, though not reduce, questions of historical productivity of cultural forms to formal patterns or semiotic codes. It goes without saying that the ultimate object of cultural studies, or of any form of culture after the ruin for that matter, is not so much the text as *the social life of subjective forms* (Johnson 1986: 62) realised in particular instances of their circulation, mediated by but not limited to their textual embodiments.

Critiques of lived cultures – the third major kind of research found in cultural studies – is often associated with a politics of "representation." From a critical point of view, textual analysis and material cultural production must eventually be linked to the study of lived cultures in their divergent forms of representation. Again the primary task here is to capture the more *concrete* and *private* moments of cultural circulation in social realities (Johnson 1986: 69, 73). To the extent that it takes the cultural worlds of others as the main object, this kind of social inquiry also involves the dominant, globalizing tendencies that are implicated in the treatment of minority cultures and non-western cultures. Consequently, any serious research on local politics of culture is inevitably tied to an understanding of the global cultural economy of values, texts and commodities. We can now take a second look at the ironic remark made by Readings:

> The idea of culture in Cultural Studies is not really an "idea" in the strong sense proposed by the modern university. *Cultural Studies, that is, does not propose culture as a regulative ideal for research and teaching so much as recognize the inability of culture to function as such an "idea" any longer.* (Readings 1995: 487)

This echoes strongly indeed with Johnson's positive representation of culture through cultural studies: "Culture is neither an autonomous nor an externally determined field, but a site of social differences and struggles" (1986: 39). In other words, when ideas are in crisis, opportunities arise for the multiplication of collective, fragmentary cultural-political struggles for identity and for difference.

As we know, non-western cities (e.g., Bombay, Istanbul, Shanghai, Taipei, Tokyo) have been represented in past scholarship as a cluster of relatively unrelated local cultures measured by their differences from Western Modernity. They are often seen as local reactions to "global" (i.e., "Western") modernity, while globalization becomes the product of the hegemonic West. Recent approaches have shifted their focus to the transnational flows of peoples, values, commodities, as well as forms of cultural representation, without losing the focus on the specific local production, circulation and transformation of texts and contexts (Chen 1998, Chambers & Curti 1996, Harvey 1989, Lash & Friedman 1992, Niranjana, Sudhir & Dhareshwar 1993, Wilson & Dirlik 1995, Wilson & Dissanayake 1996). The unique situation of Hong Kong now offers new questions of critical concern not only for local scholars, but also for regional and international experts from across a range of disciplines. The rapid spread of political system and ideology, capital and mass-mediated popular culture on a global scale since the late 1980s have generated a series of challenges for scholarship in contemporary studies. Thus, situated at the juncture of complex flows and counter-flows of cultural values, commodities, and forms of representation, Hong Kong cultural studies are in a position to conceive of our educational project in the light of a more dynamic model of interdisciplinary, even transdisciplinary, studies in contemporary culture. Clearly, our focus has to be set, among other things, on the specific historical patterns of cultural imagination, social representation and ideological sources of identity in a cosmopolitan, postcolonial urban site undergoing significant transformation.

Pedagogic Challenge, Institutional Change

> Just what is the modern university?... the university is what its members do. (Damrosch 1995: 16)

> [T]he problem for the intellectual is to try to deal with the impingements of modern professionalization... by representing a different set of values and prerogatives. These I shall collect under the name of amateurism, literally, an activity that is fueled by care and affection rather than by profit and selfish, narrow specialization. (Said 1994: 82)

The stage for a new politicization of teaching and scholarship has been set by the new shift of intellectuals in academia. In *We Scholars: Changing the Culture of the University*, David Damrosch points out that "every argument about the material scholars should study, and every argument about the methods to be used, is at the same time an argument about the nature of the community that is to do the studying" (1995: 5). From our point of view in cultural studies today, we may look forward to institutionalization. Perhaps pragmatism will always be a part of the institution, whatever the latter may turn out to be. But in order to keep our feet firmly on the ground of the culture in which we live (outside of the ruined institution), we shall have to address ourselves ultimately to the works of cultural practitioners of all sorts in the community, including journalists, writers, critics, film-makers, playwrights, teachers, editors, as well as academics. In short, we shall have to move from an institution that is ruined (University) to another that is equally so (Culture). Limiting our concern today to possible changes in the university, we can say that this kind of transdisciplinary work requires, in the long run, critical cultural sophistication and sensitivity that exceed what present day academic models in Hong Kong are ready to provide within their existing institutional structure.

Creating dynamic forms of cultural-historical understanding of contemporary issues requires us to develop new forms of cross-disciplinary scholarly collaboration and academic programmes, in which the examination, coordination and integration of multiple perspectives will be seen as a presupposition of all core work in the study of culture, rather than as supplementary or even unnecessary. The basic problem is that our institutional structures have not been adapting as much as they can to the processes of cross-fertilization, and not merely co-habitation, of academic disciplines that affect them. For our views of others' lived cultures (here our objects of study) will surely influence our views of ourselves (our roles as scholar-educators), and in an internationalizing world, any grasp of the cultural-historical processes will depend upon an informed response to this interplay of intellectual perspectives. Without bringing difference and struggle back to the ordinary field of culture, we would indeed have to accept that, as they are, academic knowledge-forms now look more like part of the problem than part of the solution (Johnson 1986: 41).

Much may eventually have to change in the current institutional practice and structure, but for now, let us focus on the (minor) postmodern mode of intellectual orientation that hinges on new institutional transformation. Damrosch devotes a whole book to an overall assessment of our institutional status as scholars today, suggesting that "the basic responsibility for our difficulties in communication lies with the institutional structures within which we work, and with the organizational culture that our institutions foster"; these structures, if left unchanged, will no doubt ruin "the ways in which we can bring together differing perspectives and the people who hold them, even as we continue to develop further the strengths of specialized work and individual identity" (1995: 9, 8). In other words, ruined as it is, today's university poses a fundamental threat to the understanding of dissent, which as we have said, is basic to the core of cultural studies. Likewise, Edward Said (1994) attributes the cause of the contemporary loss of the intellectual (in the West) to "professionalism" as an attitude. In *Representations of the Intellectual*, he seriously recommends all of us to find a solution in "amateurism"; he contends, "as a way of maintaining relative intellectual independence, having the attitude of an amateur instead of a professional is a better course" (Said 1994: 87).

Being trained pragmatists, however, we know that we cannot help the fact that "academic specialization is as much a fact of life as the complexity of modern society, and it can hardly be wished away" (Damrosch 1995: 3). This much we know for a fact about the form of our postmodern institution. Professionals that we are, we know exactly what it means to live by the kind of protectionism or aggression that has come to typify our institutional existence. Hence, any naive attempts to address the basic difficulty in communication within the university, such as suggestions for collaborative teaching or collaborative learning (Damrosch 1995: 134, 139) may materialize only with an organizational culture that promotes extended dialogue and open, committed negotiation. For through this alone can the challenge of difference and dissent be re-invested into our lived, non-intellectual pragmatism as academic specialists. Said does seem to be very skeptical when he writes: "Everyone today professes a liberal language of equality and harmony for all. The problem for the intellectual is to bring these notions to bear on actual situations where the gap between the profession of equality and justice, on the one hand, and the rather less edifying reality, on the other, is very great" (1994: 94). One might prefer the straightforwardness of a Noam Chomsky: "If it is the responsibility of the intellectual to insist upon the truth, it is also his duty to see events in their historical perspective" (1969: 352-3). Today, it would seem that a strong sense of radical historical orientation is precisely lacking in our deliberation on post-liberal education in this context of post-modern "professionalism".[8]

BA (Hons) in Cultural Studies at Lingnan University

> The question of the postmodern is a question posed to the university as much as in the university. (Readings 1995: 465)

> [T]he denunciation of the University as an institution within Cultural Studies is a problem not merely for the University but of the University. (Readings 1996: 91)

Cultural studies, as part of the institutionalized postmodern culture, is in need of radical disciplinary and pedagogic re-orientation through what I have just described as strategic border re-alignment. What follows is a case in point.

The *B.A. (Hons.) in Cultural Studies* at Lingnan University, the first of its kind in Hong Kong and perhaps in the Chinese-speaking societies at large, was launched in 1999-2000 by its School of General Education. Today, the programme is housed within the new home of the Cultural Studies Department set up in September 2000. Before this relatively smooth process of institutionalization at Lingnan, the curriculum had been planned and written by a multidisciplinary team of scholars drawn from a range of disciplines and departments from the Humanities and Social Sciences. After months of intensive discussions, the proposed programme now has a basic structure. It consists of (1) a **Foundation Year**; (2) a **Core Module** of interdisciplinary courses; and (3) a **Stream of Study** in a disciplinary focus, to be chosen by all students after their first year. In the Foundation Year, students take a set of 7 wide-ranging courses as a broad-based background to their (specialized) degree in Cultural Studies. In order to provide the groundwork necessary for advanced courses, key humanities courses are included as part of the Major programme, such as *Chinese Civilization*, *Western Civilization*, *Cultural Transformation in Modern China,*

---

[8] For an in-depth look at a range of issues relating to aspects of the "postmodern university," see Smith and Webster 1997.

Literature and Cultural Studies, *Introduction to the Philosophy of Science and of the Social Sciences*, etc. They constitute a core foundation along with the 'proper' cultural studies courses like *Introduction to Cultural Analysis*, *Commodity Culture & Everyday Life*, and *The Making of Modern Culture*.

After the Foundation Year, the interdisciplinary Core Module covers the global perspectives, theoretical questions and contextual concerns in contemporary cultural studies, with an emphasis on local issues and developments. Apart from a small number of required advanced courses (e.g. *Culture Representation & Interpretation; Culture, Value & Belief; Readings in Cultural Studies*; *Cultural Policy and Institution* and *Critical Writing Workshop)*, students will take a range of optional courses from two Core Areas, "Themes and Perspectives" and "Contextual Studies" respectively. Course titles include: *Media, Culture & Society*, *Film & Cinema Studies*, *Gender & Sexual Politics*, *Culture, Power & Government, The Cultural Politics of Reading*, *Hong Kong Popular Culture*, *Narrating Hong Kong*, *Hong Kong Cultural Formation*, *Post-Colonial Studies*, *Issues in Identity & Public Culture*, etc. Along with the Core Module, students will also take 5 courses in the second and third year in a disciplinary focus, which allows them to approach society, culture and history from a well-defined set of scholarly perspectives and methodologies. Three such disciplinary streams have initially been included in the Cultural Studies degree, namely, "***Social & Political Studies***," "***Literary Studies***," and "***Cultural & Intellectual History***." These will be further consolidated into "***Literary & Media Cultural Studies***" and "***Social & Historical Cultural Studies***" in 2002-3. The streams have been identified as much for their specific ties to the understanding of the formation of modern culture, as for the specialist training they provide, respectively, in sociopolitical analysis, textual analysis, and the history of consciousness and material cultural forms. Course titles under the "Social & Political Studies" stream include: *Political Economy of Development*, *Rhetoric of Social Sciences & Business Studies*, and *Contemporary Sociological Theory*; under the "Literary Studies" stream: *Language and Power*, *Asian Voices in English*, *Modern Chinese Literature*, *Hong Kong Literature and Cinema* and *Taiwan Literature*; and under the "Cultural & Intellectual History" stream: *History of Ideas*, *Cultural & Historical Writing, Modern Chinese Intellectual Thought, Cultural Formation in Hong Kong, Marxism and After, Translating Culture* and *Contemporary Neo-Confucianism*.

Without dwelling on the details, let me offer quickly the following points relating to the design of the programme as an illustration of our pragmatic solutions:

1. A *Core-Stream model* is adopted as the main framework of the curriculum, with the Core Module embodying a transdisciplinary approach to the theory and practice of contemporary cultural studies (carrying a total of 33 credit-units), and the selected Stream of Study driving the course of study along a disciplinary route

(carrying 15 to 21 credit-units) not always heading in the same direction as Cultural Studies writ large as a self-contained "discipline."

2. Such a design anticipates tensions, encourages dialogue and allows for cross-fertilization between, on the one hand, a *trans*disciplinary core curriculum covering all the three kinds of research in cultural studies discussed earlier (with emphasis on media culture, identity politics, policy and institutionalization etc.), and on the other hand, a particular disciplinary speciality drawing on the sociopolitical, textual, and historical dimensions of cultural studies. The proportion between the cultural studies core and the disciplinary stream is managed (2:1) so as to make any easy homogenization or satisfactory translation among the various disciplinary territories unsettling, if not actually impossible. Such "border re-alignment" is a pointed reaction to the prevailing institutional practices in which arbitrarily defined modes of scholarship within closed borders have too often led to implicit devaluation of most other kinds of academic work *outside* (Damrosch 1995: 5).

3. Both the Core Module and the Streams of Study offered are prepared for by a common Foundation Year, which will be taught as common introductions to the dynamic study of culture as embodiments of value, sensibility, power and history. It is clear that the success of this kind of integrative pedagogy depends largely on progressive moves in new modes of interdisciplinary interaction and collaborative efforts (Damrosch 1995: 12). In addition, there is a dual objective here to (i) do cultural studies scholarship in a self-reflexive, liberal arts context; and (ii) develop a critical humanities perspective capable of dealing with the crisis of the subject (the subject of Humanities, in both senses of the word *subject*) often raised in relation to the state of university education today (Zavarzadeh and Morton 1986). Apart from pedagogic merits, the integrated curricular plan can also have gains from the point of view of academic administration and resource management (Readings 1995).[9]

---

[9] "A great deal of costs are saved, for example, by fusing the humanities under the rubric of 'cultural studies' (support staff, teaching credits, physical plant, and so forth), and we have to demand that university administrators plow back these savings into funding pedagogic initiatives… that allow interesting work to be done" (Readings 1995: 478); "resources liberated by the opening up of a general interdisciplinary space, be it under the rubric of the humanities or of cultural studies, should be channelled into supporting short-term collaborative projects of both teaching and research… which would be disbanded after a certain period, whatever their success" (489).

4. In view of the fact that even undergraduate curricula have increasingly been specialized nowadays, there has been a growing concern for the broad perspectives of General Education among tertiary institutions in Hong Kong. However, critical and innovative experimentations in pedagogic strategy (Giroux 1997, Straub 1994) have yet to take real form in the local educational contexts. The challenge of Lingnan's new Cultural Studies programme design is to integrate the dynamic of interdisciplinary cultural studies with the concentration of disciplinary scholarship in areas of common, though untranslatable, intellectual concerns. To develop a new language for our institution, we must question the kind of projects we do in a dynamic framework that is both transdisciplinary and international (Ferguson and Golding 1997, Pennycook 1994, Schwarz and Dienst 1996)

For benefit of long-term development, indeed, it is necessary for cultural studies scholars to collaborate with the increasing number of colleagues working on projects and initiatives of a similar nature within and across the borders of their respective disciplinary terrains. This will increase the extent to which the university as a community overlaps the hybrid cultural sectors at large, and consolidate the base upon which scholars carry out their work in dynamic collaboration with any new kinds of intellectuals involved in lifelong disputes with questions of truth. As "tenured specialists" we are all aware of our disciplinary isolation; as educators we seldom doubt whether it is a problem when the kind of alienation has become the condition of possibility of the knowledge-forms we pass on to our students (Damrosch 1995: 110, 6-7, 10).

On the secularization of the intellectual cause, Said has been asking such questions as – "How does one speak the truth? What truth? For whom and where?" Now, to be able to ask such questions to ourselves inside the ruins, we can no longer aspire to be "humanist" in the traditional sense, but see "truth" in relation to the complexity of a new form of imperial global power (Hardt and Negri 2000). A new and transdisciplinary programme in Cultural Studies will provide a base to develop the multiple perspectives needed to understand life in the university, as part of a collective process towards the shaping and constitution of a transdisciplinary *community*, certainly to be re-imagined today in the light of the changing global cultural economy. Working towards this end, we have been concerned with these questions about Cultural Studies as an educational programme: Has the language(s) of our culture been actively shaping the language(s) of the education we provide? Has agency been involved in the process? To what extent would the agency, which bespeaks the relevance of our culture, serve as the measure of the kind of scholarly activities we do within and through the institution? How often do we realize that the measuring criteria have themselves changed? And with what consequences?

In short, the minor educational objective of such a programme is to offer a focus site for studying global patterns of cultural imagination, institutions and politics in the contemporary world. Locally, such a project presents the Hong Kong Special Administrative Region in particular and China in general as a case of critical cultural studies, and allows institutional re-alignments to work towards developing the emerging field of cultural research and education on the local ground. We have cautioned how the real threat might not exactly be cultural studies as a disciplinary net, but the net of bureaucratic institution that operates aggressively in the name of Excellence. As Said would have it, "as a ranked amateur I am spurred on by commitments that go beyond my narrow professional career" (1994: 88). Dwelling in the ruins, we must see discipline not as primarily in the production of "excellent" work (Damrosch 1995: 14), but need still to envision "culture" as the field for engendering dialogue, difference, and dissent. Recognizing that the postmodern university is a complex historical institution, let us remember what it means to dwell in those ruins without recourse to nostalgia or vulgarity, and refuse "to believe that some new rationale [for Culture/University] will allow us to reduce that complexity, to forget present complexity in the name of future simplicity" (Readings 1995: 480).

Bibliography:

Appaduari, Arjun (1996) *Modernity at Large: Cultural Dimensions of Globalization*, Minneapolis and London: University of Minnesota Press.

Bataille, Georges (1973 [1957]) *Literature and Evil*, trans. Alastair Hamilton, London: Calder & Boyars.

Bennett, Tony (1998) *Culture: A Reformer's Science*, London, Thousand Oaks and New Delhi: Sage Publications.

Bhabha, Homi K. (1994) *The Location of Culture*, London and New York: Routledge.

Butler, Judith (1997) *Excitable Speech: A Politics of the Performative*, New York and London: Routledge.

Chambers, Iain, and Curti, Lidia, eds. (1996) *The Post-Colonial Question: Common Skies, Divided Horizons*, London and New York: Routledge.

Chen, Kuang-hsing *et al.*, eds. (1998) *Trajectories: Inter-Asia Cultural Studies*, London and New York: Routledge.

Chomsky, Noam (1969) "The Responsibility of Intellectuals", in: Chomsky *American Power and the New Mandarins*, New York: Pantheon.

Damrosch, David (1995) *We Scholars: Changing the Culture of the University*, Cambridge, Mass. and London: Harvard University Press.

Eagleton, Terry (2000) *The Idea of Culture*, Oxford: Blackwell.

Featherstone, Mike (1996) "Localism, Globalism and Cultural Identity", in: Wilson and Dissanayake, eds. *Global-Local: Cultural Production and the Transnational Imaginary*, Durham and London: Duke University Press.

Ferguson, Marjorie, and Golding, Peter, eds. (1997) *Cultural Studies in Question*, London, Thousand Oaks and New Delhi: Sage Publications.

Frow, John (1995) *Cultural Studies and Cultural Value*, Oxford: Clarendon Press.

Giroux, Henry A. (1997) *Pedagogy and the Politics of Hope: Theory, Culture and Schooling*, Boulder and Oxford: Westview Press.

Gole, Nilufer (1996) *The Forbidden Modern: Civilization and Veiling*, Ann Arbor: University of Michigan Press.

Hardt, Michael, and Negri, Antonio (2000) *Empire*, London and Cambridge, Mass.: Harvard University Press.

Harvey, David (1989) *The Condition of Postmodernity: An Enquiry into the Origins of Cultural Change,* Oxford and Cambridge, Mass.: Blackwell.

Jameson, Fredric (1998) *The Cultural Turn: Selected Writings on the Postmodern, 1983-1998*, London and New York: Verso.

Johnson, Richard (1986) "What is Cultural Studies Anyway?", *Social Text* 16, 38-80.

King, Anthony D. (1990) *Urbanism, Colonialism, and the World-Economy: Cultural and Spatial Foundations of the World Urban System*, London and New York: Routledge.

Lash, Scott, and Friedman, Jonathan, eds. (1992) *Modernity and Identity,* Oxford and Cambridge, Mass.: Blackwell.

Lloyd, Daivd, and Thomas, Paul (1998) *Culture and the State*, New York and London: Routledge.

Ngugi, wa Thiong'o (1986) *Decolonising the Mind: The Politics of Language in African Literature*, London: James Currey; Nairobi: Heinemann Kenya.

Niranjana, Tejaswini, Sudhir, P. and Dhareshwar, V., eds. (1993) *Interrogating Modernity: Culture and Colonialism in India,* Calcutta: Seagull Books.

Pennycook, Alastair (1994) *The Cultural Politics of English as an International Language*, London and New York: Longman.

Ray, Larry and Sayer, Andrew eds. (1999) *Culture and Economy after the Cultural Turn*, London, Thousand Oaks and New Delhi: Sage Publications.

Readings, Bill (1995) "The University without Culture?", *New Literary History* 26: 3, 465-92.

Readings, Bill (1996) *The University in Ruins,* Cambridge, Mass. and London: Harvard University Press.

Said, Edward (1994) *Representations of the Intellectual*, New York: Random House.

Sassen, Saskia (1994) *Cities in a World Economy*, Thousands Oaks, London and New Delhi: Pine Porge Press.

Schwarz, Henry, and Dienst, Richard, eds. (1996) *Reading the Shape of the World: Toward an International Cultural Studies*, Boulder and Oxford: Westview Press.

Smith, Anthony, and Webster, Frank eds. (1997) *The Postmodern University: Contested Versions of Higher Education in Society*, London: Society for Research into Higher Education and Open University Press.

Straub, Kristina (1994) "Burning the Commodity at Both Ends: Cultural Studies and Rhetoric in the First-year Curriculum at Carnegie-Mellon University", in: Isaiah Smithson and Nancy Ruff, eds., *English Studies/Culture Studies: Institutionizing Dissent*, Urbana and Chicago: University of Illinois Press.

Taylor, Charles *et al.* (1994) *Multiculturalism: Examining the Politics of Recognition,* ed. and intro. Amy Gutmann. Princeton: Princeton University Press.

Tomlinson, John (1999) *Globalization and Culture*, London: Polity Press.

Wilson, Rob, and Dirlik, Arif, eds. (1995) *Asia/Pacific as Space of Cultural Production*, Durham and London: Duke University Press.

Wilson, Rob, and Dissanayake, Wimal, eds. (1996) *Global-Local: Cultural Production and the Transnational Imaginary*, Durham and London: Duke University Press.

Zavarzadeh, Mas'ud, and Morton, Donald (1986) "Theory, Pedagogy, Politics: The Crisis of 'The Subject' in the Humanities", *Boundary 2* 15: 1-2, 1-21.

BRITISH/CULTURAL STUDIES "MADE IN GERMANY"

SEBASTIAN BERG

The purpose of this essay is twofold: it gives an overview of how three different varieties of British/Cultural Studies (Area Studies, Cultural Studies, British Studies) were developed in Germany and in what ways they were influenced by Cultural Studies. It then argues that British/Cultural Studies in Germany (or indeed anywhere outside Britain) must have specific starting points in order to allow insights into a society as a whole while simultaneously considering its diversity. Only then can it hope to achieve what is currently accepted to be its overall aim, namely "increasing intercultural competence". This cannot be attained without analyses of concepts of "culture" and how these are related towards "nation states". The essay concludes by offering a concrete example for investigating cultural practices in Britain, in which the nation is regarded as one category of collective identity formation among many.

Introduction

"Area Studies" (*Landeskunde*), "British Studies", "Cultural Studies", "Social and Cultural Studies" are short terms for diverse concepts within English Studies departments in Germany to integrate into research and English Language Teaching questions that reach beyond Literature and Linguistics. This article cannot provide a comprehensive summary of the debate on Cultural Studies in Germany.[1] It does not give a complete account of matters of contention. While some aspects have been thoroughly discussed (especially the Area Studies vs. Cultural Studies problem), others deserve further attention. Among these is the question why and how to investigate, and teach, cultures of a particular nation state[2] (i.e. Britain) if it is agreed that nation states are "multi-cultural", "regionally diverse" and "hierarchically structured" (Hoerder 1995: 76). This

---

[1] For example, it does not consider the "Area Studies/Area Science" approaches developed in the former GDR. Although there was some dialogue between the East and West German scholars involved, Area Studies in the GDR followed very different trajectories.

[2] With "state" I describe the institutional organisation of a society and the debates that help change or preserve these institutions. "Nation state" is used because in these debates "nationality" is often employed as an ideological device to legitimate certain institutions and procedures. Nation States are viewed as holding together one "nation" (e.g. Germany) or several "nations" (e.g. Britain).

question is particularly important for researchers and teachers approaching Britain from elsewhere, because an external perspective invites to viewing a nation-state-defined society (with its cultural practices, social relations and institutions) as a monolithic whole. I think, the British state *must* be considered through British/ Cultural Studies. But rather than regarding it as an overall analytical framework on what is called the "macro-level", it should be understood as one of several configurative categories on the "meso-level".[3] To illustrate my point, I will firstly juxtapose the different concepts of British/Cultural Studies and show how they try to define "culture", and how they relate "culture" to the "nation state". I will suggest a way of dealing with diversity within (British) society without completely dismissing the (British) state as *one* category that influences cultural practices, social relations and material conditions, thus shaping the life of (British) society.

The Development of British/Cultural Studies in Germany

Three strands within British/Cultural Studies in Germany can be identified. The first is a social- or political-science-based approach to Area Studies, focusing on the British state and its institutions. The second, closer to Cultural Studies in Britain, concentrates on cultural practices in British society and their material conditions, and has a particular emphasis on "texts". The third and most recent strand can be seen as an attempt to reconcile the other two through combining the aim of analysing British society and its institutions with categories and questions derived from Cultural Studies (Mountford and Wadham-Smith 2000: 2-3). The three approaches have a common goal: increasing "(inter-)cultural competence". How they intend to achieve this goal will be explained in the following paragraphs.

*Area Studies (*Landeskunde*)*

Area Studies became a part of foreign language learning in secondary and tertiary education after the Second World War. Because of the collaborative role German Cultural Science varieties (*Kulturwissenschaften*) had played in nationalist interpretations of "foreign cultures" in Nazi-Germany, re-educationists sought for "ideology-free" concepts of teaching and avoided culturalist terminology. They preferred a political education limited to "facts and figures" that implicitly propagated the acceptance of Western democracy. Area Studies as it was taught

---

[3] Dirk Hoerder and Jürgen Kramer both suggest to distinguish between three levels of cultural analysis: the micro-level of individual action and identity formation, the meso-level of given or chosen social units like, for example families, sociocultural groups, communities ("configurations"), and the macro-level of whole societies (Hoerder 1995: 76) or systematic categories (Kramer 1997: 77).

at schools, and at the English Studies departments of a few universities, understood itself as neutral and pragmatic. However, it tended to draw a biased and selective picture of a timeless, rural, middle-class Britain (Davids 1981: 40; Kramer 1997: 21).

Area Studies was modified with the political changes of the late 1960s. On the one hand, the scope and content of English Studies at German universities was questioned. In Literary Studies this led to the problematising and contextualising of the traditional canon. The functions of literature within capitalist societies were debated. Interest in didactic questions increased: "communicative competence" replaced "linguistic competence" as the major goal in English Language Teaching. Protagonists of Area Studies argued that as a precondition for communicative competence a more systematic knowledge of institutions and life in Britain was needed. This implied a more important but still an ancillary role for Area Studies. On the other hand, this subservient function was seriously challenged during the 1970s. Several protagonists of Area Studies hinted at a tension between the didactic goal of communicative competence and the more far-reaching goals of an Area Studies based on the political and social sciences (Buttjes and Kane 1978). Prominent among these goals was "emancipation". Reflecting such a politicized Area Studies in detail, Davids defined "emancipation" as the process which develops the abilities inherent in humans to overcome all psychological and social obstacles. Human beings should be empowered to shape social reality in accordance with their wishes and needs. Within society they need an orientation that enables them to form their own identity (Davids 1981: 33). Davids pleaded for a systematisation of Area Studies towards a more complete "Area Science". Based on materialist historiography, it should provide both facts, for orientation in society, and opportunities, for identification. The approach was deliberately partisan and suggested to concentrate on working-class life, working-class politics and social movements. This focus was seen as a corrective to the middle-class bias of textbooks and the limits of traditional historiography.

Such a project facilitated the incorporation of the "classics" of "British" Cultural Studies. However, the social factors, influencing if not determining life and cultural practices, were for Davids still solidly founded in the process of production, and thus played an important role. For many protagonists of Area Studies this is still the case today, although elements of the Marxist framework and parts of the liberatory project have been abandoned. People became more sceptical about the possibility of organised and collective emancipation programmes. The result was a period of stagnation and rethinking within Area Studies (Stinshoff 1989: 14); it arguably also constitutes a partial retreat into the sub-disciplines the protagonists had originally started out from (social history, political science, literary studies). Those working under the banner of Area Studies today hope to achieve "intercultural competence" through a comparative approach, i.e. through evaluating historical, structural, and institutional backgrounds of cultural and social practices different from the learners' personal experience (Kastendiek 1994). This echoes a belated debate in Germany about multicultural society in the early 1990s after a dramatic, and still continuing increase in acts of racist violence. However, overall Area Studies has become more modest. While Davids wanted to construe "transnational solidarities", authors nowadays are content with changes of individual behaviour towards tolerance, acceptance and understanding.[4] Whereas Cultural Studies is sometimes accused of having lost the social dimension of cultural practices, Area Studies has undoubtedly maintained its materialist core.

Cultural Studies

The emergence of Cultural Studies in Germany, beginning in the 1970s, was the result of the reception of the Cultural Studies debates in Britain. The proponents' arguments are based on the theoretical concepts developed within Cultural Materialism and (Post-) Structuralism. Additionally, they suggest ways of achieving cultural competence different from those favoured by Area Studies. The goal of Cultural Studies in the context of English Studies is more ambitious than that of Area Studies.[5] While Area Studies tried to establish itself next to Literary Studies and Linguistics (apart from the articulation of some more far-reaching goals in the 1970s), several proponents of Cultural Studies claim to initiate a whole-scale reform (or replacement) of Literary as well as Area Studies.

The materialist view assumes a relation between cultural practices and social relations. Cultural Studies thus deals with the subjective side of social relations (to express it in the terminology of Cultural Materialism). It deals, in other (more postmodern) words, with the negotiating, communicating and contesting processes that take place in the context of collective and individual identity formations. Cultures exist as processes and are pluri-vocal and fragmented. For describing collective cultures, proponents of Cultural Studies isolate specific categories of ascriptive differentiation (modes of being, modes of domination, modes of oppression) like class, ethnicity, gender, nation, age group etc. The resulting analyses of a "politics of identity" must be included in, or should even replace, Area Studies, which, otherwise, would have an insitutional bias (Riedel 1995).

The idea that cultures and identities are constructed through, and exist in, discourse leads to an increasing interest in (post-) structuralism and semiotics. Cultural Studies tries to evaluate the processes in which cultures are communicated. It reads cultures as signifying practices, and consequently as

---

[4] This at least seems to be the general agreement among a number of didactic contributions to Area and Cultural Studies (cf. Klippel 1994, Nünning and Nünning 2000).

[5] The interest in Cultural Studies is not limited to English Studies departments. It has made inroads into Ethnology, Media Studies and the few existing Cultural Science departments (Göttlich and Winter 1999: 32). The majority of people coming into contact with Cultural Studies, however, probably do so in an English Studies context.

texts. Important for Cultural Studies from a German point of view is that cultural texts are generally and most easily available not while they are produced but *after* they have been completed. This facilitates a kind of persistent "retreat" into the study of literary texts. For many, Cultural Studies means above all a new way of dealing with literature. Understanding cultures as multi-faceted and plural leads necessarily to the rejection of literary canons in the traditional sense. "New" literatures (and other fictional texts like movies) have to be included: e.g. working-class, women's and post-colonial literatures. Different questions are posed towards such texts: historical, political, psychological questions (Bassnett 1994; Riedel 1995). Literary texts, to summarise, are used as cultural sources and as expressions of processes of identity formation. As such they offer opportunities for an understanding of cultures that Area Studies with its emphasis on structures and institutions cannot provide. Proponents of Cultural Studies are strongly convinced that their approaches with their affective and subjective elements are more promising in terms of promoting an increased intercultural sensitivity (Riedel 1995: 72-3).

British Studies

British Studies contains elements of both, Area and Cultural Studies. Alan Mountford and Nick Wadham-Smith, although admitting that there is no unified "theory" behind British Studies, claim as its distinctive feature a "commitment to the centrality of the nation state as an object of study" (2000:6). Unlike Cultural Studies in Britain, British Studies is not primarliy concerned with "low cultures" (Bassnett 1994: 64). There is less emphasis on the institutional dimensions of public life than in Area Studies. Configurative categories developed in Cultural Studies – and used especially in its materialist version (class, ethnicity, gender, generation) – are employed in British Studies, too. Mountford and Wadham-Smith define it as a multidisciplinary study of contemporary Britain (but with a strong emphasis on history), which also includes theoretical concepts from Literary Studies and the social sciences. The aim of British Studies is to explore the distinctive features of British culture(s) and society (2000: 1). Similarly, Susan Bassnett suggests to elaborate through the examination of "key texts" (written, spoken, musical, visual) not only the social, economic and political realities of contemporary Britain (1994: 64), but also attempts of British society to (re-)define itself (Bassnett 1994: 66). British Studies thus is Cultural Studies applied to foreign perspectives, or a methodological extension of Area Studies.

This "dual character" of British Studies is not without problems, however (Mountford and Wadham-Smith 2000: 2); the question remains whether both parts (the socio-political and the cultural) should be approached as an integrated (Klaus 1995), complementary (Kramer 1997: 57), or hierarchically structured programme (i.e. Area Studies as subordinated, or as supplement to Cultural

Studies; see Riedel 1995: 64), or whether they should be entirely separate (Kastendiek 1994: 10).

There is another problem: namely whether to achieve "(inter-) cultural competence" either through implicit or explicit comparisons between the society of and cultures in another nation state and one's own. Although (inter-)cultural competence is regarded as a precondition, integral part and fundamental goal of both, language learning and the approaches outlined above, it is here, I think, where the concepts of Area, Cultural and British Studies have so far remained least convincing. Until now, there has been a debate on cognitive vs. affective approaches to cultural learning, where cultural knowledge or cultural awareness were favoured respectively. Area Studies has been associated with cognitive approaches and Cultural Studies with more holistic ones.[6] While the knowledge *versus* awareness question may still be important, I think that another more basic point is in danger of being omitted: the actual relation between culture and the nation state.

Culture and the Nation State

"Culture" is of course a difficult term. It is often employed in ambivalent or even contradictory ways. To demonstrate this, I will give a brief summary of a recently published article entitled "*British Cultural Studies konkret*" (Nünning and Nünning 2000).[7] Under the heading "From Culture to Cultures" the authors point out that among the most important insights of Cultural Studies is the realisation that there is no "culture" but only "cultures" (7). Thus English Language Teaching should make students aware of the multiplicity of British and American cultures and the differences between various national, regional and sub-cultures. Admitting that this can be done in an exemplary way only, the authors nevertheless stress the importance of avoiding too homogeneous and stereotypical presentations. They go on to argue that while students may be informed about some differences between "the" British and "the" [definite article in the German original] US culture, they often do not have the same knowledge about regional, social or ethnic differences within these countries. There might well be ignorance about other English-speaking cultures or hybrid "mixed cultures". The authors, claiming that in times of internationalisation and globalisation teaching must

---

[6] Unfortunately, the debate is marred by prejudices and stereotypes. See for example Riedel's claim that Area Studies will necessarily affirm the established order through reproducing hegemonic knowledge and does not cover marginal topics, while investigations of subjectivities (Cultural Studies) *necessarily* hint at the "darker side" of that established order (1995: 65).

[7] In my paraphrase the use of inverted commas and of "culture" and "cultures", in the singular and plural, is exactly as in the original. I would like to emphasize that my criticism is strictly limited to the use of the term "culture" here. It is *not* a general critique of the article's ideas.

address all these aspects, suggest as starting points analyses of expressions of popular culture or youth sub-cultures, which are as different to "the" particular high culture in English-speaking countries as they are in Germany (*ibid.*).

I am not concerned with practical proposals her but would like to point to the use of the term "culture" in this paragraph, especially in relation to the nation state. Of course I agree that there is no single, unified British or US-American culture. But the question is to what degree are cultures in Britain (or the United States) British (or American)? Do working-class and middle-class cultures (if one accepts this distinctions at all) in Britain have more in common than e.g. British working-class culture and, say, German working-class culture? If they do, how can these common elements be related to Britain? And, concerning the differences between "national cultures" within Britain and the United States: does this mean in this context that one should emphasize the multiplicity of British cultures but at the same time the unity of national cultures within Britain (a Welsh, Scottish and English culture)? And, to complicate things even further, what is a sub-culture, after all? Does the term imply that there is an overarching culture with several derivative cultures "below" it; does the term primarily refer to the subversive, oppositional potential of such a culture – or both? Are these (sub)cultures shared by regions, social classes, ethnic groups? To what extent is language the defining principle of these cultures? Are cultures only "mixed" or "hybrid" if they are based on more than one language? Would a Welsh culture (supposing, again, something like Welsh culture exists) be a hybrid culture? Finally, there is also the term of "popular culture" (in the singular) with its problematic relation to youth sub-cultures. Is there really something like a scale to measure the "highs" and "lows" of cultures? Given this irreducible polysemy of the term "culture", how can Nünning and Nünning possibly define the "target culture", whose comparison with one's own should improve one's intercultural competence?

Ambiguities like these often arise when cultures are investigated as those of "foreign nation states". What constitutes a state, is a specific form of organisation. As such it is, in the words of Walker Connor, a "major political subdivision of the globe" (1994: 36). A state relates to a society and to citizens rather than to one or several nations. States are structures that link together people, not "a people" or "peoples".[8] This has repercussions for investigating cultures: the idea of the nation clearly exists and constitutes an imagined community based eventually on a variety of the myth of co-sanguinity. But there is no reason why such a discursively constructed mode of being should be regarded as an analytical framework that is more relevant than others. Categories like gender, ethnicity, class, region are as important as the nation, rather than being mere sub-divisions within it. The "commitment to the nation state as an

---

[8] Walker Connor supposes that the interchangeable use of "nation" and "state" stems from the idea that all political power starts from the people (who often regard themselves as a nation).

object of study" must not lead to confusing the nation state with a clear-cut cultural entity. Thus, to summarise:

- It is not sufficient for promoting (inter-)cultural competence to compare the target culture with one's "own" culture.

- A state is shaped not by a nation but by institutions, even though these might mirror cultural practices, collective identities, and self-images of particular groups.

- Within and beyond nation-state-based societies there are hierarchies of different cultural practices. These should be explained not in terms of high vs. low but in categories derived from Cultural Materialism and/or theories of hegemony.

The easiest way to consider these suggestions is to change the levels and perspectives of investigation. There already are proposals to combine micro-, meso- and macro-level analyses (Hoerder 1995; Kramer 1997). What I want to suggest in the last part of this essay is that there needs to be more attention given to developments and frameworks at once below and beyond the nation state level.

Liverpool: A Case Study

Mountford and Wadham-Smith suggest that we continue using traditional categories of Cultural Studies like class, gender, ethnicity but apply them to wider contexts. In order to show the multiplicity and interrelatedness of cultural practices these categories should not only be used for analyses of British society as a whole but also of smaller entities, for example cities, regions, neighbourhoods, organisations, movements etc. If looking at a city like Liverpool as an object of study, it would soon become obvious that, on the one hand, its contemporary situation is influenced by historical developments relevant for the British state and British society as a whole and other societies in Europe: colonialism and the slave trade, industrialisation and de-industrialisation, immigration, the rise and fall of the labour movement, the emergence (and decline) of working-class cultures. On the other hand, these developments also constitute *particular* consequences for Liverpool's history and its present situation:

History and culture

Liverpool was at the heart of the triangular trade. Slaves and African sailors formed an early minority population in the city. For a long time (even after the abolition of slavery and the slave trade) the (former) slave merchants ruled the city. For many, the particular involvement of Liverpool's population in the slave trade, to whom the city owes its growth, explains the persistence of racism and colonial stereotypes among the local population (Law 1981; Christian 1995).

Economy and Culture

The city's industries were organised around the port. Port labour has its particular organisational features: workers for a long time were employed on a casual basis (and increasingly are again these days). This generated certain types of industrial relations, characterised by informality and high levels of strike action. In the late 20th century, social conditions became extremely difficult because a high percentage of the workforce depended on a collapsing port-related and manufacturing labour market. This again led to high degrees of social unrest (Lane 1987).

Ethnicity and Culture

Liverpool's geographical proximity to Ireland attracted a high number of Irish migrants to the city. Catholicism plays an important role within the city to this day. But Liverpool received migrants from many parts of the world. Liverpool's black population, however, lives relatively isolated and is poorly represented in local politics (Liverpool Black Caucus 1986; Ackah and Christian 1997).

Politics and Culture

On the one hand, Liverpool's labour movement developed comparatively late and remained fractured (because of antagonisms between Catholics and Protestants). The Labour Party is weak and has a patchy history in the city (Dye 1998). On the other hand the local workers became famous or notorious for their militancy, especially during their anti-poll tax campaign, or the dockers' strike.

Popular Culture

The city is famous for some of its popular cultural products: football, music, local novels and TV-soaps dealing with working-class life. A lot of local people have a strong affinity to their city. Elsewhere, there is a specific "Liverpool myth": the city is often regarded as a violent, run-down, dangerous working-class area. It is supposed to be different from other parts and cities of Britain (Lane 1987).

Liverpool can thus be investigated as a case of its own. It can be an example for specific "British" issues (for instance the social and cultural consequences of the de-industrialisation process in the 1980s). But it can also be an example for (post) industrial cities, port cities, slave trade cities, cities in peripheral regions, cities with religious antagonisms all over the world. This reveals the overdetermined and complex situations to which cultural practices relate. This understanding of the complex factors shaping cultural practices and collective as well as individual identities are crucial to achieve "cultural competence". Moreover, these complexities can be shown in both, contextualised literary and other texts, but also through social-scientific projects. The "commitment to the nation state as an object of study" seems as useful as it is unavoidable when investigating from "outside". However, the nation state as a concept should be placed where it belongs: on the configurative meso- rather than on the analytical macro-level.

Bibliography:

Ackah, William and Christian, Mark, eds. (1997) *Black Organisation and Identity in Liverpool: A Local, National and Global Perspective.* Liverpool: Charles Wootton College Press.

Bassnett, Susan (1994) "Teaching British Cultural Studies. Reflections on the Why and the How", *Journal for the Study of British Cultures,* Vol.1 No.1, 63-74.

Buttjes, Dieter, and Kane, Lawrence (1978) "Theorie und Zielsetzung der Landeskunde im Fremdsprachenstudium", *Anglistik und Englischunterricht* No.4, 51-61.

Christian, Mark (1995) "Black Struggle for Historical Recognition in Liverpool", *North West Labour History,* No.20, 58-66.

Connor, Walker (1994) "A Nation is a Nation, is a State, is an Ethnic Group, is a...", in: Hutchinson, John, and Smith, Anthony D., eds. *Nationalism,* Oxford: Oxford University Press, 36-46.

Davids, Jens-Ulrich (1981) "Orientierung und Identität. Stichworte zu einer emanzipatorischen Landeswissenschaft", in: Buttjes, Dieter, ed. *Landeskundliches Lernen im Englischunterricht*, Paderborn: Schoeningh, 30-49.

Dye, Jim, ed. (1998) *150 Years in Struggle. The Liverpool Labour Movement 1848-1998,* Liverpool: Liverpool Trades Union Council.

Goettlich, Uwe, and Winter, Carsten (1999) "Wessen Cultural Studies? Die Rezeption der Cultural Studies im deutschsprachigen Raum", in: Bromley, Roger *et al.*, eds. *Cultural Studies. Grundlagentexte zur Einführung*, Lüneburg: ZuKlampen, 25-39.

Hoerder, Dirk (1995) "Cultural Studies. Problems and Approaches", *Journal for the Study of British Cultures*, 2: 1, 75-80.

Kastendiek, Hans (1994) "British and American Studies. Proposals for a Comparative Landeskunde Approach", *Journal for the Study of British Cultures*, 1: 1, 9-19.

Klaus, Hans Gustav (1995) "An Agenda for British Studies", Unpublished paper at the 3rd Berlin English Studies Conference.

Kramer, Jürgen (1997) *British Cultural Studies*, München: Fink.

Lane, Tony (1987) *Liverpool. Gateway of Empire,* London: Lawrence and Wishart.

Law, Ian (1981) *Race and Racism in Liverpool, 1660-1950,* Liverpool: Merseyside Community Relations Council.

Liverpool Black Caucus (1986) *The Racial Politics of Militant in Liverpool. The black community's struggle for participation in local politics 1980-86,* London: Runnymede Trust.

Mountford, Alan, and Wadham-Smith, Nick (2000) "Introduction", in: Mountford and Wadham-Smith, eds. *British Studies – Intercultural Perspectives.* Harlow: Pearson/Longman, 1-9.

Nünning, Vera, and Nünning, Ansgar (2000) "British Cultural Studies konkret. 10 Leitkonzepte fuer einen innovativen Kulturunterricht", *Der fremdsprachliche Unterricht: Englisch*, 43: 1, *Teaching Cultural Studies*, 4-9.

Riedel, Wolfgang (1995) "Cultural Studies. Positions and Oppositions", *Journal for the Study of British Cultures*, 2: 1, 61-73.

Stinshoff, Richard (1989) "Einleitung", in Stinshoff, ed. *Die lange Wende. Beiträge zur Landeskunde Grossbritanniens am Ausgang der achtziger Jahre,* Oldenburg: Zentrum für pädagogische Berufspraxis, 5-16.

ACCOMMODATING DIFFERENCE: CULTURAL STUDIES, TRANSLATION AND THE LIMITS OF INTERDISCIPLINARITY

LAURENCE RAW

This essay focuses on how cultural studies has been translated into the Turkish context, in terms of its modernising framework, and how this has given rise to very particular (and often defiantly held) opinions on the interdisciplinary limits of the discipline. The first part concentrates on how translation as a concept has been perceived as a means to develop the national culture, especially in the education and publishing fields. Through a case study of one version of cultural studies, practised in departments of humanities, the following part discusses how the preservation of the national culture has been instrumental in determining the ways in which the discipline has been imported and subsequently developed. The conclusion suggests that the future of cultural studies in Turkey is intimately related to the material technologies of power and cultural policy.

In recent years, numerous books and articles have appeared, focusing on how cultural studies has emerged in different countries such as France, Germany, Austria, Australia, Britain, the United States, the Nordic countries, Finland, and Mexico.[1] With so much material appearing on the subject, one might be prompted to question the validity of writing about the Turkish context, other than to demonstrate that each country has its own version of cultural studies, which may be worthy of sustained empirical analysis.

Nonetheless, perhaps the subject may be of interest, on the grounds that, while being a comparatively new discipline (the first cultural studies-related courses only began to appear on university curricula in the mid-1990s), the subsequent progress of cultural studies been shaped by a continuing commitment to modernisation – in other words, the kind of cultural experience associated with notions of progress and development, especially in the West. Cultural studies has also been linked to a certain type of politics – democracy, citizenship, the nation-state. In the Turkish context, such values are especially important to the Kemalist project (instigated by Kemal Atatürk on the creation of the Republic in 1923) which has endeavoured to create a new national culture, combining Western models with local traditions. Even today, there is a noticeable reluctance by

[1] See, for example, Turner (1993, 1996); Forbes (1995); Burns (1995), Carey (1997), Ferguson and Golding (1997), Denzin (1999), Horak (1999).

many academics from all disciplines to discard the idea that modernisation will, one day, lead to a fulfilment of Turkey's destiny. There is a parallel suspicion of globalisation (and postmodernity) and the fragmentation of political and cultural identity that it is thought to entail (Rumford 2000: 140).

In this essay, I want to focus on how cultural studies has been translated into the Turkish context, in terms of this modernising framework, and how this has given rise to very particular (and often defiantly held) opinions on the interdisciplinary limits of the discipline. Firstly, I should like to concentrate on how translation as a concept has been perceived as a means to develop the national culture, especially in the education and publishing fields. Through a case study of one version of cultural studies, practised in departments of humanities, I shall subsequently discuss how the preservation of the national culture has been instrumental in determining the ways in which the discipline has been imported and subsequently developed. I shall conclude by suggesting that the future of cultural studies in Turkey is intimately related to the material technologies of power and cultural policy, demonstrating how, in Tony Bennett's words

> the relations of culture and power which most typically characterise modern societies are best understood in the light of the respects in which the field of culture is now increasingly governmentally organised and constructed (Bennett 1998: 61)

Translation and Modernisation

Following the creation of the Republic of Turkey, Ataturk introduced a wide-ranging programme of cultural reforms. The Turkish language underwent radical changes; in 1928, the Roman alphabet was adopted in place of the Arabic script, and throughout the 1930s, thousands of words of Persian and Arabic origin were replaced by newly-created terms borrowed from Turkic dialects, or technical terms derived from ancient and modern Western languages. The Ministry of Education published a series of Western classics in translation, using up-do-date Turkish; these were designed to reduce the Ottoman influence over Turkish culture (and thereby encourage people to support the Kemalist Republic and its aims), as well as providing the kind of education which was perceived as common to most advanced European nations. In 1941, the Ministry of Education established a Translation Office, with the participation of leading critics, writers and lecturers, who were responsible for the production of unabridged translations from original sources. A year later, the Ministry collaborated with the British Council in a scheme to render 'selected English classics' into Turkish; by 1945, the first of these – Shakespeare's *Coriolanus* – had appeared (Raw 1995: 92-3).

Most translators of the 1940s wanted to eliminate cultural differences between the original text and their own translations, so acculturation (or call it domestication) was employed as the main strategy. Lawrence Venuti has suggested that this kind of policy is characteristic of Anglo-American cultures, which are "aggressively monolingual, unreceptive to the foreign, accustomed to fluent translations that invisibly inscribe foreign texts with English-language values and provide readers with the narcissistic experience of recognizing their own culture in a cultural other" (Venuti 1995: 15). The translators in Turkey adopted the acculturation policy, in an attempt to persuade their readers that they were part of Western culture and civilisation. In other words, they were endeavouring to implement the modernisation programme of the young Republic. This also helps to explain why the classics, perceived as the primary sources of Western culture, were translated first. What most translators and critics of that period were arguing for was a notion of an ideal of Western culture to be accommodated into the Kemalist Republic – a canon of so-called "great works" which contained, in true Arnoldian fashion, "the best which has been thought and said in the world". The acculturation strategy helped to "humanise" such material, making it intelligible to the widest possible readership. A translator who was successful in this domesticating process could be considered "a great author", whose works deserved to be considered on a par with the original text.[2]

But translation is not only a linguistic process, but involves more formal operations. In other words, translation is a mode, as well as a specific act, whereby fundamental structures are reproduced and/or reinvented in different contexts. To ensure that translators acquired the kind of cultural literacy, that would enable them to engage with great works of Western literature, several university departments of foreign languages – known as philology departments – were created; and with government support produced an impressive output of research and publication, together with new curricula based on western models. In the Department of English Philology at Ankara University, the origins of the four-year undergraduate programme could be traced back to Oxford University, combining basic literature courses (Shakespeare, the Romantics, the eighteenth and nineteenth century novel) with courses in English grammar and philology, Latin and Greek (Raw 2000b: 3). Such initiatives have been characterised by Akbar Ahmed as part of the "Muslim modernist phase", in which the leaders of many Muslim states adopted a policy of acculturation – reinterpreting Western cultural values in what they perceived as the best interests of the communities they represented (Ahmed 1992: 30).

In the decades since the creation of the first departments of foreign languages and literatures, there has been a gradual tendency towards specialisation. English Philology departments have been transformed into English Language and literature departments, concentrating mostly on literature. English language teaching is currently undertaken in a variety of institutions – private language schools, secondary schools, and university preparatory schools, which are designed to prepare undergraduates for the rigours of their four-year degree courses. In at least two universities, new departments of translation and interpretation have been established. What is most striking, however, is the extent to which departments are still influenced by the kind of values established over

[2] I am indebted to Özlem Berk of the University of Muğla for many of these observations.

half a century ago. Learning a foreign language – particularly English – is important, as it makes an important contribution to "the process of modernisation" in Turkey (König 1990: 90). Through exposure to the best works from the West – even if one does not intend to translate them into Turkish – students can arrive at an "objective and holistic understanding and a sound judgement", which should equip them well in their future careers (Akbulut 1998: 7). However, any approaches to foreign language learning, which might have been developed with Western learners in mind, should be subject to a process of acculturation. Thus it may be more advantageous to teach "the English language through local contexts which learners are familiar with", as well as through exposure to materials derived from the West, to avoid the possibility of "serious socio-psychological problems" arising if learners have "to develop a new identity through the target culture" (Özögül 1998: 25).

Case Study: Cultural Studies in Humanities Departments

It is against this background of a continuing commitment to modernisation based on a respect for Western values, coupled with an emphasis on acculturation, that we should consider how cultural studies has been translated into the Turkish context. On the face of it, it seems that one of the chief attractions of the discipline has been an interdisciplinary mode of study, which, according to one professor of English Literature, permits lecturers to "expand the [literary] canon by including texts of popular culture and other types of cultural texts … Students … must be helped to understand the forces involved in the production, distribution and consumption of works of both high and popular culture, as well as the forces at work in the construction of meaning and identities in a culture" (Menteşe 1998: 88). Unlike cultural studies in Britain, which sought at the outset to challenge established notions of the canon (understood, in this case, as a corpus of literary texts, promoting an aesthetic and élitist conception of culture), cultural studies in English Literature departments rests on a particular notion of interdisciplinarity, in which the value of the English literary canon is re-emphasised through the study of texts drawn from other disciplines, for example, media studies. This form of interdisciplinarity enables students to appreciate the value of the arts and learning, helping them to make informed judgements on the values of everyday life. The process of "doing cultural studies" is thus inherently Arnoldian in character, helping to sustain and defend the best of culture:

> My first [cultural studies] course was "Canon and the Media", in which we compared the film versions of 19th and 20th century literary texts. The first thing to do was to understand the two different languages – the language of literature and the cinema. We also looked at how a literary work changes when it is filmed – for this, the students brought in videos of the novels we studied, and compared them with the texts. I learned a lot about film language, film technique, and what decisions a director has to make when adapting a novel for the cinema (Menteşe 1999: 2).

To describe this version of cultural studies as interdisciplinary in nature might seem a contradiction in terms (after all, English Literature is still perceived as the most important ingredient in the course). Nonetheless, we have to understand that the term interdisciplinarity has been subject to a process of acculturation – in other words, it has been translated into a form perceived by Turkish scholars as the most appropriate for their students. By studying the literary canon of a Western (in this case, English) culture, students are exposed to the kind of values which contribute to their development as human beings (Doğramaci 1999: 15):

> Students of English Literature are much more understanding, much more tolerant, and open to new ideas. In general, they do not like violence.... [Literature] should bring people together ... and to be open to criticism.

Yet this knowledge is only important insofar as it enriches "the [Turkish] state, [and] … nationality" (Doğramaci 1989: 11). Thus students should be encouraged to develop practical skills – not only improving their spoken and written English, but acquiring the kind of critical and inter-cultural competence which will guarantee future prosperity in the world of work (Doğramaci 1999: 15):

> Literature can … contribute to students' development as human beings, understanding the ways in which people behave and react in given situations, as well as being made aware of the social and economic conditions of a foreign country. Students become much more open to the world as a result of literature and language; it enriches their life and their experiences of life.

If this is what can be achieved, then it is hardly surprising that most English Literature departments adopt what might be perceived in other contexts as a very restricted view of interdisciplinarity.

The importance of maintaining the tradition of translating Western values into Turkish terms, and thereby contribute to the modernising process, cannot be underestimated. Talât Halman, a former Minister of Culture, now Professor of Turkish Literature at Bilkent University, Ankara, insists that one should not mimic what has already been theorised in the West, but to find a voice of one's own (Halman 2000a: 1-2):

> My concern is not for people over-relying on theories, but rather becoming over-enamoured of theory, without absorbing or digesting it properly. Then they simply repeat it, parrot-like, and then translate it, thereby giving the impression that they are doing new and interesting work, when clearly they're not ... We have to look at Turkish culture in all its facets… using the best and most advanced ideas from the West and elsewhere… We have to create a synthesis of such theories with our own methodologies to study our own culture, as well as form new independent opinions of foreign cultures.

In looking at cultural studies in Turkish humanities departments, it is important to stress the concern – shared by many scholars – to maintain a commitment to modernisation and Western values in the face of what have been perceived as the twin "threats" of globalisation and Islamism. In a recent paper, Chris Rumford has suggested that "Modernity [understood, in this case, as a commitment to progress and gradual development] and nationalism are under threat from 'the globalizing trends and high technologies of the market ... [which] ensnarl the country with all their energy and unruliness'" (Rumford 2000: 143). The commitment to Western values is also perceived as being challenged by a new form of Islamic modernism, combining industrial and cultural expansion with a regulation of social life "that would ultimately guarantee the constitution of a 'virtuous' society'" (Atasoy 1996, Magnarella 1998). To counteract these possible dangers, many Kemalist-oriented groups, including literature departments, have endeavoured to forge "a new consensus that makes communication across social, political and theoretical divides possible while upholding the universal [i.e. Western-oriented] principles of truth and justice" (Bozdoğan and Kasaba, quoted in Rumford 2000: 146). It is this belief in consensus which determines the limits of inter-disciplinarity in literature departments: students may study texts drawn from other disciplines, but ultimately they should all be able to appreciate the value of literature, both as a cultural product of the West, and as a means to sustain the Kemalist national culture.

In recent years, however, there has been a concerted effort by universities – especially in the private sector – to restructure their humanities departments. A two-semester basic English course for first-year students at Bilkent University, including what is described as a substantial cultural studies element, advertises itself as genuinely "inter-disciplinar" in nature, offering programmes in non-research based writing in the first semester, and research-based writing in the second. The university itself is "committed to a 'liberal arts' approach in education, meaning that students should have the opportunity to study areas outside of their own faculty". They can take a variety of courses, ranging from the Holocaust to film and media studies (Hodson 2000: 1). In the academic year (2000-1) the university implemented a more extensive programme of humanities education for engineering students, organised by American faculty members, which seeks to broaden students' understanding of Western culture and their own culture through exposure to a wide variety of material, both literary and non-literary (Komins, 2000). Another programme run by the Department of Cultural Studies at Sabanci University, Istanbul (currently the only humanities department in Turkey to call itself a cultural studies department), invites students

> to explore a range of theoretical models and methodologies for studying the critical relationship between culture, knowledge and power. It is designed to introduce students to the related disciplines of Anthropology, Literary Criticism and Cultural History, and to familiarise them with the scholarly norms, practices, and ethics necessary to investigate the conditions of production, reception and use of

> contemporary forms of symbolic representation and communication (Sabanci University 1999: 1).

On the face of it, such programmes aim to establish an interdisciplinary model quite different from that of English Literature departments. Here the emphasis is on freedom of choice; on students being able to transcend disciplinary boundaries and create their own combination of subjects. By doing so, they might become better equipped to investigate the "conditions of production and reception", both in their own culture and other cultures, and thereby acquire a more developed sense of intercultural competence.

This new approach to interdisciplinarity, I suggest, could not have been possible in Turkey, were it not for the economic reforms of the 1980s instituted by the then President Turgut Özal. He was implacably opposed to what he called the "deification of the state", arguing that "development was no longer the prerogative only of the state". The objective was a new liberalised economic order, open to foreign investment and trade, while at the same time "inculcating a sense of freedom and responsibility to ... ordinary people" (quoted in Robins 1996: 73-4). In the educational sphere, Ozal's policies led to the establishment of private universities set up by entrepreneurs with government help (Bilkent University was the first in 1985; now there are some 15 universities, concentrated in Istanbul and Ankara). Students were now treated as both learners and customers, with the freedom to choose whether to pursue further education in the state or private sectors. Even if they could not pay the fees, the private universities offered scholarships, in order to attract the most academically gifted students. Since the mid-1980s, most private universities have continually tried to market their supposedly unique qualities – a web-based education, or an interdisciplinary approach to cultural studies which provides a flexible alternative to the traditional (one might say rigid) subject-based education at state universities.

Yet perhaps this model is not as radically different as it pretends to be. A web-based education – particularly if it encourages students to interact with lecturers and teachers from other cultures, or with Turks living abroad (for example, the *Gastarbeiter* in Germany) – might prompt questioning of those "universal principles of truth and justice", which lie at the heart of the Turkish national culture. Consequently most private universities have introduced humanities education as a way of disseminating these principles. The inspiration for this can be traced to post-1945 America, where many educational curricula were designed to promote a belief in "the principles of a free society… the definition of democracy in a world of totalitarianism, the effort to fortify a heritage of Western civilisation, and the need to provide a 'common learning'… as a foundation of national unity" (Russo 1979: 486).

The educational philosophy here is very similar to that of the American conservative E.D. Hirsch jr., who wrote in the late 1980s that "if we had to make a choice between the one and the many, most Americans would choose the principle of unity, since we cannot function as a nation without it." America may be proud of its pluralist traditions, but nonetheless its culture contains shared values, such as "altruism and self-help... equality, freedom, truth-telling and respect for the national law" (Hirsch 1987: 95, 98-9). Humanities education may incorporate cultural studies, but it should be translated into Turkish terms – in other words, subject to an acculturation process which enables students to appreciate the "universal principles of truth and justice" lying at the heart of the national culture. Like their counterparts in English Departments, members of the cultural studies department at Sabanci define their objectives in developmental terms: whereas they might not be exposed to the entire English literary canon, students should make use of cultural studies to become "'cultured' and culturally sensitive". "Cultured", in this sense, can be defined as the acquisition of sufficient linguistic and/or inter-cultural competence to pursue careers "informed by culture (ranging from journalism, advertising, public relations, art and literary criticism to politics, diplomacy or administration)" (Sabanci University, 1999: 1).

This case-study raises certain interesting questions about the purpose of interdisciplinarity. Should one depart from established subject areas, and introduce more radical curricula? Can the notion of interdisciplinarity be translated (or more precisely, acculturated) in a context where a homogenous national culture is promoted over pluralism? Is the term simply a marketing tool, imported by Turkish university departments from the West to demonstrate their commitment to modernisation, and at the same time attract the interest of potential undergraduate students? Such questions might equally be asked of cultural studies within the Turkish context: does it represent an effective alternative to established disciplines; should it be interdisciplinary in focus; and what exactly is its purpose? Perhaps the answers might be found if we bear in mind that, unlike many versions of the discipline in the West, which question establishment values (particularly the various manifestations of power), cultural studies in Turkey is perceived as a vehicle for promoting such values, especially the national culture. Any future progress in the discipline has to be viewed in terms of cultural policy, involving scholars who have set the educational agenda for many years, and who still have an important role to play in forming the images that the Turkish nation presents both to itself, and within the international arena.

Cultural Studies and the Policymakers

Major debates over cultural studies in Turkey are comparatively recent: until the late 1990s, with the growth of private universities offering new curricula, most departments (in common with English Literature) were content to accommodate certain aspects of cultural studies into their existing programmes. It was only with the establishment in 1996 of an annual cultural studies conference at Ege University, a state university in Izmir, with the financial support of two foreign cultural agencies, the British Council and the United States Information Service (now part of the State Department), that the purpose of cultural studies as a separate discipline came under scrutiny.[3] In a keynote speech to the 1999 conference, Talât Halman (whom I have referred to earlier on) challenged Turkish colleagues to "turn [their] attention to [their] Turkish culture and bring [their] accumulated knowledge and expertise in terms of new perspectives, new analytical strategies to the field... It is very rich, waiting to be discovered by its own people" (Halman 2000b: 11).

Within six months, a new group had been formed, comprising twelve academics from various departments, in both the state and private sectors, calling itself the *Turk Kültür Araştirmalari Grubu* (Group for Cultural Studies in Turkey). Its main aims, as set forth in a mission statement, were as follows:

> Cultures generated over centuries in what is now Turkey and by Turks ... constitute an invaluable heritage. Yet studies pursued in this field of culture... often do not go beyond descriptive work that merely transcribes or reports documentary material. Devoid of a critical perspective and failing to offer any synthesis, these studies have fallen behind cultural studies done currently in the West... [which] have evolved in an interdisciplinary direction...

The Group has defined its aim as "using an interdisciplinary scholarly approach, to develop methodology and theoretical formulations by carrying out research in cultural history and comparative cultural studies; and to conduct and support applied studies" (Cultural Studies Group 2000: 1).

In June 2000, the Group held a major two-day seminar, supported by the Ministry of Culture, on "Migration on our Culture", in which members spoke briefly about different facets of cultural studies, both in Turkey and elsewhere. Topics included a brief history of the discipline in Turkey, popular culture, cultural studies in anthropology, architecture and cultural studies, literature and cultural studies. The seminar participants (around 75 in all) were subsequently divided into discussion groups, organised by subject area (literature, social science, fine arts, etc.), and debated the future of cultural studies in Turkey, before coming together for a final panel.

Press reaction to the event tended to be divided into two camps. On the one hand, there were those who believed that existing subjects – such as literature – already covered much of the theoretical and methodological ground mapped out by cultural studies. If this is the case, then there is very little need for extensive educational reform (Onaran 2000). On the other hand, there were others who stressed that cultural studies could contribute to the process of modernisation, through an analysis of the workings of power in Turkish society (Kahraman

[3] It should be noted that I have been intimately associated with organisation of these conferences, as a member of the British Council in Turkey; and subsequently participated in the Group for Cultural Studies in Turkey's activities. In a sense, therefore, I am writing from the point of view of a cultural policymaker.

2000), or through the regular publication of short essays on the topic, in both Turkish and English (Kirtunç 2000).

Leaving aside the question of the press for the moment, perhaps we might look more closely at the Group for Cultural Studies, its purpose and its aims, in the light of the preceding discussion on translation, cultural studies and interdisciplinarity. It is evident from the name "Group *for* Cultural Studies", that the group perceives itself as acting in the national interest, and has the support of the Ministry of Culture to prove it. There may be conflicts between individual group members, but such conflicts are mitigated by a shared belief in progress and/or modernisation. The *ends* are the same; it is the *means* that differ. This creates a paradoxical situation, in which the Group for Cultural Studies' activities are informed by the principles of certainty (a shared concern for the national culture) and doubt, wherein all knowledge is formed as a series of hypotheses open to challenge (Giddens 1990). The Group, as an institution, provides a classic example of the workings of power, as described by Stuart Hall:

> Instead of thinking of national cultures as unified, we should think of them as a discursive device which represents difference as unity or identity. They are cross-cut by deep internal divisions and differences, and 'unified' only through the exercise of different forms of cultural power. (Hall 1992: 297)

Sixty years ago, the Ministry of Education created a Translation Bureau, with the specific purpose of translating canonical works from the West into Turkish, and rendering it accessible to the widest possible readership. It seems that history has repeated itself: the Ministry of Culture has chosen to sponsor a group whose stated aim is to translate cultural studies into new Turco-centric forms. If successful, the creators of such forms would be considered (both within Turkey and abroad) the equals of, not inferior to their colleagues in the West; and because their work is written in Turkish, rather than English, they could encourage future scholars and students towards a deeper understanding (and appreciation) of the indigenous culture.

At the most basic level the Group for Cultural Studies' work is interdisciplinary, in the fact that its members are drawn from different disciplines – literature, sociology, anthropology, architecture. On the one hand, this represents a radical departure from established educational practice – apart from isolated instances (such as the cultural studies programme at Sabanci University), academics have restricted their focus of attention to their own subject discipline. On the other hand, the limits of interdisciplinarity are clearly defined: as the mission statement suggests, it exists to promote a synthesis of material drawn from different disciplines, helping academics to formulate a "critical perspective", which will enable them to emulate the kind of "cultural studies done in the West". Only then will they be able to carry out effective research into their own culture. Again the emphasis is on progress, development and modernisation: interdisciplinarity will help to broaden the scope of research into Turkish cultural studies.

The Group provides a good example of the workings of the public sphere in what Habermas has described as "social-welfare-state democracies". Representatives from diverse subject constituencies negotiate and compromise among themselves and with government officials (representatives of the Ministry of Culture), while excluding the public from their proceedings. Public opinion – as expressed at the June seminar – is, to be sure, taken into account, but not in the form of unrestricted public discussion (Habermas 1989: xii). The limits are clearly defined, both through the Group's mission statement, and through the papers accepted for presentation at seminars. Press coverage serves less as a means of providing a forum for information and debate, and more as a means for promoting the Group's message about the importance of creating a new cultural studies *for* Turkey. Of the four reviews that appeared following the seminar in June 2000, two were written by Group members themselves (Halman 2000c, Kirtunç 2000), one was authored by a member of Sabanci University's cultural studies faculty (Kahraman 2000), while the remaining review was written by a literary critic (Onaran 2000).

Given this background, it might be wondered whether there are any opportunities for resistance; to look at cultural studies not from an interdisciplinary but rather an anti-disciplinary perspective, permitting radical intervention in the debates over the future of the national culture, or how educational curricula should be restructured. Certainly there has been a good deal of research on cultures of displacement and transplantation; cultures which might be described as internally diasporic. Recent analyses of Istanbul's rapidly expanding upper-middle class suburbs (Daniş 2000) and gypsy culture (Yumul 2000), have revealed the existence of hybrid identities, which may undermine the belief – lying at the heart of Kemalism – in a homogenous Turkish culture.

Yet it is also true to say that it is because of the strength of the national culture that anti-disciplinary cultural studies has been allowed to flourish. Researchers are free to write (and publish) whatever they wish; they may choose to be "radical" in their approach, but such radicalism is legitimated by the fact that it is (mostly) confined to state and/or private university departments. Moreover, what may appear "radical" from one point of view might well be considered "progressive" from another – in other words, helping to advance the progress of cultural studies, both as a separate discipline within universities, and as a means to investigate (and hence ensure the survival of) Turkish culture.

Bibliography:

Ahmed, Akbar (1992) *Postmodernism and Islam*, London: Routledge.

Akbulut, Ayşe Nihal (1998) "The Archeology of Translation Excavations Into The Multiple Layers of Text Sites", *Litera* 12, 1-19.

Atasoy, Yildiz (1996) "Islamic Revivalism and the Nation-State Project: Competing Claims for Modernity", Internet site www.epas.utoronto.ca

Barker, Chris (2000) *Cultural Studies: Theory and Practice*, London: Sage.

Bennett, Tony (1998) *Culture: a Reformer's Science*, London: Sage.

Burns, Rob, ed. (1995) *German Cultural Studies: an introduction*, Oxford: Oxford University Press.

Carey, James W. (1997) "Reflections on the Project of (American) Cultural Studies", in: Ferguson and Golding, *Cultural Studies in Question*, 1-24.

Cultural Studies Group (2000) "The Aim of the Group", Internet site www.cstgroup.org/eng/amac/ana_metin.html.

Daniş, Asli Didem (2000) "The upper middle class suburbs of Istanbul: Identity or Diversity", in: Raw and Kirtunç, eds. *Dialogue and Difference*, 123-31.

Denzin, Norman K. (1999) "From American sociology to cultural studies", *European Journal of Cultural Studies* 2:1, 117-36.

Doğramaci, Emel (1989) "Turkish Cultural Values: Identity and Religion", unpublished lecture, Hacettepe University, Ankara.

Doğramaci, Emel (1999) "Interview with Laurence Raw", *British Council Newsletter*, May, 15

Edgerton, Susan Huddleston (1996) *Translating the Curriculum: Education and Cultural Studies*, New York and London: Routledge.

Ferguson, Marjorie, and Peter Golding, eds. (1997), *Cultural Studies in Question*, London: Sage.

Forbes, Jill, ed. (1995) *French Cultural Studies: an introduction*, Oxford: Oxford University Press.

Giddens, Anthony (1990) *The Consequences of Modernity*, Cambridge: Polity Press.

Habermas, Jürgen (1989) *The structural transformation of the public sphere: An inquiry into the category of bourgeois society*, trans. Thomas Burger, London: Polity Press.

Hall, Stuart (1992) "The question of cultural identity", in: Hall, Stuart; Held, David; and McGrew, Trevor, eds. *Modernity and its Future*, Cambridge: Polity Press.

Halman, Talât Sait (2000a) "Interview with Laurence Raw", 14th March.

Halman, Talât Sait (2000b) "A Monologue on Indifference", in: Raw, Laurence, and Kirtunç, Ayse Lahur, eds. *Dialogue and Difference, Proceedings of the fourth Cultural Studies Seminar, Ege University, Izmir, May 1999*, Ankara: The British Council, 3-15.

Halman, Talat Sait (2000c), "Kültür genlerimiz" [Our cultural genes], *Milliyet Pazar*, 2nd July, 15.

Hirsch, E.D., jr (1987) *Cultural Literacy: What every American needs to know*, Boston: Houghton Mifflin.

Hodson, Daren (2000) Letter to the author, 10th April.

Horak, Roman (1999) "Cultural Studies in Germany (and Austria) and why there is no such thing", *European Journal of Cultural Studies* 2:1, 109-15.

Kahraman, Hasan Bülent (2000) "Kültürel araştirmarlar kavrami ve bir toplanti" [The concept of cultural studies and a meeting], *Radikal*, 19 June, 9.

Kirtunç, Ayse Lahur (2000) "Fazla cilt kültürü bozar!" [Excessive works on culture are superfluous], *Radikal*, 30th June.

Komins, Benton Jay (2000) "Interview with Laurence Raw", 22nd March.

König, Güray Çağlar (1990) "The Place of English in Turkey", in: Bozer, Deniz, ed. *The Birth and Growth of a Department*, Ankara: Hacettepe University, 85-95.

Magnarella, Paul J. (1998) "Desecularisation, State Corporatism and elite behavior in Turkey", in *Anatolia's Loom: Studies in Turkish Culture, Society, Politics and Law*, Analecta Isisiana XXX, Istanbul, The Isis Press, 233-57.

Menteşe, Oya Batum (1998) "The experience of British Cultural Studies in Turkey", *Journal for the Study of British Cultures* 3, 85-94.

Menteşe, Oya Batum (1999) "Interview with Laurence Raw", *British Council Newsletter*, July, 7-8.

Onaran, Mustafa Şerif (2000) "Kültür arastirmarlari" [Cultural studies], *Hurriyet Ankara Bolgesi*, 2nd July.

Özögül, Esra (1998) "Turkish students' perceptions of American Culture: implications for target culture learning", M.A. thesis, Bilkent University, Ankara.

Raw, Laurence (1995) "Translating Theatre Texts: *As You Like It*", *Shakespeare Worldwide* XIV/XV, 91-102.

Raw, Laurence (2000a) "Perspectives on British Studies at Turkish Universities", in: Mountford, Alan, and Wadham-Smith, Nick, eds. *British Studies: Intercultural Perspectives*, Harlow: Pearson Education Ltd., 21-35.

Raw, Laurence (2000b), "Reconstructing Englishness", paper presented to the 6th University of Warwick/ British Council conference on British Cultural Studies, website www.britishcouncil.org/ studies/england/raw.htm

Robins, Kevin (1996) "Interrupting Identities: Turkey/ Europe", in: Hall Stuart, and Gay, Paul du, eds., *Questions of Cultural Identity*, London: Sage, 61-87.

Rumford, Chris (2000) "Turkish identities: between the universal and the particular", in: Raw, Laurence, and Kirtunç, Ayse Lahur, eds., *Dialogue and Difference, Proceedings of the fourth Cultural Studies Seminar, Ege University, Izmir, May 1999*, Ankara: The British Council, 139-49.

Russo, John Paul (1989) *I.A.Richards: his life and work*, Baltimore: Johns Hopkins University Press.

Sabanci University (1999) Department of Cultural Studies, undergraduate curriculum, Internet site http://www.sabanciuniv.edu.tr/english/ssb/cult.html

Turner, Graeme (1993) *Australian Cultural Studies*, London: Routledge.

Turner, Graeme (1996) *British Cultural Studies*, 2nd edn., London: Routledge.

Venuti, Lawrence (1995) *The Translator's Invisibility: A History of Translation*, London: Routledge.

Yumul, Arus (2000) "Representations (Images), Counter-Representations (Counter-Images) and Identities", in: Raw and Kirtunç, *Dialogue and Difference*, 111-23.

THE PHANTOM MENACE STRIKES DOWN UNDER

MANDY OAKHAM

In 1995 the opening shots of the so-called Media Wars were fired. This alleged great battle was between the forces of the purist Empire of journalism education and the dark forces of cultural studies. The struggle took place against the backdrop of the modern university in Australia a corporate terrain where the contours are marked out by self-interest, territory and bitter politics. This chapter examines the aftermath of this war and its implications for the future of any genuine interdisciplinarity in the modern university context. The author argues for a rapprochement between the two disciplines stressing their commonalities as opposed to their differences suggesting that the real lesson of the Media wars is that new or disputed disciplines hold to notions of authentic, untainted knowledge at their own peril.

Once upon a time in a land far, far, away villains and heroes battled in a great struggle for territory inspired not only by a claim to power but a claim to righteousness. This imperialistic struggle took place against the backdrop of the modern university in Australia, a corporate terrain where the contours are defined with markers of self-interest, territory and bitter politics. Although this mighty battle was fought out within the Australian context, there are universal disciplinary lessons to be learnt.

In the dark galaxy of Australian education there is the evil Empire run by a government intent upon slashing university funding. There is a constant stream of refugees and escapees who flee to other systems where intellectual activity still has value. Those left within the system do daily battle with their own Supreme Vice Chancellors fighting for funding, student load, research points and ultimately for survival. This essay will examine the aftermath of one battle where the two "enemy" camps could have gained much from seeking alliances rather than aggression. While this battle is certainly not the only interdisciplinary struggle to take place in the new corporate education sphere in Australia it was certainly one of the most public and understandably, given its questioning of the teaching of journalism, became the focus of much media attention.

A headline featured in *The Australian's Higher Education Supplement* at the height of the battle in March 1998 perhaps said it all, "Journalism versus culture a pointless game" (41). Cunningham and Flew's article under the headline told a slightly different story. They described this interdisciplinary struggle as a:

> subset of the wider debate about the relationship between vocational and generalist or liberal arts education in an Australian higher education sector under pressure to deliver vocational relevance as much as intellectual stimulation to its student clientele. (41)

This essay intends to use this struggle as a case study to demonstrate commonalities between the disciplines as opposed to difference. It should be noted that analysis is premised on acceptance of both cultural studies and journalism as disciplines in the sense that both can be identified as working with identifiable sets of knowledge and a designated project or object of study.

The opening shots of the Media Wars, as they were dubbed in Australia, were fired in 1995. As always in every great battle there were conscripts forced into confrontation by virtue of their location within the perceived journalistic ranks. Some conscripts found themselves in "no-man's land" and this was a battle fought out in a mostly masculinist terrain with the loudest wails coming from pierced egos.

The great battle down under was fought out between the forces of the Republic, the Jedi Knights of Journalism flashing their lasers of factual empiricism against the massing dark forces of the Federation, some disguised as media studies exponents, but most were wearing their eclectic uniforms of cultural studies flashing their own light savers of radical contextualism and other sinister linguistic devices. These dark forces were led by the biggest Darth Vader of them all… John Hartley.

War was declared by Hartley in his article "Journalism and Modernity" published in the *Australian Journal of Communication.* Among the "shots" fired by Hartley was his claim that journalism "has never achieved stability as an academic discipline with its own institutional apparatus of courses, professors, methods of inquiry, specialist language, findings and debates; its own books, journals and conferences" (1995: 23). His attack continued with the allegation that:

> Journalism is not taught as a branch of learning, not even as a distinct research field but as a professional qualification which foregrounds the technical skills of producing journalistic output in words and (sometimes) pictures. Rarely do journalism courses ask their students to consider the conditions for journalism's existence: where it comes from, what it is for, and how it works in the context of modernity. Students are simply asked to do it without understanding it. (1995: 23)

Journalism he dismisses as "a 'profession' which cannot police its own boundaries, personnel standards or price which has no essential (defensible) body of knowledge and practice" (1995: 24).

Some of Hartley's accusations were just simply wrong. A simple glance at the statistics for the study of journalism in Australia shows how wrong he is. It is a fast growing discipline with its own books, journals such as the *Australian Journalism Review*, as well as its own conferences organised by the Journalism

Education Association of Australia and the South Pacific. There are professors and associate professors in journalism schools and programs. A glance at the subjects covered in the key journal for the discipline, the *Australian Journalism Review*, show an increasing emphasis on building the theoretical basis for the discipline.

But what exactly is the size of the disputed territory? Does the teaching of journalism in Australia constitute a spoil worthy of the ferocity of the Hartley attack? In a 1996 survey Patching estimated that there were around 5,000 students across the country studying journalism in some format at around 18 institutions. That number has now increased to around 22 programs. Today you will not find one program which does not contain some subversive theory even if it is hidden under the non-threatening banner of something like "Journalism and Society".

It should have been enough to point out the inaccuracies and move on, however, Australian academic Keith Windschuttle, who owns and operates his own journalism training centre, Macleay College in Sydney, declared all-out war. At the end of 1995 in his address to the Journalism Education Association's annual conference in Christchurch, New Zealand he thundered that there should be "no more theory" in the teaching of journalism.

He received support from some within the ranks of the Journalism Education Association and various volleys and outbursts appeared in many outlets reaching a crescendo with the publication of the book *Journalism: Theory and Practice* in 1998 by Windschuttle's privately-owned Macleay Press.

The general aims of this book, according to editor Myles Breen, was "to put together a wide variety of theories that can be applied to practical situations"(1998: 2). In the same introduction Breen is honest enough to admit the self-interest which motivated the book and in so doing identifies the cause for the seemingly unnecessary violent reaction to Hartley's original, mostly inaccurate taunts:

> As the training of journalists has moved to a university setting in Australia, more than a century later than in the United States, the imperatives of higher education structure have demanded that journalism educators rethink their professional role. The reality of the academy is that 'theory' is a saleable commodity when the monetary grants are distributed by the administration. A discipline without a written body of theory (literally a 'literature') is unthinkable in a university culture. (2-3)

Elsewhere in the same introduction Breen identifies the continuing problem for some, who while employed to teach journalism within a university context, still have problems in accepting it as an academic discipline. Breen talks about the eyes of journalists (that is the client group): "eyes glazing over whenever the word theory is applied to their craft" (1998: 2). This attitude, which still exists in the world of Australian journalism education, was apparent in an article by Rees published in the right wing magazine *Quadrant* in March, 1999.

The same magazine had earlier published what Rees referred to as "Windschuttle's brutal disrobing of the cultural theory emperor" which he believed was worthy of the "highest commendation" (21). Rees' tirade continued:

> My problem is not with cultural theory; as long as it is quarantined where it can do no harm, it and its adherents should be free to worship as they wish. But when the cult-theorists unleash their contumely on journalism there is danger of contagion. (1999: 22)

The declaration of hostilities obviously found some fertile ground within the ranks of journalism educators. The battle hymn in the Breen book, however, as expected was found in the chapter written by the war lord himself, Windschuttle.

He declared, "Journalism, in other words, upholds a realist view of the world and an empirical methodology" and "media theory does not deserve the academic standing it has" and that "it has no place in the professional education of journalists" (1998: 17-18). His chapter also includes attacks on the main enemies of English literary critics like Hoggart; the Frankfurt School and Althusser, the French structuralists and the postmodernists. Further he argues that:

> While journalism educators are trying to teach students to use active voice, short sentences, concrete nouns and verbs, precise grammar and clear meaning, they are faced with cultural studies courses that reward students who ape the passive voice, arcane abstractions, long and turgid expressions and grammatical howlers that characterise the latter. (1998: 31)

Most students, he claims, "…come to regard media theory as a largely incomprehensible and odious gauntlet they must run in order to be allowed to do what they really came to the institution for, to study media practice" (1998: 32). Cultural studies is further damned because of its "linguistic idealism" (1998: 24) and "supercilious illogicalities" (1998: 27).

In chapter eleven another journalism educator Martin Hirst launches his own attack on Hartley. Donning a protective guise of new journalism Hirst writes, "For Hartley the appearance of an edition of *Vogue* magazine in French (of course) edited by Nelson Mandela, 'marks a decisive shift from modernist to postmodern journalism…' I'd like to take Hartley by the throat, shake him like a wounded animal and chew on the meagre evidence he offers to defend his thesis. I want to rip the heart out of Hartley's claims for this 'new', 'postmodern' journalism" (1998: 200). Unbelievably it appears that Hartley appears to take these threats seriously.

In his 1999 reply he warns that within the book edited by Breen and published by Windschuttle were an "armed rabble plotting an ambush by disguising themselves as scholars, lying in wait among the branches of knowledge… for some unsuspecting cultural studies fop... to happen by…" (1999: 227).

Hartley was right in his response to Hirst's "death threat" that it is not enough to simply mark up your practice as theory, and he was also right in labelling the Winschuttlian push as an attempt to "see off the theorists" (1999: 228), or, as Tomaselli and Shepperson described it: "Windschuttle's valiant attempt to transfer cultural and medial studies into a conceptual trash heap" (1999: 237).

He should have stopped there. He then continues on to conclude that "journalism is a violent profession" (1999: 232). It is in his description of the cadetship process described as "young cadets have the crap kicked out of them by overbearing and unsympathetic supervisors whose job it is to prepare them for the factory system of news production"(1999: 232), that we may find some of the psychological motivation for Hartley's original attack on journalism. It is alleged that Hartley in an earlier, pre-academic life, spent a short time as a cadet on a newspaper. Clearly he did not find it a pleasurable experience. Despite the diversion Hartley does arrive at the right conclusion. He warns that the "hard-won and still limited acceptance of journalism studies is put in jeopardy" (1999: 235) if a sound theoretical base for the discipline is not fixed and nurtured.

The Breen/Windschuttle eclectic collection received mixed reviews overall even within the Australian journalism education ranks. Many however agreed with Wendy Bacon's review of the book in the *Australian Journalism Review* when she concluded:

> While most of the contributors would agree that journalists should be 'committed' to attempting to tell 'the truth', most also understand that the practice of journalism is much more complicated than suggested by realist philosophy. (1999: 162)

Further she concludes that, "What this book should show is that the Media Wars have run their course. There never were two camps in Australian journalism research – those with Windschuttle and those with the textualists led by Hartley. Rather there is a range of approaches, which in time will develop and cross-fertilise" (1999: 167).

That cross-fertilisation is clearly ongoing. Oakham (2000) in a new book on Journalism theory suggests that current theoretical thinking on journalism in Australia could be divided into four camps identified as being:

- journalism as commodity
- journalism as autonomous consciousness
- journalism as cultural activity
- journalism as empirical facts

Drawing on the work of C.Wright Mills outlining the three key questions that social analysts have asked Oakham (1998) suggested that the fundamental questions that journalism theory must interrogate are:

- What is the structure of journalism in relation to our wider society? What are its essential components and how are they related to each other? How does it differ from other professions in the social order? Within the profession, what is the meaning of any particular feature for its continuance and for its change?

- Where does journalism stand in relation to its own history and the history of society in which it is performed? What are the mechanics by which it is changing? What is its place within and its meaning for the development of humanity as a whole? How does it affect and how is it affected by any particular historical period? What are the characteristics of its history making?

- What are the varieties of journalism which now prevail in society?

- What other varieties have come into existence or have not prevailed? What are the factors operating here? (1998: 26)

If this is the task for those developing journalism's theoretical base then clearly some cross discipline engagement must be on the agenda. While the disciplines may rage at each other at the level of rhetoric what is actually happening at the level of practice in journalism programs across Australia? Those working at the white board face are clearly not as antagonistic to theory, and indeed to cultural theory, as the "Windschuttlians" would like.

Ian Richard is the head of the postgraduate journalism program at the University of South Australia and clearly recognises the need for some engagement between the two disciplines:

> Obviously the media are a major component of 'culture' and journalism is an important part of the media. Accordingly cultural studies should be able to inform the process of analysing aspects of what journalism is about. There is a strand of cultural studies which is extremely relevant to answering the fundamental question 'what is journalism' (epitomised by the work of James Carey). All of this suggests that there are grounds for collaboration between some of those working from a cultural studies perspective and some of those working from a journalism perspective.

Lynette Sheridan Burns is the former head of department of communication and media arts at Newcastle University and shares similar views:

> I think cultural studies has a crucial role to play in helping journalists understand the impact of the cultural context on their work. Putting it simply, cultural studies helps to explain why some revolutionaries are 'freedom fighters' and others are 'anti-government rebels' and why a single group of people gathered in a public place may be variously described as 'hooligans' or 'citizens'.

Burns said that the concept of journalism as "cultural practice" underpins the university's journalism program. She argues that for the program to produce "critically reflective practitioners", students must understand "their own cultural perspective and the effect of the dominant culture on the way they work."

Michael Meadows heads up the journalism program at Griffith University and is even acknowledged by Hartley as being "among those Australia media academics with whom I share many theoretical and disciplinary assumptions, and with whom I am personally on cordial terms" (1999: 227).

Meadows identifies the five themes underpinning his journalism program as being "news and news judgement; reporting or evidential method; linguistic technique; narrative technique; and method of interpretation or meaning..." (1998: 16). He further argues that journalism can adopt a "principle of articulation" (1998: 4) from cultural studies which will allow it to look at the way in which relationships are produced in particular social, cultural and historical contexts.

Journalism "might be theorised as a set of cultural practices... It is a key cultural resource that plays a pivotal role in the strategic management of cultural goods, like the media, in the process of the formation of the 'imagination' and thus, consensus and culture" (1998: 8). He further draws on Gramscian notions of hegemony alongside his proposal for an integral journalism that can have a transformative impact on commonsense. Finally he urges to look at journalism as a cultural resource and examine its role in the formation of culture.

We are obviously now in territory very far removed from that alien, hostile world of journalism studies described by Hartley. What the Media Wars did demonstrate was the folly of interdisciplinary war and the views of the journalism educators quoted above surely point us to the fruits of genuine interdisciplinarity. The most superficial glance at the current development of the journalistic discipline in the Australian context can see overtures and alliances and unions being formed with other disciplines like sociology, applied ethics, philosophy, politics, psychology. The war also highlights many of the present tensions and future trajectories within the terrain of the new academy. The alleged battle between cultural studies and journalism is actually about the battle for survival, the common problem for new entrants and old hands alike in the hostile academy. An article in *The Australian* in July, 2000 begins with the statement that it was only three years ago that the "prestigious Australian Academy of the Humanities bowed to the inevitable setting up a new division for communications and cultural studies. They did so 'because the level of scholarship in those areas was achieving such prominence,' says Graeme Turner, the director of the Centre for Critical and Cultural Studies at the University of Queensland" (22).

The article then goes to outline the dismal scenario that Turner is one of the two last inaugural fellows elected to the academy to remain within the Australian education system. In the same article another of those fellows, John Frow, who has left the Australian system for a post at Edinburgh University is quoted as saying, "There is a real sense of demoralisation in the Australian university system" (22).

Marginson (2000) sets out the dismal statistical profile of tertiary education in Australia. In the mid 1970s Australia had 270,000 higher education students and spent 1.4per cent of gross domestic product in public funding of education.

At the start of the 90s he estimates 500,000 higher education students with 1.1 per cent of GDP in public funding. Ten years later he estimates 800,000 students with public funding now running at less than 0.8 per cent of GDP. Faced with this as context then surely alleged "enemy" disciplines must look for common ground to make their stand.

The Common Ground

Within the Australian context both journalism and cultural studies have demonstrated that they can be both pragmatic and adaptive within the academic environment. They both have *had* to be.

Both disciplines have shown that they can respond to shifts in student or "client" demand. Both could also be described as holding out the promise of popularity which can encourage the lowering of institutional drawbridges within the academy. Enrolments in journalism programs across Australia have been consistently high, certainly exceeding the demands of the profession.

Both journalism and cultural studies work with the aim of deconstructing and articulating the process of some forms of culture. The study of journalism of course may have a more specific focus, for example, the acculturation of journalists and their specific domains, that is the newsrooms, but the framework is still the broader culture. As Zygmunt Bauman (2002) argued culture is becoming the prism through which other traditional disciplines are now fracturing and examining their knowledge bases.

Turner in addressing a 2000 seminar at Deakin University in Melbourne, Australia argued that cultural studies has been "less concerned with internal health" than other traditional disciplines. The same could also be said of the journalism discipline. Both, it could be argued have focussed more on the objects of their study at the expense perhaps of truly critical, reflexive appraisal of how they and others within their discipline carry out that study. At the same seminar Turner argued that cultural studies is "multily formed" and seeks to problematise reality. Likewise journalism problematises the process of news production and current developments within the discipline also testify to it being "multily formed" in the sense that it draws on broad theoretical and methodolgical frameworks. Both "theory shop" to have academic credentials and both could be said to have employed promiscuous methodologies. A collection of cultural studies essays, as indeed a collection of work in journalism, reveals threads of sociology, philosophy, semiotics, ethnography, textual analysis and engagement with the discourses of economics, politics, and history; and within these discourses there are as summed up by Frow and Morris, "incompatibilities, divergences and edges of disagreement as well as resonances between them..." (1993: xi).

Turner speaks of cultural studies being appealing to the academy because it could be done with "existing knowledges", that is, no new paradigm was needed before the discipline could begin its work. The same could be applied to journalism.

Both also in their quest for university recognition such as tenure, promotion, grant getting, face the real possibility of being institutionalised in a way they would reject, or at least regret. Both cultural studies and journalism would contend to have "ethical" positions. If British cultural studies as epitomised by Hall *et al.* was developed with the intent of a political intervention it could be argued that journalism as a discipline was also developed with a partially political interventionist base. Most journalism educators would see themselves as playing a role in intervening in the ever-increasingly, concentrated commercial circles of news production and inserting those non-commercial concerns like social responsibility and the public interest.

Both face or have faced institutional marginality. Both have had to face up to the academic sneer, that sneer being what place does the study of the everyday, the mundane, the routine of life, be it the content of the tabloid page or the essence of soap operas, have within the academy? Both have had their objects of study questioned as well as their methods of study. Hartley himself wrote that journalism "entered the realm of formal learning late, reluctantly, and without much of a welcome from the existing inhabitants" (1995: 23).

Both gain value through incorporation from other disciplines. Both have sometimes hidden within the skirts of the other more traditional disciplines such as sociology. This is surely ironic given that sociology experienced the same breech birth into the academy.

Both disciplines contain within them their own, to use the Marxian term, kernel of contradiction – a kernel which in turn could threaten their continued existence. For both academic approval may mean a loss of some aspects of their perceived projects. Journalism educators face the continual dilemma of instilling critical thinking about the practice of journalism in their students while fully acknowledging that students adopting such a critical line with the major employing news groups will rarely find a permanent position. Milner acknowledges the problem for Australian cultural studies and for all cultural studies, that the "mythic history" surrounding the founding fathers of Hoggart, Williams, Thompson and Hall make it clear that each would "have been opposed to the notion that Cultural Studies should ever become a formal academic discipline. They appear to have imagined it either as a political intervention into the academy and its existing disciplines or alternatively as the paradigmatic instance of interdisciplinary studies" (1999: 272-273).

If Windschuttle is to ever to be seen as one of the founding fathers of the journalism discipline, at least in Australia, then it is clear that he would have shared the anti-disciplinary attitude attributed to these other "godfathers."

The frequent use of the word "craft" at least by Australian journalism educators, but also in evidence when reading both British and American journalism texts, reflects the continuing ambivalence to the rigour imposed by both professionalism and discipline. As Morgan 1998 argued from the journalistic perspective:

> Theory is, of course, always tentative and provisional. It is also disciplined by actuality... Yet in many fields theory is often seen as the antithesis of practice. Many practising journalists see journalism as a lively occupation, organically responsive to and intimately entwined in the social and cultural milieux in which it is undertaken... For them theory is all too academic... For others it threatens their mystique and their autonomy. (54)

Having identified the commonalities between the disciplines, how then build the rapprochement towards interdisciplinarity so clearly needed in the current terrain of university life?

Clemens (1998) identifies what he calls the four "commonplaces" or "ages" or "motifs" of contemporary cultural studies. These are "universal reportage", "bricolage", "vagabondage", and "anecdotage". Here Clemens gives us at least the linguistic bridges between these two disciplines, and, perhaps more significantly, provides the future project for both. Clemens quotes Mallarme's definition of this reportage as consisting of:

> ...revealing only the monotonous outward aspects of the world, as news-boys do... All that is vulgar which receives no more than the stamp of immediacy (1998: 109)

Surely both journalism and cultural studies have turned their attention to the monotonous, outward aspects of the world and in so doing have revealed the vulgarity in such aspects. In so doing they have also earned themselves the jibes of doing the work of "news boys" or as Clemens calls it " bad rock journalism" (1998: 109). But also having done this work as disciplines they reveal the heroic, the nobility, the poetry and the beauty in everyday existence. There is always more in this monotony than just the "empirical facts" much loved by Windschuttle.

The next motif as described by Clemens is "bricolage". He quotes Lévi-Strauss's description of the *bricoleur* as someone who works with his hands and is "adept at performing a large number of diverse tasks" (1998: 110). The *bricoleur* works with a set of tools or a knowledge base which is the "contingent result of all the occasions there have been to renew or enrich the stock or maintain it with the remains of previous constructions or deconstructions" (1998: 110-111).

Both in their development of theory and their practice those who work within the cultural studies or the journalistic frameworks clearly have to be *bricoleurs* and should be applauded as such. Clemens argues bricolage "constitutes an affirmation of the supposedly irreducible and heterogeneous multiplicity of cultural and sub-cultural practices themselves" (1998: 111). Here again we have confirmation of the project common to both disciplines.

The next motif, "vagabondage", Clemens defines as the "perambulatory antics" which provide cultural studies with a theme and a model of practice. "For cultural studies not only loves to walk – it abhors and repudiates sedentary or immobile entities and cultivated sites" (1998: 111). There is also in this notion of vagabondage an element of skirting, if not direct violation, of state imposed laws. Again it would seem if both disciplines are to carry out their projects there should be such opposition to absolutism and to prescription.

Finally Clemens moves to "anecdotage" which he suggests rather than being the stories of the "interminable rattling bores" he says should be seen as the:

> attempt to present the construction of the subjectivity that presents within the presentation itself in order to – and despite appearances to the contrary – arrest the absolute dissemination and mobility of form and content to which this subject seemingly assents and to which it is responding. (1998: 112)

One of the continuing problems in the development of a viable theoretical base to journalism has been the struggle to articulate the role of the subjective in a daily practice which clings to a cloak of threadbare objectivity. Critical reflexivity maybe the goal of some who teach journalism but rarely is it shared or practised by the practitioners.

Clemens argues that if these motifs were fully recognised then cultural studies would be not as "dispersed or as undefinable as it so often seems" (1998: 113). Cultural studies would also be able to differentiate itself from other disciplinary formations. Clemens believes that the four motifs or "knots" can also be reconfigured to lead to cultural studies' undoing but I would argue that they can still be used to provide linguistic frameworks for identifying the commonalities between this discipline and that of journalism.

An incorporation of these motifs by both would result in dynamic, engaged disciplines delighting in their promiscuous methodologies and theoretical strands, articulating the overlooked or suppressed narratives of their designated cultural milieux. Reprimands from their designated objects of study they would wear as confirmation of their project.

The Media Wars and their focus on interdisciplinary challenges have made many Australian journalism educators question their role, their pedagogy, their methodologies as well as the content of their programs. Disciplines must engage and contest and, as Tomaselli and Shepperson identify, this engagement must move beyond that point which they describe as "importations" which "tend to be canonical, derivative and cut-and-paste into local conditions" (1999: 248). Adoptions of the Clemens motifs should avoid such perfunctory introductions. As Cunningham and Flew conclude:

> Journalism educators, while quite properly maintaining the necessity of professional qualifications for staff teaching the core skills of the field, often strongly endorse the need for their students to be exposed to the broad range of ideas and concepts found in liberal arts education. Similarly, if journalism is the 'sense making practice of modernity' to use cultural and media studies theorist John Hartley's phrase, then media and cultural studies have much to gain from a serious engagement with its professional codes and practices (1998: 41)

Also as Frow and Morris argued there is some worth in identifying "methodological insecurity, perhaps with a certain fruitful insecurity about… legitimacy as a discipline, but perhaps too with the way it conceives its object as being relational rather than substantial" (1993: xix).

They of course were referring to cultural studies but I would argue the position would also hold for journalism. Both disciplines while maintaining this "fruitful insecurity" should hold onto the security of their designated projects and an insistence on the role of agency in both their projects.

Frow and Morris also described culture as a "a contested and conflictual set of practices of representation bound up with the processes of formation and reformation of social groups" (1993: xx). They could just as easily have been describing the news production process and again reinforce the closeness between these two disciplines and their projects.

There is also another struggle which can be identified here and it is the disciplinary struggle with the notion of authenticity. Authentic is defined by the dictionary as being "real, genuine, true" and such words immediately raise journalism's long-running struggle with the spectre of objectivity. The struggle is further clarified when this definition is contrasted with that of synthetic as being "artificial" or that which is "put together or combined." Looking at the words we can perhaps see that the obstacle to true interdisciplinarity lies in those journalism educators who see synthesis as dilution rather than strength.

What perhaps the Media Wars exposed more than anything else was that new or disputed disciplines hold to notions of their own claim to some authentic, untainted knowledge as their own at their peril. Chemistry has taught the lesson that compounds can deliver strength and stability.

Conclusion:

Birch argues that "creating an ethic of dissent has been a crucial part of the cultural studies agenda in the West" and claims that all associated with it should continue to maintain a "counter-hegemonic position" (2000: 143):

> This core – this demand for interrogation, for dissatisfaction with comfortable solutions, for exploring the alternatives, for recognising that scholarship and criticism are political acts, for insisting on establishing new answers, new knowledges, new ways of thinking – this core should be at the heart of all scholarship, every discipline. (2000: 151)

The above should be the ultimate brief for both journalism and cultural studies.

Our energies should not be wasted in interdisciplinary squabbles but we need to work again the real threats to intellectual work. What should be clear from this case study is that the confrontation between the two disciplines was prompted from outside. There were obvious individual issues of ego at stake but there were also potentially more damaging structural catalysts at work here. It is only because of the reconfiguring of tertiary education systems that both were so clearly ready to respond to challenges to their perceived weaknesses by accentuating their perceived strengths. Both perhaps should consider this proposition. Were the claims of the cultural studies camps based on their alleged academic strengths but fueled perhaps by the challenge of lack of vocational relevance? And does journalism on the other hand need to consider its own deficiencies as it basks in its vocational strengths and frets over its perceived lack of academic antecedents.

Our role as academics is being constantly figured and reconfigured by the number crunchers as we speak. The expansionary economic and political forces operating within and without of universities… these are the real dark forces. If cultural studies is to provide some of the critical weapons to support the consolidation of journalism within the academy then so be it, and if cultural studies can benefit from the large numbers of students attracted to the vocational journalism then so be it. Survival has to be the first concern of all disciplines in the current climate.

To return to Hartley and his original assault, if the journalism discipline is a "*terra nullius* of epistemology, deemed by anyone who wanders by to an uninhabited territory of knowledge, fit to be colonised by anyone who's interested" (1995: 27) then let the colonisation begin. Hartley said that journalism as discipline "has attracted no Foucault to analyse its power relations, no Derrida to unthink its presumption of the innocence of its writing, no Williams to historicise its mode of cultural production" (1995: 29-30). It is time to prove him wrong!

There is clearly mutuality within both the designated projects of these two disciplines. Both share the responsibility to challenge the centre, as well as the margins. The emphasis of both disciplines should be on the lived culture, be that in a newsroom or on the football terraces. Here both disciplines will find their genuine constituents. As the Jedi Knight Master says to his pupil in *The Phantom Menace*: "Your focus is your reality."

Milner argues that cultural studies "will therefore find itself sooner or later to negotiate some sort of accommodation between itself" and what he describes as "contagious socio-discursive formations" (1999: 279) which take place within the university context. Surely the crucial issue is not that this accommodation takes place but rather the terms under which this occurs. What is crucial is that it must occur as the result of genuine intellectual exploration and engagement and not under the economic compulsions of the new corporate university capable of inducing the schizophrenia and paranoia so transparent in the Media Wars.

May the force be with us all!

Bibliography:

Bacon, W. (1999) "Review of *Journalism Theory and Practice*, *Australian Journalism Review*, 21: 1, 161 –168.

Bauman, Z. (2002) see "Postscript" in this volume.

Birch, D. (2000) "Transnational Cultural Studies: What Price Globalisation?", *Social Semiotics*, 10:2, 141–156.

Breen, M., and Windschuttle, K , eds. (1998) *Journalism Theory and Practice*. Sydney: Macleay Press.

Burns, Sheridan L. (2000) Interview with Oakham, March 2000.

Clemens, J. (1998) "A report to an academy in Cultural Studies and New Writing", *UTS Review* 4: 1, 107-122.

Cunningham S., and Flew T. (1998) "Journalism versus culture a pointless game", *Higher Education Supplement, The Australian*, March 25, 41.

Frow, J. and Morris, M. (1993) *Australian Cultural Studies; A Reader*, St Leonards, NSW: Allen and Unwin.

Hartley, J. (1999) "Why Is It Scholarship When Someone wants to kill you?: truth as violence", *Continuum* 13: 2, 227-236.

Hartley, J. (1995) "Journalism and Modernity", *Australian Journal of Communication* 22, 20-30.

Hirst, M. (1998) "Journalism Theory and Practice" in Breen, M., ed. Marginson, S. (2000) "Cash cure for campus blues." *The Australian* May 9, 13

Meadows, M. (1998) "Making Journalism: The Media as a cultural resource", *Australian Journalism Review* 20: 2, 1–23.

Milner, A. (1999) "Can Cultural Studies Be Disciplined? Or should it be punished?", *Continuum* 13: 2, 271-281.

Oakham, K.M. (1998) "Kick it, Karl: A jump start for journalism theory", *Australian Journalism Review* 20: 2, 24-34.

Oakham, K.M. (2000) *Journalism: Beyond the Business in Journalism: Theory in Practice,* South Melbourne, Australia: Oxford University Press.

Rees, T. (1999) "In Defence of Journalism", *Quadrant Magazine*, March 1999, 21-22.

Richards, I. (2000) Interview with Oakham, March 2000.

Tomaselli, K. and Shepperson, A. (1999) "The poverty of journalism: media studies and science", *Continuum* 13: 2, 237-253.

Turner, G. (2000) Address to Deakin Faculty of Arts on the formation of a new cultural studies major. Melbourne, Australia, April 2000.

CROSSING THE 'THRESHOLD OF INTOLERANCE': CONTEMPORARY FRENCH SOCIETY

KARIMA LAACHIR

Contemporary debate around immigration and asylum seekers, xenophobia and new varieties of racism, and social tensions rising in different parts of Europe would greatly benefit from an intervention by Cultural Studies. This essay explores the paradoxes of post-colonial, post-industrial France where cultural and ethnic cohabitation has recently been put in jeopardy. It can be argued that while the increased presence of the Maghrebi ethnic communities (the major "visible" ethnicities in France) has been blamed for crossing the French '*seuil de tolerance'*, French society itself has crossed a certain 'threshold of intolerance' by its widespread rejection of 'foreigners' or outsiders whose culture and values are considered as incompatible with 'Frenchness'. This, of course, runs against the egalitarian and humanitarian principles of French Republicanism itself, which has welcomed large numbers of immigrants throughout its history. This somewhat paradoxical situation calls for a new response to the recent transformations in cultural and national identity. Summoning the interdisciplinary and international field of cultural studies, this contribution attempts to read the specific post-colonial and post-modern French cultural and social context with its conflicts between the Republican tradition of universalism and the delayed negotiation of its plural and multicultural social reality.

Cultural studies is itself a 'diasporic' field of research which flexibly allows its 'practitioner' to migrate from one discipline to another. Since its establishment in the eighties, its main purpose has been to promote scholarship that will render the humanities politically effective and intellectually 'useful' to the analysis of social, political and economic tensions.[1] Its trajectory set off with the analysis of 'local' cultural struggles[2] and has since moved towards a more trans-national dimension

[1] The question whether Cultural Studies' 'political effectiveness' has been eroded by its institutionalisation is beyond the scope of this essay, but I fully agree with John Mowitt that Cultural Studies must "pose and live up to" the question of how it can re-think the question of political organisation and the role of academic intellectuals considering especially "the intellectual fallout of capitalism's abandonment of the nation-state" and how to think of a "radically democratic practice" (see Mowitt, in Alessandrini 1999: 89).

[2] Cultural Studies pioneers such as Raymond Williams and E.P. Thompson for example claimed that the field provides an academic umbrella for the "increasingly muted protest embodied in 'traditional' British working-class culture" (Mowitt (1999): 91-2).

to contribute to the analysis of issues relating to the recent historical displacement of individuals and whole communities, as one of the far-reaching consequences of colonialism and post-colonialism. This accounts for the increased interest in the 'diasporic', the subaltern and the post-colonial within Cultural Studies.

Contemporary and controversial issues of the social and political implications of immigration, the international division of labour, and the economic and cultural forces of neo-colonialism can be said to constitute our present 'state of emergency'. Julia Kristeva (1991, with special reference to France) argues that at a time when the world becomes a melting pot of different races and cultures, the question that imposes itself is how to live with others without neither absorbing nor rejecting them. Kristeva suggests that the first step towards accommodating the difference of the other is to admit that this 'other' or 'foreigner' is always already 'within' us, or part of us, and we must therefore learn how to cohabit with him/her and his/her difference. She stresses the importance of considering the personal psychology of the human subject in his/her social context as an important step towards the analysis and the 'cure' of xenophobia.[3]

The issue of immigration, the contemporary debate about the political and social status of 'foreigners', and the political and cultural climate of this historical juncture, which continues to witness outbreaks of xenophobia and racism all over the world, must become more prominent in Cultural Studies. Cultural Studies needs to *actively* address the current revival of extreme nationalist and xenophobic movements. In many European countries for example, the popular imagination is currently being haunted by images of a Europe swept by foreigners, economic and political refugees perceived as 'welfare-scroungers', 'job-snatchers' and 'threats to security' (*Economist* 2000: 25, 26 and 31). Some politicians have started to propagate these fears in order to increase the number of their votes, especially politicians of the extreme right.[4] However, the 1951 Geneva Convention states the right of asylum seekers to be received in Europe without restrictions; nevertheless, many European governments believe that the numbers of those seeking asylum, which has considerably risen since the Eighties, simply represent an increase in economic refugees 'in disguise' (*ibid.*). Tough immigration laws have been introduced to deter these 'potential' economic

---

[3] For an analysis of Kristeva's preoccupation with the issue of foreignness and the relationship she establishes between the concept of the nation and psychoanalysis, see Mowitt (1998) and Kristeva (1991).

[4] But even the centre right for example in the UK and Germany are trying to "play the immigration card". William Hague, the conservative leader in the UK claims that "bogus asylum seekers" are flooding the country and that Britain should keep them in detention till their status is "sorted out". The German conservative leader Jürgen Rüttgers has expressed the same view claiming that Germany should take care of its own children instead of "importing Indians". This was his response to the German Chancellor's (Gerhard Schröder) call for recruiting around 20,000 high-tech specialists from India (*Economist* 2000: 19, 25).

refugees and have helped to construct an image of a Europe as an impenetrable 'fortress'.

Today more than ever, in the West, the ethical question of 'hospitality' towards the foreigner is answered by a suspicious silence on the part of individuals, by political violence on the part of the nation states and by repressive (European) legislation. The immigration issue is of course ethical, as well as political, and needs to take into consideration the economic inequalities between rich Northern and poor Southern countries. To that effect, the migratory phenomenon needs to be perceived not as a 'fatality' or a 'danger' but as a result of historical developments and economic transformations.

This essay addresses some of the contradictions and conflicts with the current, historically specific, 'French' context.

' The Threshold of Tolerance?"

France's trajectory in terms of immigration is somewhat different from that of other European countries in what can be seen as its early positive embrace of foreigners as immigrants, settlers and as citizens. This willingness to accept and integrate foreigners as citizens is founded on the Republican tradition inherited from the French Revolution whose universalising 'Declaration of Human and Civic Rights' (*Déclaration des droits de l'homme et du citoyen*) and the belief in 'Liberté, Fraternité, Égalité' were initially proclaimed in 1789. Nevertheless, this tradition of openness has not been without rules and restrictions: alongside an idea of a certain (invisible) 'threshold of tolerance' has evolved that immigration or 'immigrants' must not cross. This was referred to for example by François Mitterrand, in a television interview in 1989, when he announced that the 'threshold number' of immigrants in France had been reached (Silverman 1992: 95). A strong debate in the French media followed which focused on the 'problem of immigrants'[5] and the risk of crossing this 'threshold of tolerance' (*ibid.*). The phrase implies the 'belief' that strong concentrations of immigrants or ethnic minorities in specific places (or ghettos) constitute an obvious reason for social conflict. This argument is based on the (so far unproven) hypothesis that ordinary people become racists as a reaction to the increased visibility of immigrants around them, an attitude usually exacerbated in times of economic crisis (King 1995: 187, Silverman 1992: 97-98).

Max Silverman argues that Mitterrand's declaration was not very 'diplomatic'; it came at a time when public opinion was divided due to 'the headscarf issue' (i.e. the argument whether it was right to prevent two Franco-Maghrebi Muslim girls from attending the strictly 'lay' public school while

[5] My own use of the word 'immigrants', referring in particular to the Maghrebi ethnic communities, is strategic and reflects French usage in which the word '*immigré*' is rather negatively connoted (e.g. with employment-seeking), as opposed to the more positively connoted '*immigrant*'.

wearing their headscarves; see Silverman 1992: 96). Moreover, the term *'seuil de tolérance'* (threshold of tolerance) had previously been identified by the Left as a racist expression, used by the Right to describe 'ethnic relations' (*ibid.*). Mitterrand's use of the phrase, according to Silverman, therefore evokes a consensus between Left and Right about some ideas relating to this threshold, and thus contributed to establishing consensus about immigration as being a major problem for French society in general. But what is this threshold that immigrant communities have allegedly crossed? And what does this 'threshold' represent in relation to the Republican principles?

Traditionally, French Republicanism[6] is based on egalitarian principles that defend social justice and equality, stress the sovereignty of the people and encourage their participation in public life (Hayward 1983: 88). However, as Jim House points out (1997: 50), the political environment that led to the 1789 *Déclaration* has changed, which means that it has become problematic to see the *Déclaration* as 'the application of universal rights'. Rather, the it may today be seen as an opening of a space, a horizon, for the values of freedom and equality that remain to be implemented (*ibid.*). This explains the constant tension within French society, between, on the one hand, the reference to and belief in those principles and, on the other hand, their continued 'non-realisation' (*ibid.*).

The tension between the ideals of the Republic, which as a political ideology strongly endorses the concept of a nation not based on ethnic exclusiveness (as opposed for example to the case of Germany; see Silverman 1992), and the actual implementation of these ideals, has been clear in France ever since the Revolution. The core of French Republicanism is "its emphasis on citizenship rather than race or ethnicity as the defining condition of membership of the national community"; thus, it is the *'jus solis'* and not the *'jus sanguinis'* which determines the conditions for acquiring French citizenship (Hazareesingh 1994: 87). However, the French State and its institutions have been promoting 'a dominant identity', by "secreting norms of cultural belonging" and by "also acting to shape the identities of dominated groups" (House 1997: 58).

Republicanism also claims, of course, that principles of universality lead to the abolishment of all privileges based on rank, blood or birth and instead promotes an 'inclusive' rather than 'exclusive' concept of citizenship based on universal rights (Hazareesingh 1994: 72). Fraternity and equality are supposed to offer all members of society the same rights and privileges and juridical protection (Hazareesingh: 87). Moreover, "the Republic's principle of equal citizenship rested on an 'open' conception of national identity" in the sense that "membership of the national community was available not only to those who had

[6] Republicanism as a political ideology was, of course, highly controversial during the Nineteenth and the beginning of the Twentieth century and went, during its process of consolidation, through a number of changes; it has triumphed in the Twentieth century and has received wide-spread support among the French public mainly because of its egalitarian principles, its respect for the rights of 'man', individualism and citizenship (see Berstein and Rudelle 1992: 11).

been born in France (or had lived there for several generations), but also to those who had elected to make France their *patrie*: for example, citizens of its colonies and immigrants" (*ibid.*).[7] However, in practice, Republican France has been developing a political culture that considers rights to be "exclusive of the membership of one nation-state" (House 1997: 54). As a result, from the Third Republic onwards, the access to these 'universal' rights has been restricted to nationals.

From the late Nineteenth Century onwards, Republicans introduced exclusionary practices in the colonies (House: 41). These practices paved the way for a Republican discourse that directed aggression towards specific cultural and ethnic 'differences' (especially towards the Muslims of North Africa). The effect was the creation of new processes of differentiation "through social practices of categorisation, ... which would increasingly be perceived (and experienced) in 'racial' or ethnic terms" (House: 42).

Republicanism stresses national unity in the name of conformity and rejects any form of communitarian or cultural identities. It collapses 'French nation', universalism and homogeneity. It is precisely these ideas that have come under scrutiny, and which have started yielding their contradictions hitherto used to sanction the exclusion of ethnic minorities. Republican universalism is increasingly questioned, and 'demythologised' as having been a process of 'simplifying' the complexity of the past and 'homogenising' French identity in order to legitimise the exclusion of 'others' (Silverman 1995: 254). It is therefore high time for the Republican model to be 'revised' in terms of recognising the cultural and ethnic multiplicity of French society.

Already Roland Barthes, in 1954, 'denaturalised' what he called the French myth of a multi-racial unified French nation by referring to a by now famous picture on a *Paris-Match* cover. This photograph shows a young black soldier saluting the French flag, a gesture which according to Barthes signifies French colonial ideology. It represents 'the greatness of the French Empire' and that "all her sons, without any colour discrimination, faithfully serve under her flag, and that there is no better answer to the detractors of an alleged colonialism than the zeal shown by this Negro in serving his so called oppressors" (Barthes 1972: 116).

Barthes's interpretation of the French myth of a unified nation is still revealing in today's French society where immigration has become another name for 'race', and 'immigrant' a term that 'legitimates' strictly speaking racist classifications (Balibar and Wallerstein 1991: 223). At a time when the French Republican tradition speaks again about the unity of its population and about

[7] It must be noted here that anti-republican conceptions of nationality are usually based on race and not on citizenship. They usually reject the idea of cultural integration and thus normally support the idea of withholding citizenship from those groups who are suspected of 'disloyalty' to France (this is one of Jean-Marie Le Pen's main arguments; see Hareesingh 1994: 87-8).

universalism, French citizens of immigrant origin, more than ever, find themselves categorised as outsiders. Children of North African immigrants born in France are still usually referred to as 'second-generation immigrants' and the debate on whether they can be integrated into French society is still ongoing. Most of them, however, think that they already *constitute* a part of French society. The problem is the resistance to recognise that the ideal of integration, namely the belonging 'to a *de facto* historical and social entity' does not normally correspond to 'a mythical national type' (*ibid.*). The debate about how to define 'integration' has been ongoing in France since the 1980s. Xenophobia and racism are on the increase, especially against the Maghrebi immigrant communities, the largest ethnic minority in France (and the one believed to be causing most social 'trouble'), even though, for decades previously their presence has gone almost unnoticed.

It is important to note (as Tahar Ben Jelloun argues in *L'Hospitalité française*, 1997: 24) that immigration did not become a part of political debate in France until the petrol crisis of 1973, or perhaps the Paris events of 1961 (demonstrations and riots by Algerians calling for Algeria's independence). Ben Jelloun argues that the problem is not that of immigration as such but rather the recognition of the mistakes committed in France's colonial past, and the constant attempt to disavow this past rather than its public 'working through'. The historical wounds, the massacres and usurpations that took place in France's colonial history continue to haunt and cause confusion, fear and hatred. France has developed amnesia towards its colonial past. Ben Jelloun argues that though colonialism, post-colonialism and their consequences have been the object of many studies, they still are repressed in the social and political collective consciousness (22). The repression of its history means that France is in need of a "politics sustained by a philosophy, a thought that puts the self and the other in a face-to-face relation that is creative, healthy, without rancour and without resentment" (Jelloun: 16).

The French historian Gérard Noiriel argues that the phenomenon of immigration in French society should not be seen as external to 'French history' but as an integrative and constitutive part of that history (Noiriel 1988: 4-7). Looking at the origins of the French nation, Noiriel argues that all members of today's French population (by which he means the population resident on French national territory) are in fact the product of an historical process of immigration (Noiriel 1992: 43-44). The country had been known for its tradition of hospitality, and immigration has always been an important factor in the construction of the modern French nation (see Stasi 1984, and Corderio 1984). Thus, according to Noiriel, the differentiation between *les Français de souche* (seen as the 'real' French, 'belonging' to the country as the 'true' descendants of the Gauls) and others, seen as 'false' French, immigrants and thus of 'foreign' origin, is rather arbitrary (Noiriel 1992: 43-44).

Throughout the late Nineteenth and the early Twentieth Century France welcomed a large number of immigrants from surrounding European countries such as Belgium, Italy, Portugal, Poland, etc. After the Second World War, it opened its doors to non-European immigration from countries of its former colonies, especially in North and West Africa. The previous influx of immigrants from European countries is thought to have led to successful integration within 'French culture', whereas the most recent wave of immigrants from the former colonies, especially from North Africa, have been branded 'un-assimilable' in nature, mainly because of their Islamic cultural background. In contemporary France, the use of the term 'immigrant' has thus come to refer solely to those migrants of non-European origins. 'The problem of immigration', thus, in fact, names a specific community (i.e. North Africans) which is represented as a threat to national culture and identity (Silverman 1992: 3).

This new form of racism that is sweeping Europe in general and France in particular is therefore related to what Balibar calls 'external groups', the ones blamed for crossing 'the threshold of tolerance', immigrants from non-European countries, some of whom have been living and integrating (despite their cultural difference) in Europe for a long time (Balibar 1997: 326). Of all European countries, however, France seems to resist the historical and social transformations of migration most strongly. This is manifested in its refusal to recognise the ethnic and cultural plurality of its society as part of what constitutes 'Frenchness' today. The idea of a 'threshold of tolerance' clearly reflects the fear within French society of a multi-cultural, multi-racial national identity. It illustrates the refusal to recognise the transformations that have taken place and thus constitutes a refusal to acknowledge France's colonial history and its responsibilities.

Why Intolerance?

In trying to establish the reason for this specific form of intolerance I do not intend to determine the causes for the spread of racism in France. Instead I want to further explore the paradoxes of a post-colonial, post-industrial society in which cultural and ethnic cohabitation is today in jeopardy. I would argue that if the Maghrebi ethnic communities have been blamed for crossing the French '*seuil de tolerance*', French society itself has crossed a certain 'threshold of intolerance' by adopting, on a collective level, negative attitudes towards the 'foreigner' (Balibar 1997: 327-8). France therefore has turned against its 'own' egalitarian and humanitarian Republican principles. This situation calls for a new round of negotiations with regard to the recent transformations in French cultural and national identity.

Contemporary French society is torn between its egalitarian principles on the one hand and its everyday racism on the other. The latter presents itself today in the form of a prolonged political, moral, cultural and economic crisis. The rise of xenophobia poses a major threat to the future of the country's multi-racial and multi-cultural reality. However, the phenomenon of a racist 'epidemic' is, of course, not new (neither is it peculiar to France), but what is striking is the appearance of a 'neo-racism' marked by the intensification of violent and *collective* racist acts. What Etienne Balibar calls the "*passage à l'acte*" which publicly and collectively authorises what was hitherto unthinkable: physical violence against people, 'justified' as acts exercising an historical right (Balibar 1997: 325). This is a crucial 'threshold of intolerance' to be crossed. The increase of verbal and physical violence, hatred, and worst of all, the appearance of organised movements whose purpose is to institutionalise discrimination and exclusion, is taking new forms, gains more active support and includes more targets. Moreover, the increasing popularity of the extreme right wing party, the Front National, which uses immigration as a way to rally support, results in the adoption of the immigration 'issue' by other, more 'moderate' political parties and discourses, that aim to 'please' and 'appease' the electorate (Balibar and Wallerstein 1991: 217) – a situation mirrored in other European countries (see for example the rise of Austria's Freedom Party).

On the contemporary French political scene, contradictions exist, on the one hand, between the belief in universalism, secularism, a clear distinction between the private and the public spheres, individual assimilation, the integration of difference, and the hostility towards the creation of communal identities, and, on the other hand, the undeniability of cultural and ethnic differences which characterise post-colonial France and which put the Republican model aimed at confining difference to the public sphere into question.

The rise in populist xenophobia in the last two decades which almost exclusively blames the Maghrebi immigrants and their children for the social and economic problems of the country, has resulted in the erosion of French national identity and culture in general (see Blatt 1997: 40). David Blatt argues that: "the increased political saliency of immigration issues helped revive a traditional French discourse on integration and the nation-state that insists on the preservation of republican principles of undifferentiated citizenship and a firm rejection of any public recognition of ethnic and cultural identities" (Blatt 1997: 40-1). It appears that for 'the French' it would mean to lose their 'national identity' if they were to adopt the Anglo-Saxon model of multiculturalism – a model that certainly is not without its own problems.

Racism is usually legitimised, by all social classes, as a kind of defensive reaction that wants to preserve a 'threatened' national identity and defend security. The presence of numerous foreigners or immigrants is believed to threaten the well-being of the state because it seemingly causes chaos on the level of employment and public order, in the sense that some cultural differences can hinder cohabitation and thus force the 'natives' to question their national identity (Balibar 1997: 325-326).

There are two important factors that need to be taken into consideration with regard to the crossing of the 'threshold of intolerance' in France today. First, the hegemonic proliferation of collective attitudes and ideological formations directed against 'the foreigner' – to the extent that one may even speak of a 'social movement'. It is the passionate and hysteric denial and rejection of 'foreignness' and their cultural and historical functions that transpire in popular and academic discourses alike, which reveal a profound fear of a multicultural society and cultural '*métissage*' (Balibar 1997: 327-8). The focus, however, is specifically on the increase of racism within the working-class, caused by the dismantling of trade unions, economic insecurity and globalisation, the latter of which, in turn, has exacerbated the problem by depriving the nation state of its control over domestic cultural and economic conflicts. Second, the formation of what Balibar and Wieviorka respectively call, "the immigration complex" and "imaginary racism" or "racism of fear and status", which all refer to the strong belief that immigrants are to be seen as a 'problem', which then results in intolerance and xenophobia.

The recent spread of racism among the population, but especially among the French working-class, takes the form of excluding immigrant workers from the negotiations of employment issues. This does not mean, however, that other forms of racism in other social classes and among intellectuals do not exist. The – maybe exaggerated – attention given to popular racism is due to the fact that the rise of this particular form of racism immediately threatens institutionalised ideas of anti-racism that are strongly associated with the exploited classes. In other words, although the working-class is not believed to have itself initiated anti-racist struggles, it, nevertheless, has always contributed to its promotion by its commitment to anti-racist programmes and policies (Balibar and Wallerstein 1991: 224). A change of policy in this context could therefore strengthen racism and contribute to its spread across the social spectrum.

The phenomenon has to be examined in depth in relation to the history of the French working-class. Xenophobia towards immigrant workers is not simply a matter of competition on the labour market but rather it is the result of the state and the employers' policies that lead to the hierarchization of work by reserving skilled jobs for the 'French' and unskilled work for immigrants. This in turn leads to a focus on industrialisation processes which require further unskilled labour. The result of which is to rely on immigration to provide the cheap labour, which today is effectuated by employers actively encouraging clandestine immigration. Racism within the French working-class is therefore related to keeping social privileges. However, the phenomenon of de-industrialisation, insecurity of work, poverty and dropping standards of living have eliminated high-skill jobs while creating a large number of un-skilled jobs, which has forced 'nationals' (or *Français de souche*) and immigrants to increasingly experience the same form of exploitation, now deprives 'nationals' of their former privileges. Such 'reproletarianization' necessarily overturns class practices and ideologies (Balibar and Wallerstein 1991: 225; Wieviorka 1992). Racism is exacerbated when civil rights and social rights are looked upon as a form of privilege that needs to be protected and reserved for 'natural beneficiaries'. However, 'Rights *grow* of themselves qualitatively through the increasing number (and power) of those who enjoy and claim them', whereas 'privileges can only be guaranteed by the defence of an exclusiveness that is as restrictive as possible' (Balibar and Wallerstein 1991: 226). This is what accentuates the crisis within the working-class and what contributes to the uncertainty and insecurity they experience in their existence and their 'collective identity'.

The working-class, in fact, is faced with very similar problems of social exclusion as the immigrant communities. Many critics perceive the reasons of exclusion in the *'expansion regressive du Marché'* in the sense that the globalisation of market economy and its corresponding social norms have not only led to economic growth, but also to de-industrialisation and growing structural unemployment (Balibar 1997: 329).

Immanuel Wallerstein argues that in a system based on the accumulation of capital and the maximisation of (short term) profit, racism provides the best formula to guarantee minimum costs of production through a cheap labour force while, at the same time, minimising the costs of 'political disruption' through reinforcing the 'ethnicization' of this labour force. Wallerstein argues that the pattern of ethnicization has been constant but the details have varied according to time and space and according to the 'hierarchical needs' of a particular economy (Wallerstein 1991: 34).

The breakdown of modern institutions within industrial society and the weakening of the Republican traditions such as state education, secularism, trade unions, political parties and the failure of those institutions to bring people together around issues of equality and solidarity have widened social gaps (Wieviorka 1992: 31). These economic changes would, in fact, require an expansion of social representation and collective participation, which in turn demands finding a social balance that can accommodate individual initiatives and collective activism in workers (Balibar 1997: 330). Both political and workforce organisations, however, have so far failed to embrace this fact, with the result of further excluding workers, and further contributing to the decline of the nation state and its social security system. The nation state finds itself torn between the world financial market and its incapacity to control social domestic conflict. In other words, as a result of globalisation, the state has lost its traditional role of making economic and social decisions, and is now incapable of defining for itself a social basis founded on the representation and the mediation of collective conflicts similar to those that gave the democratic nation-states their legitimacy in the first place (Balibar 1997: 330). This 'paradox of social nation states that have become anti-social, of nation states that have become anti-national and finally supra-national states that are resistant to the development of all forms of popular or collective internationalism', has to be critically examined if one wishes to understand the current themes of exclusion, corruption and political disenchantment (*ibid.*). Thus, paradoxically, it is the social and political impotence of the state whose apparatuses are almost absent when it comes to discussing issues of collective insecurity, the integration of immigrants or offering 'hospitality' to refugees, that has contributed to the rise in popular racism (Balibar 1997: 331).

Unlike racist ideologies in some countries (e.g. the US), however, it seems that racism today is no longer determined by class; class differences no longer are a main factor in attitudes towards immigrants, there now seems to be a consensus in all social classes about the necessity to exclude and discriminate against 'foreigners'. Thus, with the collective 'formation of an immigration complex', an important threshold of intolerance has already been crossed which threatens the peaceful co-existence of communities in France. Etienne Balibar defines this development as "a racism typical of the era of 'decolonization'", referring to the movement of people from the old colonies to the metropolis, leading to what he calls "a division of humanity within a single political space" (Balibar and Wallerstein 1991: 21). He claims that:

> Ideologically speaking, current racism which in France centres upon the immigration complex, fits into a framework of 'racism without races' which is already widely developed in other, in particular Anglo-Saxon countries. It is a racism whose dominant theme is not biological heredity but the unsurmountability of cultural differences, a racism which, at first sight, does not postulate the superiority of certain groups or people in relation to others but 'only' the harmfulness of abolishing frontiers, the incompatibility of life-styles and traditions; in short, it is what P.A. Taguieff has rightly called a *differentialist racism.* (Balibar and Wallerstein 1991: 21)

Even if theoretical discourses on the equality of cultures exist, no-one can deny that for immigrants (for example 'blacks' in Britain and '*Beurs'* in France) the assimilation demanded of them before they can attain integration within the target society is normally perceived as 'progress'. Progress, however, is already modelled on the European 'universalist' idea of cultural superiority, with 'non-European' cultures still seen as 'particularist' and 'primitive'. Therefore, a paradox emerges within this culturally differentialist form of racism which means that arguing for the preservation and 'respect' of all cultures (cultural relativism) *de facto* is used to protect the European cultures from what Balibar calls a "third Worldization" (Balibar and Wallerstein 1991: 25). Moreover, and contrary to what traditional Republican ideals claim, House (1997: 63) suggests that "there has never been any real 'model' of openness for certain social groups" and that "assimilation has never been considered a real possibility for Maghrebians".

The 'formation of an immigration complex' certainly does not simply refer to variant immigrant groups being harassed or targeted, but to the increasing belief and acceptance of the idea that immigrants in general constitute a 'problem'. Subsequently every other social issue, e.g. schooling, housing, social security, public health, unemployment, delinquency and crime, is perceived as being either caused or aggravated through the presence of immigrants. Thus, the state adopts the policies of restricting immigration on the basis of the yet unproven assumption that the concentration of ethnic minorities in specific places is a strong reason for the rise of social tension (see King 1995: 182). Although there may be a relation, in fact, research has shown that the racist feelings are not restricted to those places where immigrants tend to live. The *Front National* received many of its votes from people who do not have many direct contacts with immigrants and to whom they represent a 'merely' symbolic threat (Wieviorka 1992: 160).

The anxiety of preserving one's social status and the obsession with 'insecurity', are a matter of lived experience, as Michel Wieviorka argues, which means that they are not necessarily linked to the actual presence of immigrants. In fact, the real problem is that people from diverse environments develop what Wieviorka calls an anti-immigrant 'syndrome' which is neither based on daily contact with immigrants nor on 'objective insecurity', or a real danger, but rather on a common feeling or perception of a crisis in the existing social and cultural order, the breakdown of institutions and the weakening of traditional community life (*ibid.*). In her research about *Front National* voters, Nona Mayer claims that those who vote for the *FN* do not tend to co-habit or share the same space with the immigrants; they are usually not victims of theft or crime attributed to immigrants, but their votes are rather the result of a diffuse fear and feelings of insecurity. In fact, daily contact rather tends to reduce anti-immigrant feelings. However, other, non-residential, contacts, e.g. in schools, at work, media representation, do of course also have an influence (Mayer 1995: 102-3).

FN votes can be said to be a result of 'situational and personal factors' (Mayer 1995: 107) in the sense that *FN* voters are prone to fears generated in big urban places with a high rate of unemployment, crime and a high concentration of immigrants. These urban agglomerations are usually economically and socially not well equipped to deal with these fears. These feelings are linked to the insecurity of some classes, especially the working-class (Mayer 1995: 105-6). These (urban) fears existed of course even before the *FN* became an electoral force, and before the issue of immigration began to be seen as a problem. The *FN*, however managed to establish links between these issues, and encouraged, politicised and legitimised these fears. As a result other parties had to follow suit and address these social phenomena under the agenda and representation dictated by the *FN* (Mayer 1995: 107-8).

However, if popular fear of immigrants and delinquency are often irrational, it would be wrong to say that this fear bears no relation to social reality, as Wieviorka argues. This assumption would only lead to a disjuncture between everyday-life reality where fear is formed and the targets on which this fear is then projected (Wieviorka 1992: 161). Even for the middle-class or those who live in 'safe' places, factors like social, cultural and economic crises, the decline of state power, and the appearance of different cultures and forms of 'modernity' of which they may not be a part, and which may threaten the notion of a national identity, contribute to a generalised state of 'anxiety'. The most obvious solution always seems to be the closure of borders and the expulsion of immigrants. The first paradox of this anxiety complex in Balibar's words is that "the less specific the social problems of 'immigrants', or the social problems that most affect immigrants, the more blame is put on immigrants" (Balibar and Wallerstein 1991: 220).

Another paradox here is, of course, that the immigrant community is not a homogenous entity, but is rather heterogeneous in its variety of countries of origin, cultures, religions, histories and their degrees of assimilation or integration. Thus, the word 'immigrant' is a unifying principle by which heterogeneous groups of people can be labelled. The *Français de souche* does not usually differentiate between Algerian, Tunisian, Moroccan or Lebanese; for the average French person these usually are 'Arabs'. In fact, strong stereotypes often prevent a social mixing with immigrants, enhancing the view that North African immigrants cannot or 'do not want to be' assimilated. These stereotypes always run into problems and paradoxes as soon as they are required to set up criteria – whether religious, cultural, racial, or ethnic – by which Arabs, Blacks, Asian, etc. can be clearly identified and thus 'located' – controlled and confined to designated social 'spaces' (*ibid.*).

Therefore, "the category of immigration structures discourses and behaviours, but also, and this is no less important, provides the racist – individual and group – *with the illusion of a style of thinking, an 'object' that is to be known* and explored, which is a fundamental factor of 'self consciousness'" (*ibid.*). In other words, it is the danger of racist 'effective thinking' directed towards 'an illusionary subject' (immigration as a problem). For Balibar, whoever can be classified or categorised (in racist terms), only 'exists collectively', or 'causes to exist in practice that illusion that is collectively based on the similitude of its members' (*ibid.*). Anti-racist movements, therefore, must discard the view that racism is a matter of absence of thinking and that it is only a matter of making people reflect upon it that can make racism disappear. In fact, racism is a mode of thinking, and thus its prominence constitutes another sign of the crossing of the threshold of intolerance, namely its taking root in the mentality of people. The most difficult task in this context consists of changing people's strategies of thinking and reasoning (Balibar and Wallerstein 1991: 222).

Related to the formation of the immigration complex is what Michel Wieviorka calls 'imaginary racism' or 'racism of fear and status' which does not only work in the form of a discourse but is also active in keeping the immigrants 'at a distance'. It aims at protecting the image of the self by setting irreducible boundaries (Wieviorka 1992: 162). Wieviorka argues that this type of racism operates on three levels. First, it works on the level of individual behaviour, leading to boycotting the immigrants and whatever is associated with them. For example, if the immigrants or their children frequent a certain place it will be avoided by the *Français de souche* and their children (an example is Marseille which is virtually split into the 'ethnic' Northern part and the 'rich' South of the city). This type of behaviour attempts to undo any effort of bringing together different communities and thus enhances social intolerance (Wieviorka 1992: 162-3).

A second level on which imaginary racism operates is the public sphere. Fears are politicised, that is, prejudices, fears, and hatred enter the political discourse of all parties (not only the *FN*, as explained above). Anxieties thus 'translate' into political promises to restrict the movement and space of immigrants, which, in fact means segregating them in housing and schooling. Therefore, political and municipal life is usually marked not only by a generally anti-immigrant discourse, but also by specific demands for segregation at local levels of community politics (Wieviorka 1992: 164).

A third level involves collective actions of inhabitants of a specific area promoting exclusion and isolation (for example excluding immigrants from participating in social events). This type of racism aims to ensure (in Wieviorka's words) the ethnic homogeneity of a certain territory by actively expulsing an 'undesirable' part of the population. Moreover, this barrier further contributes to keeping the 'other' at a distance, a form of "practical ignorance and lack of knowledge of those situated 'on the other side' [of the social barriers]" (*ibid.*).

Thus, racism becomes an 'imaginary' discourse based on fictional representations and imaginary constructions of difference that, however, lead to real instances of hatred and violence unrelated to any form of practical understanding or lived experience with the other. Wieviorka reminds us that in history, the worst forms of racism were not necessarily based on direct contact with concrete 'others' (1992: 164-5).

Conclusion

One has to admit that the Republican ideals with their call for 'uniformity in the name of equality' are not without a certain appeal, but it seems that it is high time to question the dualistic model of particularism and universalism on which they are based. Silverman suggests that a re-examination of the history of 'past models for formulations of rights' may be a good start and would point towards a reformulation of the Republican concepts, especially in view of a more 'inclusive' notion of citizenship. The Republican ideals nowadays are being exploited politically by the *FN* and employed to enhance the cultural difference of (in particular North African) immigrants in order to legitimise French nationalism. The current discussion about Republicanism seems to prevent, in fact, any serious attempts to institutionalise a rational discussion about 'difference' and 'ethnic minorities'. It therefore seriously restricts any efforts to reconsider the issue of the citizens' rights on the basis of difference and ethnic identity (Silverman 1998: 258).

What is needed is a radical renewal and re-foundation of democratic practices, as Balibar puts it, which have to be accepted collectively. Attention must also be given to the specific historical moment, within the process of European integration, at which these political developments occur. The question of racism will be crucial for the required democratisation of European institutions and for the necessary discussion on 'citizenship' (Balibar 1997: 332). It is also important to develop ethical and intellectual alternatives to traditional forms of anti-racism that would no longer be based on the simple 'refusal of the refusal of the other'. Equally crucial will be overcoming symbolic barriers within 'national' cultures, as inscribed in state apparatuses and institutions. This involves recognising and addressing current forms of 'institutional racism' (in France, for example the institutionalised discrimination against Islam under the name of Republican secularity; Balibar 1997: 335).

Moreover, it has to become clear to a future European public consciousness, that even in simple terms of general economic welfare and growth, statistics show that the European Union will need at least 1.6 million migrants a year to ensure the continuity of its workforce in the next fifty years or so (*Economist* 2000: 19). Europe's economy though prospering relies on an ageing population.[8] The contemporary wave of anti-immigrant feelings in Europe has made the acceptance of these facts very difficult. Europeans, however, will have to face that for their future prosperity and indeed their survival, immigrants are necessary and 'desirable' and that xenophobic fears of the 'other' must be overcome.

I would agree with Saskia Sassen who argues that both policy makers and the general public must understand that immigration is not only caused by poverty or persecution in poor countries. Such a narrow perception can only cause the spread of xenophobia, intolerance and fears of 'mass invasion' (Sassen 1999: 2). Moreover, host countries must embrace their responsibilities within the very processes of migration and the 'mapping of their immigration structures' (Sassen 1999: 1). Geopolitical and economic factors need to be acknowledged as much as the individual fates of migrants 'searching for a better life' (*ibid.*). Sassen argues that "when persecution, poverty, and overpopulation are seen as no longer sufficient explanations in themselves of migration flows, then images and metaphors based on invasion will no longer satisfy us, and policy-making concerned with immigration could be more innovative, because it would address a confined event, a shaped experience, a manageable process" (1999: 3).

In the French context, this implies a re-thinking of the ideas of the 'threshold' and of the Republic which, as history teaches us, have always been in flux. The potential for development within the Republican idea becomes clear by looking at the five successive Republics, and the adaptations each of these constitute with relation to their specific historical circumstances (Berstein and Rudell 1992: 10). There is no reason why Republicanism today should be seen as a rigid political ideology that cannot include the recent changes in French society

---

[8] *The Economist* on May 6th 2000, page 25, states that "In order to keep its working-age population stable between now and 2050, at current birth and death rates, Germany would need to import 487,000 migrants, according to a recent report by the United Nations' population Division. France would need 109,000 and the European Union as a whole 1.6m. To keep the ratio of workers to pensioners steady the flow would need to swell to 3.6m a year in Germany, 1.8m in France and a staggering 13.5m a year in the EU as a whole."

this essay has outlined. So far the response by Republican politicians to the rise in racism has been rather unimpressive. Many questions about the relation between the existing Republican principles of social freedom, civil equality, and the fight against discrimination against French citizens on the basis of ethnic, religious, cultural or racial difference remain to be addressed. The political institutions of the French Republic have to be opened for reforms to increase their efficiency in their fight against racism today. Cultural Studies – as a 'diasporic' field that aims to be politically effective and intellectually 'useful' for the analysis of social, political and economic tensions – 'carefully' translated into the French intellectual scene, could contribute to the kind of open debate on the Republican heritage, on social solidarity and egalitarianism and on the issues of race and citizenship that are needed today.

Bibliography:

Balibar, E., and Wallerstein, I (1991) *Race, Nation, Class: Ambiguous Identities*, London: Verso.

Balibar, Etienne (1997) *La Crainte des Masses*, Paris: Galilee.

Barthes, Roland (1972) *Mythologies*, trans. Annette Lavers, London Jonathan Cape.

Ben Jelloun, Tahar (1997) *L'Hospitalité Francaise*, Paris: Le Seuil.

Berstein, Serge, and Rudelle, Odile, eds. (1992) *Le Modèle Républicain*, Paris, Presses Universitaires de France.

Blatt, David (1997) "Immigrant Politics in A Republican Nation", in: Hargreaves and McKinney, eds., *Post-colonial Cultures in France.*

Economist *(2000) The Economist*, May 6th 2000, 19-31.

Hargreaves, Alec G. and Leaman, Jeremy, eds. (1995) *Racism Ethnicity and Politics in Contemporary Europe*, Hants: Edward Elgar.

Hargreaves, Alec G. and McKinney, Mark eds. (1997) *Post-Colonial Cultures in France*, London and New York: Routledge.

Hazareesingh, Sudhir (1994) *Political Traditions in Modern France*, Oxford and New York: Oxford University Press.

Hayward, J.E.S. (1983) *Governing France: The One and Indivisible Republic*, London: Butler and Tanner.

House, Jim (1995) "Contexts of Integration", in: Hargreaves and Leaman, eds., *Race, Ethnicity and Politics in Contemporary Europe*.

House, Jim (1997) *Antiracism and Antiracist Discourse in France From 1900 to the Present Day*, Ph.D. Thesis: University of Leeds.

King, John (1995) "Ethnic Minorities and Multilateral Institutions", in: Hargreaves and Leaman, eds. *Race, Ethnicity and Politics in Contemporary Europe*.

Kristeva, Julia (1991) *Strangers to Ourselves*, trans. Leon Roudiez, New York: Columbia University Press.

Mayer, Nona (1995) "Ethnocentrism and the Front National Vote In the 1988 French Presidential Election", in: Hargreaves and Leaman, eds. *Race, Ethnicity and Politics in Contemporary Europe.*

Mowitt, John (1998) "Strangers in Analysis: Nationalism and the Talking Cure", *Parallax* 4: 3, 45-63.

Mowitt, John (1999) "Breaking Fanon's Voice", in: Alessandrini, A. C., ed. *Frantz Fanon: Critical Perspectives,* London: Routledge.

Noiriel, Gérard (1988) "Enseigner l'histoire de l'immigration", *Expression Français-Immigrés* 56, 4-7.

Noiriel, Gérard (1992) *Population, Immigration et Identité Nationale en France – XXe Siècle,* Paris: Hachette.

Sassen, Saskia (1999) *Guests and Aliens*, New York: The New Press.

Silverman, Max (1992) *Deconstructing the Nation: Immigration, Racism and Citizenship in Modern France*, London and New York: Routledge.

Silverman, Max (1995) "Rights and Difference: Questions of Citizenship in France", in: Hargreaves and Leaman, eds. *Racism, Ethnicity and Politics in Contemporary Europe.*

Silverman, Max (1998) *Facing Postmodernity: Contemporary French Thought on Culture and Society,* London and New York: Routledge.

Wieviorka, Michel (1992) *La France Raciste* , Paris: Seuil.

Section E:

Cultural Studies: Translation and Globalisation

TRANSATLANTIC FEARS: RE-CONFIGURATIONS IN A GLOBAL CONTEXT

HOLGER ROSSOW

The transatlantic dialogue between Europe and America has been characterised by competing discourses and an uneven distribution of negotiating and agenda-setting power. The terms Europe and America are used to refer to culturally constructed products of our minds rather than to clearly defined spatial entities. This analysis focuses on the most recent period of the dialogue - the age of rapid processes of globalisation and growing interconnectedness. The relationships between Europe and America are placed in the wider context of the contemporaneous phenomena of globalisation, Americanisation and Europeanisation. Central questions addressed are the balance sheet of globalisation, the complex relation between Americanisation and globalisation, the European dimension of the globalisation process, and the prospect of a new world order. This analysis endeavours to de-construct and remove the mythology of contemporary notions of "America", "Europe" and the triumphant rhetoric of globalisation while, at the same time, to avoid its depiction as an exclusively negative and disruptive process.

> I do not want my house to be walled in on all sides and my windows to be stuffed. I want the cultures of all the lands to be blown about my house as freely as possible. But I refuse to be blown off my feet by any. (Gandhi, in HDR 1999: 5)

> Despite the claims to a spurious rhetoric of 'internationalism' on the part of the established multinationals and the networks of the new communication technology industries, such circulations of signs and commodities as there are, are caught in the vicious circuits of surplus value that link First World capital to Third World labour markets through the chains of the international division of labour. (Bhabha 1988: 6)

The oceans could be envisaged as a medium of exchange of sets of ideas and concepts of political, economic and cultural diversity or homogeneity that might be considered as dangerous, imposing, enlightening – or just negligible – between different parts of the world. In today's world, the view seems to prevail that this cultural exchange has turned into a one-way street from the USA to Europe and, indeed, the rest of the world, a process of globalisation based on American models primarily founded on and fuelled by free-market liberalism. This monodimensional and mono-directional view tends to obscure the fact that we *might* only observe yet another (perhaps passing) period of political, economic, military and cultural hegemony – "Europeanisation" could well be the dominant force in this century.

This essay is part of a larger project aiming at an historically dynamic perspective rather than a static photograph of the multi-faceted and multi-level relationships between "Europe" and "America." Both terms are used to refer to culturally constructed products of our minds rather than to spatially clearly defined entities. In the case of the term "America" one should be aware of what Berlant sees as an "interarticulation, now four hundred years old, between the United States and America, the nation and utopia" (Berlant, quoted in Appadurai 1993: 425). The relationship between these constructs is seen as a permanent dialogue already stretching over several centuries. It has been a dialogue that is very similar to the communication of individual people: sometimes interrupted, characterised by mutual miscomprehensions and periods of introspection in "splendid isolation" followed by intense discussions. This dialogue, and this is crucial, as I will show below, is characterised by competing discourses and an uneven distribution of negotiating and agenda-setting power.

Central to the whole project is the notion that the dialogue between Europe and America can only be understood if it is embedded in concrete historical contexts. The demystification of contemporary notions of America, Europe or globalisation can only be carried out if it is supported by an understanding of the historical processes, contexts and determinants that have produced and constructed these notions. Spivak argues that the point of the study of culture is "to negotiate between the national, the global, and the historical as well as the contemporary diasporic" (Spivak 1999: 186).

It is also vitally important to avoid the danger of what Appadurai perceives as:

> a disturbing tendency in the Western academy today to divorce the study of discourse forms from the study of other institutional forms, and the study of literary discourses from the mundane discourses of bureaucracies, armies, private corporations, and nonstate social organizations. (Appadurai 1993: 412)

The need for an interdisciplinary approach that ignores, for example, neither the economic dimension – for fear of being accused of "economic determinism" – nor studies of international relations or changing institutional structures is also emphasised by Appadurai when he argues that "[t]he complexity of the current global economy has to do with certain fundamental disjunctures between economy, culture and politics which we have barely begun to theorize" (Appadurai 1999: 221). Interdisciplinarity is understood as implied in border discourses. The inherent hybridity of border discourses helps, for example, to address the question of the meaning of America or Europe, of the intercultural relations between the two notions and, at the same time, emphasises the heterogeneity of both the cultures of America and Europe. It also offers the opportunity to move beyond the traditional notion of interdisciplinarity simply as "the (re-)combination of methods from several academic disciplines in the pursuit of an overarching research project" (Lenz 1999: 19).

Such an approach would help to keep Cultural studies an "open field" in which the endeavour to theorise should not be allowed to be taken to a point where, for example, politics and theory become mutually exclusive and where we are left with a kind of "post-political speaking-in-tongues variety" (Pfister 1996: 294) of cultural studies. To avoid losing focus, it is imperative to find at least provisional criteria to select certain periods or aspects to be examined. Lenz suggests cultural "contact zones" and "defining moments of the clash, the mixing, and the reconstitution of cultures" (Lenz 1999: 12). The war in Kosovo, for instance, could be seen as such a defining moment, highlighting international and intranational problem areas at various levels, and, at the same time, sparking off a controversial debate and proclamation of values that supposedly motivated the intervention.

The following analysis endeavours to shed some light on the most recent stage of the dialogue between America and Europe in an age of rapid processes of globalisation and growing interconnectedness. The dialogue is becoming more complex than it has ever been before. I concentrate on selected aspects of the relationship between America and Europe by placing it in the wider context of the contemporary processes of globalisation, Americanisation and, what I would like to call, "Europeanisation". The multifold implications of and interrelations between these processes will be analysed by using a multi-level and multi-issue approach. One of the major challenges of such an approach lies in the interdependence of multiple issues – economy, national politics, international relations, welfare systems, cultural phenomena and practices in a more restricted sense, to name but a few – that makes it so difficult to disentangle what can, by its very nature, not be understood in isolation.

The Balance Sheet of Globalisation

The dialogue between America and Europe is part of and embedded in manifold simultaneous and interdependent processes of globalisation and reassertions of localisms that are characteristic in the contemporary world. The most fundamental trend in recent years has been the almost universal embrace of the capitalist model by countries around the world after the collapse of communism. The analysis of processes in this global context has to go beyond simplistic notions of bi-directional relations between nations. This is arguably even more necessary now than before. And it clearly requires going beyond the nation as the major or only point of reference. Appadurai demands in "Patriotism and Its Futures" that:

> [w]e need to think ourselves beyond the nation. [...] Though the idea that we are entering a postnational world seems to have received its first airings in literary

> studies, it is now a recurrent (if un-selfconscious) theme in studies of postcolonialism, of global politics, and of international welfare policy. (Appadurai 1993: 411)

Going beyond the nation also brings postnational forms into play that already do exist and influence global and local change. Analysing the acceleration of the emergence of postnational social formations, Appadurai observes that "[t]he new organizational forms are more diverse, more fluid, and more *ad hoc*, more provisional, less coherent, less organized, and simply less implicated in the comparative advantages of the nation-state" (Appadurai 1993: 418). This notion is particularly important with regard to the issue of global actors that is taken up further below.

Hall warns with regard to the cultural impact of the globalisation process that:

> globalization must never be read as a simple process of cultural homogenization; it is always an articulation of the local, of the specific and the global. Therefore, there will always be specificities – of voices, of positioning, of identity, of cultural traditions, of histories, and these are the conditions of enunciation which enable us to speak. We speak with distinctive voices; but we speak within the logic of a cultural-global, which opens a conversation between us, which would not have been possible otherwise. (Hall 1996: 407)

Globalisation as a process has been a theme throughout the entire 20th century. *The Economist* wrote already in 1930 that "[o]n the economic plane the world has been organised into a single, all-embracing unit of activity" (*Economist* 1999a). But although globalisation is not a new phenomenon, the present era has distinctive features: "Shrinking space, shrinking time and disappearing borders are linking people's lives more deeply, more intensely, more immediately than ever before" (HDR 1999: 2).

Another difference is that the present discourse of globalisation has come to resemble a kind of all-embracing "*ersatz*-ideology". At least, it would be justified to speak of a period of hegemony of the "globalisation agenda" – widely accepted and only very rarely criticised or challenged and then often only with regard to very specific and often minor points. Why, for instance, is there so little opposition to globalisation? One answer may lie in the fact that globalisation is usually represented as the prerequisite for economic growth. Secure jobs and a rising standard of living are perceived as a function of economic growth as well as a precondition for the welfare of the people. So, if globalisation is believed to provide growth, it must be good both for employers and employees.

The dominant global discourse is further characterised by the assumption that, although there might be certain shortcomings or problems connected with the process of globalisation, on the whole the effects are positive. *The Economist* claims that:

> More broadly and over a longer period, the replacement of central planning by market-based economics and a general lowering of trade barriers have begun to lift millions of people around the world out of poverty, giving them more income, more education and more freedom of choice. (*Economist* 1999b)

One particularly interesting area to challenge over-optimistic assessments is the world-wide balance sheet of globalisation so far, i.e. the distribution of positive and negative effects. Many of the negative effects of the changes in the poor countries over the last decades are more likely to be interpreted as mistakes or exceptions that are rather consequences of the lack of enthusiasm or the insufficient implementation of the ideas of the liberal market economy than possibly of systemic shortcomings of a programme being applied fairly indiscriminately to very different countries. The question is not only whether the negative effects are systemic or exceptional, but also why there is seemingly much less opposition to or questioning of the globalisation agenda, than might be expected.

Although lip-service is being paid to the distinctiveness of the countries affected by globalisation there seems to be a widespread and dangerous belief that the same measures applied to completely different contexts may lead to similar results. Tony Blair signifies this problem when he argues that "even as between developing and developed nations, it is the similarities in the economic and social issues that often mean more than the differences. And as for within the developed world, the challenges are virtually identical" (Blair 2000a)

The analysis of the globalisation discourse reveals a sometimes astonishing readiness to perceive certain aspects of what is usually subsumed under the buzzword as *natural* and, therefore, unavoidable rather than the consequences of wilful decisions of politicians in a fairly limited number of countries, their *clubs* like the G7, managers of multinational (*trans*national) corporations, or international organisations like the United Nations, the International Monetary Fund (IMF), the World Trade Organisation (WTO) or the European Union – most of which lack any substantial democratic legitimation, or, what is more important, accountability.

Politicians are becoming increasingly aware that political, economic and social re-configurations of such a scale require the shaping of public opinion in order to get public support or, at least, minimise opposition. In Western Europe, the fears of the public are addressed by *translating* the language of globalisation into localised versions (e.g. the "Third Way") which are presented as taking the potential dangers and insecurities of the changes into consideration. One of the most outspoken propagators of the globalisation agenda in Europe, Tony Blair, claims that:

> [a]longside the advance of global markets and technologies we are seeing a new search for community, locally, nationally and globally that is a response to change and insecurity, but also reflects the best of our nature and our enduring values. With

> it is coming a new political agenda – one that is founded on mutual responsibility – both within nations and across the world. (Blair 2000a)

The de-construction and de-mythologising of the triumphant rhetoric of globalisation has to avoid the apparent danger of depicting it as an exclusively negative and disruptive process. It requires investigating the concrete effects of globalisation and the empirical evidence which is, although not always conclusive or unequivocal, available in order to highlight the differential effects of globalisation and simultaneously challenge its over-optimistic evaluation and representation.

Globalisation is a very complex and multi-faceted process that has positive and negative effects – quite a few of which are not yet discovered, hardly recognised or understood. But even this binary distinction does not go to the heart of the matter because it ignores the differential consequences in different contexts, for different countries or for different strata of society within a particular country and underestimates the enormous diversity in conditions – economic social, cultural, ecological. Moreover, certain short-term effects might change in the medium or long-term perspective. There is no space here to present the data extensively, but I would like to name at least some examples that illustrate the differential effects of globalisation and, at the same time, challenge overoptimistic assessments.

Much of the free-trade rhetoric, for instance, assumes that globalisation necessarily leads to economic progress. This view is supported by the fact that most industrial countries, the newly industrialising East Asian tigers and, for example, Chile, the Dominican Republic, India, Mauritius, Poland, Turkey and many others have managed to take advantage of the increasing global integration and technological advances and to catch up with the most advanced. Japan, for example, had scarcely 20% of US income in 1950, a figure which had risen to 90% in 1992; southern Europe has seen a similar trend – with 26% of US income in 1950 and 53% in 1992 (HDR 1999: 38) Other countries, to quote the 1999 Human Development Report at some length:

> are becoming even more marginal – ironic, since many of them are highly "integrated", with exports nearly 30% of GDP for Sub-Saharan Africa and only 19% for the OECD. But these countries hang on the vagaries of global markets, with the prices of primary commodities having fallen to their lowest in a century and a half. They have shown little growth in exports and attracted virtually no foreign investment. (HDR 1999: 2)

> More than 80 countries still have per capita incomes lower than they were a decade or more ago. While 40 countries have sustained average per capita income growth of more than 3% a year since 1990, 55 countries, mostly in Sub-Saharan Africa and Eastern Europe and the Commonwealth of Independent States (CIS), have had declining per capita incomes. (*ibid.*: 2-3)

The process of widening gaps is not exclusively a problem for the poor countries but can be observed similarly in the OECD countries: "Recent studies show inequality rising in most OECD countries during the 1980s and into the early 1990s. Of 19 countries, only one showed a slight improvement. The deterioration was worst in Sweden, the United Kingdom and the United States" (*ibid.*: 37). Interestingly, both the UK and the US are countries that have embraced the globalisation agenda most enthusiastically and comprehensively.

These and similar figures and trends do not imply that they are necessarily and inevitably a consequence of global economic integration, but rather of the failure to distribute the benefits more evenly between countries and specific strata within countries. Despite the claims of an increasingly integrated and co-operating world this co-operation continues to be characterised by clearly unevenly distributed powers to take part in the agenda-setting and decision-making processes. An increasingly globalised world will need stronger governance[1] if the benefits of it are to be more evenly distributed. The Human Development Report, quoted above, points out that the continuing and, arguably accelerating, marginalisation of many poor countries could only be addressed if the international structures and processes for global policy making became more representative and reflective of the interests and needs of those countries. The problem is not limited to representation and participation but includes the issues of transparency of the decision-making processes and accountability of the global actors. The existing and newly emerging structures, rules and practices for global governance put very few countries clearly at an advantage and prioritise the creation of a secure and beneficial environment for open markets; human rights protection and human development only come second. Self-appointed policy groups like the World Economic Forum are making "*de facto* global economic policy, outside the United Nations or any other formal system with democratic processes and participation" (*ibid.*: 34).

"Americanisation" or Globalisation?

Another central question that can only be indicated here, is how much of the adoption of the "American model" world-wide could be subsumed under the terms Americanisation, globalisation, or simply raw capitalism, set free or freeing itself from the previous, but only temporary constraints after the demise of its major opponent at the end of the Cold War. Lenz emphasises the need to avoid a simplistic equation of the terms Americanisation and globalisation:

> If "modernization" has turned out to have been, and to be, *not* identical with "Americanization," as many foreign observers had claimed earlier during this

[1] The concept of governance is not to be confused with government. It means "the framework of rules, institutions and established practices that set limits and give incentives for the behaviour of individuals, organizations and firms" (HDR 1999: 8).

> "American Century," the more recent *globalization processes* are also *not* to be seen simply as processes of "Americanization" in a new post-Fordist capitalism by the one remaining world power, but as happening and being conceived in *different* ways in a multicentered world. (Lenz 1999: 16-17)

It is, however, evident that globalisation takes place at a time when there is no serious challenge to the political, economic, military and technological leadership of the United States. So it is perhaps not surprising that globalisation is often equated with Americanisation. The fact that Americanisation has become more attractive and less threatening to many today than it might have been at other times is very much based on its very positive economic performance in the 1990s and improvements of various social indicators (the most notable exception to this partial "acceptance" of Americanisation is the case of the continuing charges of "cultural imperialism").

However, identity creating or re-configuring processes are occasionally supplemented by what could be called "negative identity formation." In the European context this draws in some quarters on distaste for and distrust of American might in business, diplomacy and arms and Asian competition, which is also perceived as a threat. The historian Dan Diner has pointed out the paradoxical function the negative projection of America has had for 200 years to bring about a European identity. America as the younger brother who has quickly outgrown Europe is ascribed all those negative characteristics from which Europe wants to separate itself (Herzinger 1999). There are, however, limits to "Othering" the USA because they are widely perceived and represented as the driving force and a positive example to follow in many ways in the "age of globalisation."

The intricacies of accepting the role model of the United States became apparent during the Kosovo war. NATO displayed a cohesion that had not been expected by many observers. During the course of the war, however, cracks in the alliance became apparent, and European commentators criticised the leading role of the United States. The doubts about the strategy of NATO were accompanied by massive anti-American emotions. Some on the far left perceived the war as a new instance of aggressive American imperialism and the attempt to impose its model, if necessary by military means. Some on the far right argued that the United States are the prototype of a universalistic multiethnic society that aims at the eradication of racial and national characteristics. The NATO attacks on behalf of the Kosovo Albanians were interpreted as part of the American strategy to destroy European ethnicities through the mixture of nations (*ibid.*). Others claimed that the United States instrumentalised NATO for their own egoistic aim of achieving global dominance – the European partners acting as "deputy sheriffs" (*ibid.*). The renewed willingness of the US to get involved in European affairs was perceived as "arrogance of power." The accusation that the USA were, once again, defeating their opponents with their technological dominance while minimising their own risks drew heavily on deeply ingrained resentment especially in Germany (*ibid.*).

Another problematic issue is the widespread attempt of politicians to "sell" unwelcome or difficult changes they would like to make themselves as *necessitated* by globalisation although national governments are finally responsible for them. Appadurai argues that:

> the simplification of these many forces (and fears) of homogenization can also be exploited by nation states in relation to their own minorities, by posing global commoditization (or capitalism, or some other such external enemy) as more 'real' than the threat of its own hegemonic strategies. (Appadurai 1999: 221)

This is perhaps most apparent in the field of labour de-regulation and cuts in or "re-structuring" of welfare systems – the blame is put on the requirements of globalisation (which is perceived by many as just a new term for Americanisation). In certain cases the recognition that the public might be against certain changes because they are perceived as forms of further Americanisation and the attempt to avoid accusations of slavish imitation of the USA might lead to very curious results, as, for instance, in the blueprint for "radical transformation of the European economy" that European leaders produced at a summit in Lisbon in 2000:

> Georges Perec once wrote a 300-page novel without using the letter e. To write a 5,000 word manifesto on the "new economy" without once using the word America, or even the words United States, cannot have been much easier, but the European Union's leaders were equal to the task when they met in Lisbon last week. (*Economist* 2000)

Americanisation and globalisation clearly raise the question of the future of national and local cultures in a context that seems to work towards a global culture. Globalisation is not necessarily going to have a negative influence on people's cultures – but the question of the specific character of the changes to come remains unanswered. Although Americanisation as a theme has figured most prominently in Western Europe over several decades, it must not be overlooked that other cases of cultural domination might be more important for individual countries. Appadurai draws up an alternative list of cultural domination exerted by other countries and concludes that "for polities of smaller scale, there is always a fear of cultural absorption by polities of larger scale, especially those that are nearby" (Appadurai 1999: 221).

The European Dimension of Globalisation

An essential aspect of the analysis of the European dimension of globalisation is the question whether we are witnessing a re-definition of Europe, the development of a new common identity which might be a step towards becoming a global player equal in weight to the USA. Arguably, this is not going to happen in the foreseeable future and it might be time to remind ourselves of Henry Kissinger's famous question: "Who do you call when you want to call Europe?" (*Economist* 2000a).

Approaching the notion of Europe, one becomes only too aware that Europe's political and economic order is by no means settled, it is rapidly shifting, and may be changing even more quickly as a consequence of EU enlargement and globalisation. Many of Western Europe's parties of the left, currently governing some of the most influential countries in the EU, have been moving towards economic structures and social models that were hardly imaginable just 15 years ago. These changes take different shapes in individual countries throughout the EU, but the general trend, despite what politicians tell their alarmed electorates, seems to be set towards what could loosely be described as the "American model" with a "European face". This is also true for those countries who expect (or hope) to become members of the European Union. In this respect the EU, although it has not been much involved in classic foreign policy until now, has already radically influenced developments towards market economies and political restructuring: "By manipulating one main instrument, the prospect of EU membership, it has transformed and stabilised half Europe, with more to follow" (*ibid.*).

The question which concerns us here is whether the strikingly successful economic and political "European Project", i.e. the striving for ever closer union, has also had an impact on the creation of some kind of a new identity going beyond national boundaries or national self-interests which hoped to be enhanced by membership. The potential of the European Union to provide a focal point for the creation of a European identity, however, has been severely undermined by the fact that many politicians have fanned voters' hostility to the EU – "Brussels bureaucrats" make easy scapegoats for almost every ill. Often these charges are not only contradictory, but they also ignore the crucial point that most of Brussels' directives require the approval of the national governments. Michel Barnier, France's minister for Europe, said in 1997 that "Brussels-bashers at home are always impressed when he points out that all EU directives require the approval of member governments – and that all these directives bar one (on summer time) have had the French government's support" (*Economist* 1997). One major reason to be an influential member of the European Union that goes beyond the boundaries of a solely European context is given by Tony Blair, who is convinced that:

> as we lost influence in Europe, it did not help us in America. Britain has close ties with America. They will remain close, no more so than under this Government. But America wants Britain to be a strong ally in a strong Europe. The stronger we are in Europe, the stronger our American relationship. (Blair 2000)

In his "Doctrine of the International Community" he also emphasised this point by saying that "[f]or far too long British ambivalence to Europe has made us irrelevant in Europe, and consequently of less importance to the United States"

(Blair 2000c). Similar to other countries playing a leading role in Europe the present British government perceives the European Union not as an alternative to the nation state but as a way of enhancing their national interests at a time when world-wide other states are forming co-operative bodies – ASEAN in Asia, MERCOSUR in Latin America, NAFTA in North America. This notion that the EU is foremost a tool to advance national self-interests within and via a power bloc could be seen as working against any future development towards a common identity beyond egoistic motives. Taking into account these possibly divisive forces it could, nevertheless, be argued that, despite internal quarrels and egoistic motivational structures, an identity defined in relation to "outsiders" and based on "European interests" in addition to national ones will emerge, which might eventually, although primarily negative, serve as a cohesive element.

For the new entrants, much more than for established members, the question arises whether the EU could, apart from offering economic and political incentives, be a new site of "belonging" (McRobbie 1996: 242) or identity that could be chosen. This notion of the opportunity to choose a site or sites of belonging could be applied to the question of potentially emerging multi-level identities or loyalties in the contexts of nation, Europe or the "Empire of Democracy", i.e. the part of the world that upholds and subscribes to the values of democracy, market economy and the need for global integration and co-operation. Politicians trying to address, create or reconcile these multiple sites of belonging regularly find themselves in a force-field of contradictory necessities and arguments. This becomes clearly apparent in the relation between national and European interests and priorities. The perceived need to strengthen the role of the European Union as a global player, for instance, immediately emphasises the relation between individual member states and the EU. Playing the national card does obviously not strengthen the coherence of the latter. Apart from political or economic questions this problem also involves issues of cultural identity and discourses that cannot take place in isolation on one chosen level without any reference to alternative discursive levels.

Although the emergence of a European identity as a result of future changes is far from certain, the prospect of membership will be crucial for the degree and speed of political and economic reforms in Eastern Europe and the Balkans. The indirect domination of the future direction of those reforms by the European Union has been compared to "remote-control colonialism". Lucas argues that "the governments of the Czech Republic, Poland, Hungary, Estonia and Slovenia look and sound independent, but in reality their freedom of action will be ever-more constrained by the requirements of their western neighbours" (*Economist* 1998). This kind of remote-control colonialism is not necessarily confined to applicants as Austria discovered in February 2000 as a consequence of Jörg Haider's Freedom Party entering the Austrian government.

The probability of the emergence of a coherent European identity is still fairly small because of the heterogeneity even within the European Union which has been working towards an ever closer union for more than 40 years and due to the persistence of nationally defined priorities both in relation to the future of the Union and towards what is perceived as national matters. If, however, the liberalisation process, hand in hand with the encouragement of convergence of European economies through the common currency, leads to less distinction between national economic interests, then there will probably be more reasons to move towards a common foreign and security policy. This could then function as the basis of a European identity defined in relation to "outsiders". The possibility of negative identity formation *against* the United States will remain limited as long as the US continue to function as an economic (and for some also social) role model. This will depend crucially on the performance of the US economy.

Towards a New World Order?

The development of the relationship between the United States and Europe through the European Union and NATO raises the question whether we are witnessing the emergence of a new Euro-Atlantic alliance, or the "Empire of Democracy", now that a continuation of the involvement of the United States in Europe is taken for granted – at least by European observers. In the USA this is less clear. Homi Bhabha, already in 1988, argued that he is:

> convinced that in the language of international diplomacy there is a sharp growth in a new Anglo-American nationalism (NATO-nalism?) that increasingly articulates its economic and military power in political acts that express a neo-imperialist disregard for the independence and autonomy of Other [*sic*] people and places, largely in the Third World. [...] I am further convinced that such economic and political domination has a profound hegemonic influence on the information orders of the Western world, its popular media and its specialized institutions and academies. (Bhabha 1988: 6)

At the World Economic Forum in the USA in 1999, Thomas Donohue, the meeting's co-chairman and then President and Chief Executive Officer of the US Chamber of Commerce, pointed out the important need for global interaction and co-operation. Specifically, he stressed "the current importance of a stronger transatlantic alliance in both the political and economic spheres" (Report 1999: 6).

The analyst of the role of the United States in the process of globalisation and the creation of a Euro-Atlantic alliance needs to be aware that it is not as if globalisation is foisted on helpless politicians around the world who simply lack the power or courage to reject it. Looking at Europe this is apparently not the case. Tony Blair and New Labour might be more willing than others to follow the leadership of the United States, but this is rather a matter of degree than principle. When Blair addressed the *Economic Club* in Chicago on 23 April 1999, he confirmed both the dominant position of the USA and the vital need for it to continue its global role. Addressing his hosts, he pointed out that "America's allies are always both relieved and gratified by its continuing readiness to shoulder burdens and responsibilities that come with its sole superpower status. We understand that this is something that we have no right to take for granted, and must match with our own efforts" (Blair 2000c).

The contours of a future Euro-Atlantic alliance or "Empire of Democracy" were sharply focussed during the war in Kosovo which also shaped the discourse about the respective roles of the USA, Britain and Europe in the global arena and an allegedly emerging world order. For both Europeans and Americans the war in Kosovo differed from other locations of ethnic strife and mass killings because it echoed Europe in the period preceding the Second World War and the war itself. Echoes of "forced migration, the separation of families and the slaughter of men, the way nationalism can trump all other arguments and emotions, and the horror of the large-scale bombing of towns and villages" (*Economist* 1999b). This reading of the war was strongly employed by those who defended the action against Serbia and Milosevic: "We have learned twice before in this century that appeasement does not work. If we let an evil dictator range unchallenged, we will have to spill infinitely more blood and treasure to stop him later" (Blair 2000c).

The World Economic Forum in the USA in 1999 raised the question whether the war had the potential to spread and disrupt the post-war peace settlement and how ethnic conflict will be handled in the future: "[I]s the world creating a new standard of action thereby changing the international legal order and creating new expectations for the future in other ethnic conflicts?" (Report 1999: 6). *The Economist* is convinced that events in the Balkans have made plain that Europe cannot keep the peace without the United States and sees a kind of "division of labour" in the making:

> In the continent's potential killing fields, moreover, there is a natural division of labour whereby America's might serves as a strategic deterrent, while artfully applied economic assistance from EU governments keeps local antagonisms from boiling over. (*Economist* 2000b)

The significance of the war in Kosovo as a "defining moment" for the move towards a new world order cannot be overestimated. The war not only provided new examples for international institutions like the United Nations being ignored but also for a revolutionary re-definition of the concept of sovereignty. The re-definition of the concept of sovereignty is potentially more important for the future course of the world than the ignoring of the United Nations in particular circumstances.

The sovereignty of states had been, at least in theory, guaranteed by the League of Nations. Though it could be argued that the United States, the Soviet Union and many other countries have militarily intervened in sovereign states, the war in Kosovo was different from all these precedents because for the first time "a coalition of respectable countries has openly said that it is prepared to use force to stop the accepted ruler of a sovereign state doing bad things to his own people" (*Economist* 2000c).

This re-defined concept of sovereignty is reflected in the new NATO doctrine that will be radically different from that of the Cold War. Beedham argues that:

> [t]he purpose is no longer for America to help the European democracies defend their borders against Russia. It is for Europe and America to march side by side to the wars they will very likely have to fight outside their borders in the century ahead. NATO, formerly an American arm round Europe's shoulder, is becoming an organisation capable of projecting global force. (*Economist* 1999)

In a statement on the NATO summit in 1999 celebrating the 50th anniversary of the organisation, Blair told the House of Commons that:

> [w]hile NATO's fundamental role will remain the defence and security of the allies, there was an equally strong consensus on the need for a more capable and flexible Alliance, able to contribute to security throughout the Euro-Atlantic area and to promote the values of democracy, human rights and the rule of law for which it has stood since its foundation. (Blair 2000b)

The war in Kosovo could be interpreted as the beginning of a new bi-polar world. One pole would be the "Empire of Democracy" with the United States as its unrivalled leader and the second formed by those countries who do not qualify for "citizenship". This Empire of Democracy would be open to new entrants who subscribe to what is defined as its core values: liberty, the rule of law, human rights and an open and democratic society.

The most pressing foreign policy problem for this Empire of Democracy would be to define circumstances in which it should get involved in other countries' affairs. Although the principle of non-interference is re-affirmed as being central to international affairs, it is argued that it can or, indeed, must be qualified in important aspects. According to Blair, whose views on this particular problem are shared by other European leaders, intervention would be justified under the following circumstances:

> Acts of genocide can never be a purely internal matter. When oppression produces massive flows of refugees which unsettle neighbouring countries then they can properly be described as 'threats to international peace and security'. (Blair 2000c)

Blair insisted with regard to events in Kosovo that "[w]e cannot allow that to happen, not on Europe's doorstep without acting" (Blair 1999a). The practical consequences of this stance in the future are open to debate, but the language clearly resembles that of the USA when justifying their interventions in Latin America. Such a view might become even more problematic with the shifting of the "doorstep" further East as a result of the NATO entry of Poland, Hungary and the Czech Republic.

The defeat of Milosevic and the concept of an Empire of Democracy also inform the possibility and contours of a European identity. Addressing the Atlantic Club of Bulgaria, Blair outlined his vision of a future Europe:

> From this time on, let us offer a common vision of the future: where nations become part of the true family of Europe, part of our security, part of our Prosperity. We are all European nations. We are all European peoples. [...] We have a common interest, in rebuilding the Balkans on the principles of peace and democracy. This is the struggle for the future. Milosevic is the past. We, the Democrats, are the future. It is our common destiny. (Blair 1999)

Three questions among many others in the future will be who is going to define this Empire of Democracy beyond seemingly uncontroversial principles of peace and democracy, who is going to become the keeper of the gates, and what is going to happen if one country cannot meet the high standards? The reaction of the European Union towards the "case" of Haider mentioned above and the "remote-control colonialism" in Eastern Europe might be indicative of things to come.

Conclusion

The major challenge of globalization is not, in the words of the Human Development Report, to stop it, but:

> to find the rules and institutions for stronger governance – local, national, regional and global – to preserve the advantages of global markets and competition, but also to provide enough space for human, community and environmental resources to ensure that globalization works for people – not just for profits. (HDR 1999: 2)

Globalisation is "too important to be left as unmanaged as it is at present, because it has the capacity to do extraordinary harm as well as good" (*ibid.*: v). This will mean that lip-service currently paid to aspects of the globalisation process and the problems particularly in developing countries will have to change to tangible actions. Emerging global NGO networks have the potential to grow in strength and ability to influence the direction of the globalisation processes towards human development, environmental protection and protection of human rights through pressure on the decisive global players. Perhaps amazingly, despite all the current problems and controversies that characterise the globalisation process:

> [t]he drift, as sceptics will have detected, is back towards the Enlightenment optimism derided earlier: that all problems are solvable. [...] But, and here is the limit to such blue-sky optimism, this does not mean that it will be: solvable problems are not always solved. (*Economist* 1999b)

Clinton, for example, genuinely seems to believe that the business leaders of the world are going to sort out the problems of the future. Addressing roughly 1,000 of the most influential business leaders he said that his most important wish is:

> that the global business community could adopt a shared vision for the next 10 to 20 years about what you want the world to look like, and then go about trying to create it in ways that actually enhance your business, but do so in a way that helps other people as well. (Clinton 2000)

There is a certain tendency to ascribe most of the changes, at least those that might hurt somebody, to some not quite tangible process of globalisation, Americanisation or Europeanisation that leaves sufficiently unclear those who work and decide behind these "conceptual smokescreens". Truly interdisciplinary and politically engaged cultural studies could play a vital role in lifting those smokescreens. Although the global economic framework increasingly defines the limits of national activities, and much of the impetus for future changes in Europe (not only in the European Union) will continue to come from Brussels, this does not imply that there is no room for public concern, opposition or pressure from the public including academics. It should be stressed again that the globalisation process itself is not a natural force and therefore open to human intervention that will have to go beyond traditional party politics.

Bibliography:

Appadurai, Arjun (1993) "Patriotism and Its Futures", *Public Culture* 5: 3.

Appadurai, Arjun (1999) "Disjuncture and Difference in the Global Cultural Economy", During, Simon, ed. (1999) *The Cultural Studies Reader*, 2nd ed., London and New York, 1999.

Bhabha, Homi K. (1988) "The Commitment to Theory", *New Formations* 5.

Blair, Tony (1999) "Speech to the Atlantic Club of Bulgaria" [17 May 1999], Tony Blair's Political Speeches, www.number-10.gov.uk/ (13.02.2000).

Blair, Tony (1999a) "Interview with NBC Today" [04 May 1999], www.number-10.gov.uk/ (15.02.2000).

Blair, Tony (2000) "Committed to Europe, Reforming Europe" [23 February 2000] The Prime Minister, Delivered at Ghent City Hall, Belgium, Wed 23 February 2000, www.number-10.gov.uk/ (27.03.2000).

Blair, Tony (2000a) "Speech at the World Economic Forum at Davos, Switzerland, 18th January 2000", Tony Blair's Political Speeches, www.number-10.gov.uk/ (24.02.2000).

Blair, Tony (2000b) "Statement on NATO Summit in Washington" [26 April 1999], www.number-10.gov.uk/ (15.01.2000), House of Commons.

Blair, Tony (2000c) "Doctrine of the International Community" [23.April 1999], Tony Blair's Political Speeches, www.number-10.gov.uk/(17.02.2000) [Blair in Chicago addressing the Economic Club.].

Clinton, William J. (2000) "Address to the Annual Meeting 2000", Davos, Switzerland, 29 January 2000, www.weforum.org/davos.nsf/Documents/ (27.03.2000)

Economist (1997) "European Union. Learning to Love the EU", *The Economist/Internet Edition*, 31st May 1997, www.economist.com/ editorial/freeforall/19970531/eu5.html (14.12.1999).

Economist (1998) Edward Lucas, "Eastern Europe: Time to Smarten Up", *The Economist/Internet Edition*, www.theworldin.com/1998/eu015.html (13.08.1999).

Economist (1999) Brian, Beedham, "All Eyes on Turkey", *The Economist/Internet Edition*, www.theworldin.com/1998/in002.html (12.09.1999).

Economist (1999a) "Survey 20th Century. A Semi-integrated World," *The Economist/Internet Edition*, 11th September 1999, www.economist.com/ editorial/freeforall/19990911/su5380.html (16.03.2000).

Economist (1999b) Emmott, Bill, "Survey 20th Century. On the Yellow Brick Road", *The Economist/Internet Edition*, 11th September 1999, www.economist.com/editorial/freeforall/19990911/su3796.html (22.02. 2000).

Economist (2000) "Europe in Cyberspace", *The Economist/Internet Edition*, www.economist.com/editorial/freeforall/current/ld2384.html (4.04.2000).

Economist (2000a) "Lots to Be Doing in Europe", *The Economist/Internet Edition*, www.theworldin.com/1999/arts/eur/eur1.htm (12.02.2000).

Economist (2000b) "The Next Balkan War", *The Economist/Internet Edition*, www.economist.com/editorial/ freeforall/current/ld2160.html (4.04.2000).

Economist (2000c) Brian, Beedham, "The Empire of Democracy", *The Economist/Internet Edition*, http://www.theworldin.com/1999/arts/lea/ lea3.htm (19.01.2000).

Hall, Stuart (1996) "Cultural Studies and the Politics of Internationalization. An Interview with Stuart Hall by Kuan-Hsing Chen", in: Morley, David; Chen, Kuan-Hsing, eds. (1996) *Stuart Hall. Critical Dialogues in Cultural Studies*, London and New York, 1996.

HDR (1999) "Human Development Report 1999", www.undp.org/hdro/ report.html (28.02.2000).

Herzinger, Richard (1999) "Feindbild Rambo. Der neue Antiamerikanismus ist ein Versuch, die europäische Verunsicherung zu überspielen", *Die Zeit* Nr. 21, 20.5.1999.

Lenz, Günter H. (1999) "Towards a Dialogics of International American Culture Studies: Transnationality, Border Discourses, and Public Culture(s)", *Amerikastudien/American Studies* 44: 1.

McRobbie, Angela (1996) "Looking Back at New Times and Its Critics", in: Morley, David and Kuan-Hsing Chen, eds. (1996) *Stuart Hall: Critical Dialogues in Cultural Studies,* London and New York.

Pfister, Joel, (1996) "The Americanization of Cultural Studies", in: Storey, John, ed. (1996) *What Is Cultural Studies*, London, New York, Sydney, Auckland.

Report (1999) "Report on the 1999 USA Meeting, Operating in a New Global Market Place", Washington DC, 14-15 April. "Committed to Improving the State of the World", www.webforum.org/pdf/USA_report.pdf (25.03.2000).

Spivak, Gayatri Chakravorty (1999) "Scattered Speculations on the Question of Cultural Studies", in: During, Simon, ed. (1999) *The Cultural Studies Reader*, 2nd ed., London and New York.

POSTSCRIPT:

CULTURAL VARIETY OR VARIETY OF CULTURES?

ZYGMUNT BAUMAN

Radical change is taking place in the way we think and talk of 'culture' – that part of human condition which is 'human made': the part, that is, which has not been determined by the no-appeal-allowed verdicts of inhuman nature, but depends on past, present and future human *choices* and could be therefore, at least in principle, different than it is.

The idea of 'culture' is modern; it was born together with the modern spirit notorious for its bold and sometimes arrogant ambition to correct, improve and otherwise remake the setting of human life so that it would serve better the cause of decent life and human happiness. The term 'culture' appeared first in the Eighteenth Century vocabulary as an exhortation, a clarion call, name of a job to be done and a declaration of intent to see that job through. The concept conveyed a message: like plants in the field, orchard or garden, human beings need to be cultivated in order to develop in full their best qualities. The humanity of human beings is not something 'given', and would not develop on its own accord. Humanity lies still ahead: it is a task – one which has to be carefully designed, resolutely executed and vigilantly monitored all along.

Since culture, unlike 'nature', was a matter of choice – a sediment of choices made in the past and outcome of choices currently made – it went without saying that the 'humanity' which the effort of cultivation (of teaching, training, educating, socialising, or whatever other name was used for the 'formative' influence) brings to bear may take various shapes and colours. There are many cultures; as Ruth Benedict famously put it, there are many cups with which different peoples drink from the stream of life.

The concept of 'culture' had an evaluating ring; it implied hierarchy – it suggested that being cultured is a matter of degree, that there could be men and women who are better, worse or not at all 'cultured' (educated, refined), who come closer or stay distant from the ideal which the labour of cultivation aimed to promote. But it had also a differentiating edge; human collectivities differ from each other depending on the 'cultural patterns' by which they shape and obey their daily routines, setting apart the proper from the improper, good from evil, beautiful from ugly, the desirable from the resented, true from false and right from wrong. Each culture has its ideal standard, but what is considered to be ideal differs, and it is this difference between selected ideal patterns that makes human groups different from each other.

Our perception of the world is as a rule 'praxeomorphic'. We tend to see the world through the prism of the tasks we set for ourselves or the 'problems' which we recognise as calling for our attention and are struggling to resolve. At the time the idea of culture was coined, the human world was viewed from the perspective of the agenda set by the ruling and the learned classes engaged jointly in the complex task of 'nation building'. While setting that task, the governments of the emergent nationstates, unlike the powers of the 'ancient regime', could not rely on the intrinsic wisdom of self-reproducing habits and routines; transformation of the many and varied types of 'locals' into the patriots of 'one nation' would not have occurred on its own accord.

Loyalty to the state claiming to embody the unity of the nation would not sprout and ripe by itself; its seeds had to be carefully selected and sown; fertilised, sheltered from inclement weather, protected against weeds and parasites. To replace the irritating randomness of the plurality of ways of life by an integrated and one-for-all national culture, not just intense indoctrination, but coercion had to be frequently used and a penal system had to be set in operation; under the French Third Republic, for instance, use of local dialects instead of standard French was prohibited, and penalised, in schools (including the playgrounds), in the army and in public offices (Warnier 1999: 69). Governments of the day treated their compatriots not unlike the populations of invaded countries were treated by their conquerors bent on colonising the captured territory and effacing its separate identity. Intended homogeneity of national culture required stamping out local customs, dialects and calendars, consigning local histories to oblivion and tearing apart local bonds and loyalties. The confused and confusing variety of locally rooted traditional forms of life had to be thrown into a melting pot and recast as the spirit of the not-yet-existing nation. 'National culture' was nowhere else but at the horizon of the long and tortuous effort of cultivation.

Protecting the shared history, serving the shared interest and securing the shared future of the nation was to become the prime legitimating formula of modern states; the formula all governments of modern states would invoke whenever demanding from their subjects discipline to the law of the country, obedience to the powers of the state and sacrifice in the name of the shared goals as set out by state authorities.

Propagation of national solidarity, of the 'us' feeling (and so of the 'us versus them' perception of the world) provided the lens through which the role of culture was viewed and the cognitive frame in which the vision of culture was plotted. Like all other legal and institutional supports of the nation-state sovereignty and of its claims to the citizens' obedience, culture had to be complete, distinctive and internally coherent and harmonious. No wonder it was visualized as a system – and a total and self-sustained system. Everything in a culture visualized in such a fashion was related to everything else, there was no room inside it for anything jarring with or unfitting the rest, 'dysfunctional' or simply useless and devoid of function. Imported items were feared to throw the totality out of balance, to disturb or even incapacitate the system as a whole. Cultures basked in the reflected glory of the nation-state sovereignty and like the state-made laws claimed monopoly over the territory under the state's sovereign rule. In Ulf Hannerz's description: cultures tended to be imagined as 'bounded, pure, integrated, cohesive, distinctive, place-rooted and mapped in space' (Hannerz 1993: 68).

It is this image which has lost by now a lot of its past credibility. And no wonder – since the powers of the nationstate (more exactly; of the modern state struggling to become a nationstate) whose practices sustained the credibility of that image and made it look like a faithful replica of cultural reality have been radically weakened while the holders of state power shed much of their previous normative-regulative ambition. Moreover, the state powers have found other, less costly yet no less efficient means to legitimise the demands of the citizens' obedience to its much reduced authority than beefing up and then harnessing their patriotic sentiments. Governments ceded a large part of the social-integration task to the seductive force of the consumer market, by its nature exterritorial and cosmopolitan; a force which unlike the state sovereignty thrives on variety and difference and could not care less about the ideological preferences of its customers.

Thanks to the failing interest of political powers (and of the nation-state in the first place) in regulating the capital and commodity movements, and its diminishing ability to constrain and channel them, the global network of economic dependencies has acquired growing independence from the territory. A new 'global void' has emerged, in which departures occur that are crucial for the life conditions of the residents of territorially circumscribed units, but which neither these residents nor their political representations can control. Even if they were the comprehensive, coherent, and self-enclosed systems as they had been imagined in the nation building and the state sovereignty era, 'cultures' would be unable under the new conditions to sustain the self-reproduction of communal, territorially plotted identities as they were supposed or imputed to do. The point is, though, that with the power-assisted intentions to secure and guard the purity of national cultures all but non-existent, and their pressures on daily life and life-prospects ever less felt, there is little in the life experience of the denizens of the globalisation era to suggest, let alone to corroborate, the 'system-like' image of culture.

Indeed, we may say that the imagery of 'culture' inherited from the nation-building era undergoes currently a veritable 'paradigm crisis'. The pile of evidence contradicting the holistic/systemic model of culture grows sky-high and can no more be set aside or dismissed as 'exceptions from the rule', anomalies or marginal disturbances of the pattern. An empirically sustainable model of culture, a model capable of incorporating and 'making sense of' current experience, needs to put paid to the idea of cultures as coherent, self-equilibrating and self-sustainable systems altogether. As Ronnie Lippens summed it up recently, the 'reading of contemporary experience comes down to a reading of impurities, of hybridities' (2000: 11). Having coined the composite concept of (b)orders which emphasises the fact that borders have been at all times by-products of ordering bustle, Lippens suggests that what we have come to realise nowadays better than ever before is that (b)orders tend to 'get thinner, while fixating'; and that 'ours is a time when (b)orders ... have exploded. There are no clear (b)orders anymore' (Lippens 2000: 78).

Let us note that in order to make the new experience intelligible Lippens had to resort to concepts and images which have acquired their meaning from an experience now left behind and no more available; for that reason, they are not well fit to embrace the experience which has come to replace it – a predicament that further testifies to the condition of the 'paradigm crisis'. The terms like 'impurity' or 'hybridity' tacitly assume what the propositions formed with their help openly deny: that there could be such thing as 'pure' (that is, free from 'foreign' intrusions) cultural totality and that each one of them could be 'of one stock', 'monolithic'. And so even when the picture is meant to represent the 'normal' state of the cultural scene, now grasped thanks to our retrospective wisdom, it looks more like a collage of 'abnormalities'. We still deploy 'ghost' terms, 'zombie terms' (Ulrich Beck), and deploy them '*sous rature*' (Jacques Derrida) – lacking the vocabulary fully adequate to the task of narrating our kind of life – a life lived 'in a flow' rather than amidst fixed objects.

Perhaps the time is ripe to abandon the term 'culture' altogether. The meanings which this term has been coined to convey have lost a good deal of their experiential grounding; the hierarchical, evaluating meaning has lost much of its sense since there are no more 'ideal patterns' to promote and no agencies wishing or able to promote them, let alone hope of the ultimate success of the undertaking, while the differential meaning has lost much of its use in view of the notorious porousness of all boundaries and glaring impotence of the border-guards. In addition, the opposition between 'culture' and 'nature' (between 'human made' parts of the world and all the rest) has lost much of its previously assumed sharpness; aspects of the world once believed to stay firmly beyond the reach of human transforming capacity, like heredity, are increasingly the objects of purposeful manipulation – while on the other hand many phenomena once considered to be unaffected by human actions, like weather patterns, are found to be outcomes of human activities – even if only as their unanticipated consequences.

All this is not meant to imply that the global flow of free-floating cultural tokens (objects as well as behavioural patterns) which are no more system-riveted nor space-bound, signals the levelling-up of cultural distinctions and demise of separate 'culturally shaped identities'. As Nigel Rapport convincingly argues, the emerging picture is ambiguous. On one hand, there is growing evidence to support Lee Drummond's suggestion that in view of the abundance of 'creolisations', cultural patterns of mixed origin and often incoherent composition, we can no longer sensibly speak of 'distinct cultures', only of 'inter-systemically connected, creolising Culture' (Drummond 1980); one could agree therefore with Ulf Hannerz that the time has arrived to conceive of culture as a 'flow', or a 'diversity' of interrelations'; and one should accept Clifford Geertz's metaphor of 'Kuwaiti bazaar' for all 'local points', which are constituted as 'global collages' (Geertz 1985). Indeed, all local or group-oriented 'condensations' are products of creolisation of heterogeneous items drawn from the world-wide pool of cultural offers and can no longer claim their uniqueness, own history independent from the 'global flow' or a separate and autonomous logic of development. On the other hand, however, Rapport points out that 'advocates of different selections' tend to be 'exclusionary if not hostile', and that the result of such an 'exclusionary tendency' is 'cultural compression', 'an insistence of socio-cultural difference'; 'a piling up of socio-cultural boundaries, political, ritual, residential, economic, which feel experientially vital, and which people seek to defend and maintain' (Rapport 1997: 71). Homogenising pressures proceed hand in hand with a new diversification. They are both effects, closely intertwined and interdependent effects, of the pressures of, and responses to globalisation.

Deprived of the protective, even if stiff and often cramping-the-moves armour of the nationstate sovereignty, no place can claim now immunity to global pressures, the right to resist them or the capacity to withstand. As the place is becoming a meeting point for shifting and restless global powers, and thus is fast losing the meaning of 'secure home' it once carried – it paradoxically acquires new and enhanced significance; however illusionary the protective capacity of the place might have become, people buffeted by forces they can neither understand nor control tend to cling, in their desperate search for security, to 'the place' as the sole entity that stands still while everything else – sources of livelihood and the skills they require, partnership and neighbourhood, objects of desire and causes of fear – seem to be on the move and change shape with constantly rising speed.

Whatever the enthusiasts of globalisation may say about the impending unification of the human kind it is bound to bring in its wake, its immediate effect is quite opposite: not only the anticipated species-wide solidarity is slow to materialise, but in many places the prospect of 'one humanity' seems to arouse a lot of anxiety and resentment. In her essay on Karl Jaspers, Hannah Arendt (1957) predicted such reaction and explained why it should happen:

> It is difficult to deny that at this moment the most potent symbol of the unity of mankind is the remote possibility that atomic weapons used by one country according to the political wisdom of the few might ultimately come to be the end of all human life on earth. The solidarity of mankind in this respect is entirely negative, it rests... on a common desire for a world that is *a little less unified* (Arendt 1996: 83; italics added).

The collapse of the 'ancient regime', the weakening of the balancing integrating powers of traditional community-based institutions, and the sudden exposure to the inexplicable, apparently haphazard impact of distant and poorly understood as well as completely uncontrolled powers, must have had exerted a similar psychological effect on the generations witnessing the birth of the modern order. But at that time a new dense network of the state-run and administered institutions was quick to fill the void and mitigate the threats it emanated – state institutions set to provide a collective and nation-wide insurance against individual and local misfortune. The modern state asserted itself as the embodiment of what since the time of the French Revolution was to be described as the 'politics of pity' and was bound to underlie the emergent sentiments of national unity and shared national home. Nothing comparable, however, is happening so far, on the global scale this time required, to fill the void opened by the demise of the state-bound warrants of existential security. Under the circumstances, there is little to prompt and add vigour to the species-wide solidarity; more often than not 'mankind' (indeed, everything 'global') is suspected to be the factory of the known and the as-yet-unimaginable risks and thereby acts as a prolific source of apprehension and suspicion, while the orphaned and unanchored hopes of security drift in the search of 'locality' small and cosy enough to offer the feeling of a home-like safety.

The dreamt of and feverishly sought stable and secure place has, however, no officially confirmed and legally protected location. Designating and manning the boundaries, once the institutionalised prerogative of the state, has now become for all practical intents a do-it-yourself job, left by and large to local initiative. Since the borders can count on no other protection except the vigilance, dedication and determination of people who draw and patrol them, the assertion and defence of borders become highly emotional affairs – manifestations of patriotic loyalty instigated by well-settled and entrenched nation-states seem bland and lukewarm by comparison. The do-it-yourself border derives whatever reality it might have and can count on from the perpetual tug-of-war with the neighbours and a never lapsing vigilance against the 'fifth column', 'the enemy inside'; not so much the admittedly alien foreigners, as those 'among us' who are indifferent to the purification zeal or not-strongly-enough committed to the cause of purity.

The urge to draw boundaries is not the result of the perception that the dear-to-heart difference is threatened and therefore needs defence. It is, rather, the other way round; the overwhelming desire to wall-off one's abode from the storms of globalising forces prompts the search of orientation points around which turrets could be erected and moats dug. Differences, genuine or putative, are given new salience, and are drawn into the focus of attention and assigned 'topical relevance' (Alfred Schütz) in as far as they promise, or are hoped, to serve as such orientation points. We may say that given the intensity of the separation-exclusion urge, were there no differences they would have to be invented. There is, however, no shortage of distinctive marks around which boundaries can be drawn and defensive lines built. The inventiveness of commodity merchants is itself more than sufficient to assure a constant supply of differences to choose from.

Imagination needs to defy the realities of life in the globalising world to endow a modicum of credibility to the cohesive 'communities of fate' it conjures. The defiance can never lapse, since the postulated communities tend to fall apart as quickly as they are assembled and the stories of unity, however long may be the stretch of history they invoke, hold only as long as they are told, heard and listened too. As Nigel Rapport puts it – community-bound identities tend to be temporary and fickle products of 'dialectic between movement and fixity. It is in and through the continuity of movement that human beings continue to make themselves at home' (Rapport 1997: 77). Identity is, like the people who seek it, constantly on the move; to use Paul Ricoeur's terms – the '*ipséité*' (the distinctiveness that makes the difference) needs constant re-negotiation, re-adjustment and re-assertion in order to secure a degree of '*mêmete'* (continuity over time); it can never stand still, it cannot be defined once for all, though this is precisely what the spokesmen of communal identities have to and do aver. One can apply to cultural identity John Berger's description of home as 'no longer a dwelling but the untold story of a life being lived' (Berger 1984: 84; quoted in Rapport 1997: 73). The story needs to be reiterated no end, and each time over in terms likely to catch the attention of the audience.

The stories are likely to change with each successive repetition, yet telling them will hardly stop, after all, as Robert Dunn points out, 'the politics of identity and difference are only a manifestation of a generalized and structurally induced *de-stabilisation* of identity in the West and perhaps throughout the world' (Dunn 2000: 110) – and since de-stabilisation is a permanent condition of the world undergoing globalisation in its present and apparently durable form, factors that add urgency and impetus to the politics of identity and difference will not be in short supply in a foreseeable future. Given that, the audibility of the message must be set at a high and rising pitch not to be drowned in the cacophony of competitive offers. The stage on which the drama of identity is played is likely to remain for a long time full of sound and fury.

There is nothing remotely reminiscent of a '*global* culture' in the sense of a cultural choice shared by the whole of the human species; neither is it certain that such world-wide 'cultural sameness', were it to become reality, would be necessarily a good thing. 'Global culture' is neither desirable nor, fortunately, on the cards, though this is what some observers, taking *pars pro toto,* imply when quoting the world-wide spread of various 'globalized localisms' like the 'basic English' of the internet addicts, car sellers and car park attendants, McDonald burgers, Coca-Cola bottles, Pizza parlours, explosive births and instant deaths of a Pokemon/Digimon craze, Princess Diana's mourning or American soap-operas and the Sydney Olympics beamed by television channels throughout the world.

There is, though, a new phenomenon of the '*globality* of culture' – world-wide 'virtual travel' and world-wide display of locally born forms of life. The totality of human cultural invention constitutes today the pool from which cultural items deployed in the construction of difference, prompted by the politics of identity and recognition, are picked. Globality of culture is sustained by the world-wide communication between locally born and bred traditions; it proves, if a proof is needed, that cultural inventions gestated in localities remote from each other and isolated are mutually comprehensible, and that the bond that tied them historically to a particular location is contingent and relative and does not bar them from being adopted and enjoyed by others. By the same token, globality of culture holds a promise that all cultural creations may, conceivably, gel into a common property of human kind and become a shared treasure chest from which the stuff of which individual and collective identities are kneaded can be drawn by all.

Globality of culture is a scene: scenes limit the range of scenarios which can be staged yet do not determine which scenario will be eventually chosen nor the style of production. Most seminal of choices is that between *cultural variety* and a *variety of cultures* (between cultural pluralism and the plurality of cultures); and between *multicultural* and *multicommunitarian* policies. The first assumes, to quote Alain Touraine, that culture stops being seen and treated as a 'system', a self-sustained order, having been recognised instead as 'orientation of individual conduct'; in other words – that it is admitted both in theory and in practice that cultural choice is the matter left to the discretion of individual men and women and that the choices individuals make are respected. To stand a chance, this scenario however needs 'breaking up the communities' formed after the pattern of social systems, that is such communities as aspire to pre-empt cultural choices by the conjunction of institutionalised power and communal consensus. A 'multicultural society' Touraine recommends is possible only if the prospect of a 'multicommunitarian society' (the second of the alternative scenarios) is rejected and resisted' (Touraine 1997: 306, 312). Multi-communitariarism is not the fulfilment of multiculturalism – but its principal adversary.

Cultural plurality carries a tacit assumption of human rights – that is, of the right of every human individual to be different and to have her or his difference respected. As Jürgen Habermas alerts, the promotion of human rights cannot be 'focused on safeguarding private autonomy' while 'the internal connection between the individual rights of private persons and the public autonomy of the citizens who participate in making the laws is obscured from view... Safeguarding the private autonomy of citizens with equal rights must go hand in hand with activating their autonomy as citizens...' (Habermas1994: 114, 116). There is no autonomy of the individual without an autonomous society, and the autonomy of society means fully-fledged citizenship. The right to be different cannot be fulfilled unless the equality of individuals as citizens is institutionally entrenched and practised. The right to citizenship is the preliminary condition of human rights to be honoured and observed: of the forms of life chosen through private autonomy to be respected and recognised.

This is the preliminary, but not the only condition, though. Political equality won't suffice if it is not supported by the capacity of citizens to act on their preferences and practice the form of life of their choice. And to do that, the citizens need more than the absence of interference and legally guaranteed tolerance – they need the resources which would allow them to make choices and to 'make them stick'. As I argued in *Liquid Modernity* (Bauman 2000), we are all now individuals *de jure* – deemed responsible for our choices and charged with responsibility for their consequences; we are praised for success and blamed for failure, and if our efforts do not bring the results we wish, we are told that it is because of the lack of trying or not trying hard enough. We are, so to speak, 'individuals by decree' – but the decree assumes, counter-factually, that we are all equally able to shape our life-trajectory, attend to life-challenges and solve life-problem on our own; and that we possess, individually, the tools allowing us to do just that.

None of these assumptions hold however much water. The era of 'liquid modernity' is the time of precarious, insecure and uncertain existence, of increasingly fragile and ineffective inter-human bonds and – last though not least – of rapidly rising inequality of individually available resources of action and the ranges of realistic choices. Perhaps a minority of 'individuals *de jure'* can practice the strategy recommended to us all; seek and find *biographical* solutions to *systemically* produced problems and eke out a satisfying and stable existence despite the endemic insecurity of our condition; or even use the uncertainties which haunt most of the people to their own individual advantage. The rest, however, may at best watch and envy. For that rest, choices are made by default rather than design. To rub salt into the wound, even if the choice happens to be satisfactory there is no knowing for how long it will stay such and how great its holding power will prove to be; and to add insult to injury enjoyment of 'good choice' is likely to be poisoned, and the pain inflicted by the wrong one made more acute, by the awareness that – whatever happens for whatever reason – it is the victim who will be blamed and that when it comes to the passing of verdict no allowances will be made on the victims' powerlessness to change the course of their fate.

The distance separating individuality *de jure* from individuality *de facto* is something relatively few people find easy to negotiate once the network of public transport has been phased out line by line, and the few remaining bridges spanning the gap carry a warning: 'entry for private cars only'. It should not come as a surprise, therefore, that the resulting anxiety and anger may turn against the lonely travel as such; against the no-choice precept to choose individually which evidently serves well a few while handicapping all the rest. The very idea of 'doing it alone', of taking decisions on one's own responsibility, becomes suspicious and off-putting.

Since the prospect of joining the privileged few who feel at home in the unstable and fluid environment (that is, the prospect of acquiring enough individual power for self-confident action) seems remote and nebulous, another ostensible remedy – cutting down on the number and reducing the gravity of choices to be individually made and simplifying thereby the equation that needs to be resolved at every step – becomes ever more alluring. 'Multicommunitarianism' promises just that: rather than to amplify the individual choice and put it in the reach of all those who have been thus far denied the capacity of practising it (and so to make the merely formal rights real and to lift the 'individuals *de jure*' to the status of 'individuals *de facto*'), it sets about sparing the individuals the trials and tribulations which have accompanied so far the necessity to choose. Instead of offering the way to bridge the gap between individuality *de jure* and individuality *de facto*, 'multicommunitarianism' suggests that the gap, and so the need to cross it, can (and should) be taken off the public agenda by the simple expedient of reducing the scope of individual choice and deleting some choices altogether from the inventory of individual rights.

John Gray (1997: 80-81) rightly points out that 'in the context of the past two decades or so... communitarian thinking is a response to the conception of the sovereign individual chooser that has been advanced, or pre-supposed, in recent liberal thought both of the Left and the Right.' Communitarianism in its present form capitalises on the increasingly evident hypocrisy of 'abstract individualism' which mistakes legal equality for the 'equality of sovereign choosers' and refuses to take account of the factual inequality of conditions under which individuals make their choices. There is little doubt that the ailments to which communitarianism offers itself as a remedy are genuine. The problem, though, is whether the remedy attacks indeed the causes of the sufferings it promises to cure, and how painful the side-effects of the therapy are likely to be.

Gray warns that 'communitarian thought will be fruitless or harmful if it engages in any project of propping up traditional forms of social life or recovering any past cultural consensus.' He is right, since even if restoration of the self-enclosed enclaves of 'cultural consensus' were feasible it would come nowhere near making innocuous or palatable the condition that prompted the search for remedy in the first place. Precariousness and insecurity that haunt individual life would stay by and large unaffected and unmitigated. The loss of individual rights which the implementation of the communitarian programme is bound to incur won't be compensated for by the gain of confidence and self-assurance. The riskiness of life won't go away while the chances that the new human freedoms may offer are lost or surrendered.

Something else is required: instead of trying to make the burden of individual rights lighter by cutting down on the right to choose, what is needed is the optimising of the conditions under which choices are made, and making those conditions available to those who have been thus far denied access. And that, in turn, calls for a number of essentially political steps of which the communitarian programme keeps silent and which 'multicommunitarianism' would do little, if anything at all to facilitate. To quote Gray once more, what needs to be assured is:

> reforming the central institutions of the free market so that they are *friendlier to vital human needs for security and autonomy...; preventing social exclusion* by enabling all to participate in productive *economy...;* developing institutions, countervailing or complementary to those of the market, *which foster common life* where the working of markets risk furthering exclusion. (Italics added)

All in all, these and other measures of this kind, unlike the multi-communitarian programme, may use the chances of communication and mutual comprehension which the present-day cultural plurality entails, for the sake of peaceful, solidary and mutually enriching coexistence of forms of life, varied and different yet united in their humanity. Cultural plurality and plurality of cultures are names of alternative political responses to the challenge of 'liquid modernity': responses which carry widely divergent consequences for the prospect of good society and humane life.

Bibliography:

Arendt Hannah (1996 [1957]) "Karl Jaspers: Citizen of the World?", in: *Men in Dark Times*, Harcourt Brace & Co.

Bauman, Zygmunt (2000) *Liquid Modernity,* Cambridge: Polity Press.

Bray, John (1997) "What Community Is Not", in: *Endgames: Questions in Late Modern Political Thought*, Cambridge: Polity Press.

Drummond, Lee (1980) "The Cultural Continuum: a Theory of Intersystems", *Man* 1980, 352-74.

Dunn, Robert G. (2000) "Identity, Commodification and Consumer Culture", in: Savis, Joseph E., ed. *Identity and Social Change*, Transactions Publishers.

Geertz, Clifford (1986) "The Uses of Diversity", *Michigan Quarterly Review,* Summer 1986, 105-22.

Habermas, Jürgen (1994) "Struggle for Recognition in the Democratic Constitutional State", in: Gutmann, Amy, ed. *Multiculturalism: Examining the Policy of Recognition,* Princeton UP.

Hannerz, Ulf (1993) "The Cultural Role of the World Cities", in: Cohen, A.P., and Fukui, K., eds. *Humanising the City*, Edinburgh: EUP.

Lippens, Ronnie (2000) *Chaohybrids: Five Uneasy Pieces*, University Press of America.

Rapport, Nigel (1997) *Transcendent Individual: Towards a Literary and Liberal Anthropology*, London: Routledge.

Touraine, Alain (1997) "Faux et vrais problêmes", in: Wieviorka, Michel, ed. *Une société fragmentée? Le multiculturalisme en débat*, Paris: La Découverte.

Warnier, Jean-Pierre (1999) *La Mondialisation de la culture*, Paris: La Découverte.

CONTRIBUTORS:

Zygmunt Bauman is Emeritus Professor of Sociology at the University of Leeds. He is one of the leading figures in contemporary social thought. His work ranges across issues of ethics, culture and politics. His books include *Culture as Praxis*, *Legislators and Interpreters*, *Modernity and the Holocaust*, *Modernity and Ambivalence*, *Intimations of Postmodernity*, *Mortality, Immortality and Other Life Strategies*, *Postmodern Ethics*, *Life in Fragments*, *Postmodernity and Its Discontents*, *Globalization*, *Work, Consumerism and the New Poor*, and most recently *In Search of Politics*, *Liquid Modernity*, *The Individualized Society* and *Community*.

Sebastian Berg teaches British and North American Studies at the University of Chemnitz (Germany). He wrote *Antirassismus in der britischen Labour Party. Konzepte und Kontroversen in den achtziger Jahren* (Anti-Racism in the British Labour Party: Concepts and Controversies in the 1980s), Frankfurt, Peter Lang 2000. He has published articles on the politics of race, social movements and methodological questions of British Studies. He currently works on the British New Left and its perspectives on British society and the British state since the 1960s.

Paul Bowman is lecturer in cultural studies at Bath Spa University College. He leads courses in cultural theory, political philosophies and culture, and deconstruction. Formerly the editor of the journal *Parallax*, he has published widely in this and a variety of other academic journals and books. He is currently working in the area of the politics of knowledge and the university, post-Marxist political philosophy and cultural studies, preparing books on the politics of cultural studies (*Interrogating Cultural Studies*, Pluto Press, forthcoming), and the ramifications of post-Marxist political philosophy for the future of cultural research (*Post-Marxism versus Cultural Studies*, Edinburgh University Press/New York University Press, forthcoming), as well as work on the practical 'uses' of cultural theory (*The Love and Hate of Cultural Studies*, forthcoming). Future works are planned on science, fiction, and philosophy, as well as on deconstruction and zen.

Duncan Campbell completed his Ph.D. at Cardiff University and currently works in academic publishing. He has published widely on issues in literary and cultural theory and is at present completing a book on time in Laurence Sterne's *Tristram Shandy*. His research interests also include the theory and practice of contemporary music, the poetry of David Jones, and questions of space, territory and subjectivity in twentieth-century literature.

Andrew Carlin (Ph.D. Stirling) is the H.W. Wilson Newman Fellow at the Department of Library and Information Studies, University College Dublin. His research interests include ethnography, ethnomethodology and research practices. His current project is on the local order of bibliographies.

Stephen C. K. Chan is Head of the new Department of Cultural Studies at Lingnan University, Hong Kong. He has also taught English and Cultural Studies at The Chinese University of Hong Kong, where he edited the bilingual *Hong Kong Cultural Studies Bulletin,* and was Director of the Hong Kong Cultural Studies Programme. He is founder of the book series *Hong Kong Cultural Studies* released by the Oxford University Press (China). He has published internationally on Hong Kong culture and literature; his books cover topics ranging from literary, filmic to cultural imagination. Currently he is interested in issues of cultural representation and urban sensibility, transnational flows and images in action cinema, and critical education through affective pedagogy and popular genres.

Michael Hayes started off his career in education by teaching juniors with learning difficulties. He went on to secondary school to teach drama and later became involved in teacher training. He joined the University of Central Lancashire where he is now teaching drama and linguistics. His first publications were on modern drama and popular fiction, more recently he has published in France, Germany and Italy on film from a semiotic/linguistic angle.

Stefan Herbrechter is Senior Lecturer in Cultural Analysis at Trinity and All Saints, College of the University of Leeds. He holds an MA in English and Romance Philologies from the University of Heidelberg (Germany), and a PhD from Cardiff University (Centre for Critical and Cultural Theory). He is the author of *Lawrence Durrell, Postmodernism and the Ethics of Alterity*. He has also published on a variety of issues in literature, cultural theory and cultural studies and is currently preparing volumes on *Post-Theory*, *Posthumanism*, *Strangers and Strangeness in Literature*, *Theory and Culture*, and *European Cultural Studies*.

David Katan is Associate Professor in Translation at the Scuola Superiore di Lingue Moderne per Interpreti e Traduttori (University of Trieste) where he teaches dialogue interpreting, specialised translation and intercultural communication. His research interests lie in the area of translation studies and cross-cultural communication in a variety of fields (business, journalism, literature and television). He is currently working on applying Neuro-Linguistic Programming techniques to his research on translation and cultural orientations. Recent publications include a book for St. Jerome (1999) *Translating Cultures: An Introduction for Translators, Interpreters and Mediators*; (2000) “Language Transfer: What Gets Distorted or Deleted in Translation”, Mostovi, xxxiv: 29-37;

and (2001) "'Look Who's Talking': the Ethics of Entertainment and Talk Show Interpreting", *The Translator*, 7: 2, 213-238.

Karima Laachir is currently finishing her PhD. entitled: "The Ethics and Politics of Hospitality in Contemporary French Society: 'Beurs' Translations" at the Centre for Cultural Studies, University of Leeds. Her research interests include post-colonial cultures, literatures and histories, ethnicity and race studies, and post-modern theory.

Karl Maton (St John's College, University of Cambridge) is currently writing up his doctoral thesis, which develops a dynamic epistemological sociology of knowledge through a case study of the conditions of emergence for cultural studies in post-war English higher education. He is also currently co-editing (with Handel K. Wright) a book on cultural studies as education in education.

Katrina Mandy Oakham is a senior lecturer in journalism at Deakin University in Victoria, Australia. She is the former vice president of the Journalism Education Association which represents educators in Australia, New Zealand, the South Pacific, Hong Kong and the United Kingdom. Katrina has worked as a journalist in both Australia and the United Kingdom and was an examiner for the National Council for the Training of Journalists in the United Kingdom. She is the editor of *Don't Bury the Lead: A Guide to Australian Newsgathering and Writing* (Deakin University Press 1996) and is currently completing her PhD on the socialisation of cadet journalists in Australia. Her current research centres around the development of journalism theory and she is a contributor to *Journalism: Theory in Practice* (OUP). Her other research interests include sociology of the journalism profession, gender and ethical issues. She will also be the co-author of *Reporting in the Digital Age* to be published by Allen and Unwin, Australia, in 2002.

Simon O'Sullivan is a Lecturer in Art History/Visual Culture at Goldsmiths College. His research interests include Art theory, Visual Culture, Aesthetics and Continental Philosophy. Has published articles in *Parallax* and *Angelaki*. He is currently working on a book on Deleuze and Guattari and Art History/Practice.

Malcolm Quinn lectures at Wimbledon School of Art and The Royal College of Art. His first book *The Swastika: Constructing the Symbol* (Routledge, 1994) was concerned with the construction of national identity and the colonisation of the visual field under Nazism. He has also written on the relationship of contemporary art, commerce and everyday life in *Parallax* and *Third Text*, *Blueprint* and in *The Independent*. He has contributed an article on cultural studies to *The Philistine Debate* (Verso), forthcoming in 2002.

Laurence Raw is Senior Lecturer in English in the Department of American Literature at Baskent University, Ankara. His publications include *Changing Class Attitudes* (1994), *The Country and the City* (1997), and five co-edited collections of essays. He is currently working on a book on contemporary Turkish cultural studies.

Holger Rossow is Assistant Professor of British Cultural Studies at the University of Rostock, Germany. His current research interests are New Labour and environmental policies, nationalism and regionalism, migration and multiculturalism, and transatlantic relations. Among his latest publications are "New Labour and Environmental Politics", in: Riedel, W., ed. (1998), *Narratives of Nature: Perspectives of Cultural Construction*, Essen, 111-129 and "Economic Considerations as the Secondary Formal Principle of Britain's Immigration Policy towards the 'New' Commonwealth, 1962-1973", in Borgmann, Ulrike, ed. (1999) *From Empire to Multicultural Society: Cultural and Institutional Changes in Britain*, Trier: Wissenschaftlicher Verlag Trier, 71-82.

Necdet Teymur is currently Visiting Professor at the University of Dundee, School of Architecture. He studied at METU, Bouwcentrum and Liverpool University, worked as an architect at Arne Jacobsen's office in Copenhagen, taught at British Universities (1978-94) and has been Professor of Architecture and Dean at METU, Ankara (1995-2001). His books include *Environmental Discourse* (1982), *Architectural Education* (1992), *Taboo Circle* (1995) and, as co-editor, *Re-Humanising Housing* (1988), *Culture : Space : History* (1990), *Architectural History and the Studio* (1996), *Basic Design / Basic Education* (1998).

Eduardo J. Vior studied History in Argentina, where he also worked as journalist. Since 1980 he has been living in Germany where he studied Politics at the University of Heidelberg. He received his PhD in Political Sciences in 1991 from the University of Giessen (the subject of his thesis was "Representation and National Identity in Brazil and Argentina"). He has taught Spanish Language, Translation and Special Communication at the Universities of Heidelberg, Worms, Heilbronn and Magdeburg. He has also coordinated and conducted training courses in "Intercultural Management". He researches and publishes on Latin American cultural identity, Latin America's "new frontiers", Globalisation, and US-hegemony.

Jen Webb is a senior lecturer in Creative Communication, and Programme Director, Professional Writing at the University of Canberra where she teaches creative writing and cultural studies. Her professional background includes art house and academic editing, and researching, publishing and teaching in the areas of communication and culture. She holds a doctorate in cultural theory, is currently a candidate for a doctor of creative arts (writing) and is an active member of a number of research and professional organisations, including the Australian Key Centre for Cultural and Media Policy, the Cultural Studies Association of Australia, the Australian Association of Writing Programs, and the ACT and Queensland Writers Centres. She is the academic editor of the literary journal *Redoubt*, the editor of *Re-Siting Theatre: approaches to regional theatre development* (1997) and the co-author of *Understanding Foucault* (2000), *Understanding Bourdieu* (2001), *Understanding Globalisation* (forthcoming, 2002), and *Reading the Visual* (forthcoming, 2003). She is also the author of a number of articles in journals such as *Diacritics* (USA), *Social Semiotics* (UK), *SPAN* (New Zealand) and *Journal of Australian Studies, Media International Australia* and *Southern Review* (Australia). She has also published short fictions and poems in literary journals such as *Imago: New Writing*, *LiNQ* and *Refractory Girl* (Australia), *SPAN* (New Zealand), *New England Review* (USA) and *The Amethyst Review* (Canada).

Russell West completed an MA at the University of Melbourne, Australia, going on to doctoral and postdoctoral research in Cambridge, Lille and Cologne. He currently teaches English Literature and Cultural Studies at the University of Lüneburg, Germany. Recent publications include *Conrad and Gide: Translation, Transference and Intertextuality* (1996), *Marginal Voices, Marginal Forms: Diaries in European Literature and History* (ed. with R. Langford; 1999), *Subverting Masculinity: Hegemonic and Alternative Versions of Masculinity in Contemporary Culture* (ed. with F. Lay; 2000), and *Spatial Representations on the Jacobean Stage: From Shakespeare to Webster* (2001).

Rem B. EDWARDS

What Caused the Big Bang?

Amsterdam/New York, NY 2001. XXII,411 pp.
(Value Inquiry Book Series 115)
ISBN: 90-420-1407-5 € 85,-/US-$ 85.-

This book critically explores answers to the big question, What produced our universe around fifteen billion years ago in a Big Bang? It critiques contemporary atheistic cosmologies, including Steady State, Oscillationism, Big Fizz, Big Divide, and Big Accident, that affirm the eternity and self-sufficiency of the universe without God. This study defends and revises Process Theology and arguments for God's existence from the universe's life-supporting order and contingent existence.

Rodopi

Editions Rodopi B.V.
USA/Canada: One Rockefeller Plaza, Ste. 1420, New York, NY 10020,
Tel. (212) 265-6360, *Call toll-free* (U.S.only) 1-800-225-3998,
Fax (212) 265-6402
All Other Countries: Tijnmuiden 7, 1046 AK Amsterdam, The Netherlands.
Tel. ++ 31 (0)20 6114821, Fax ++ 31 (0)20 4472979
Orders-queries@rodopi.nl
www.rodopi.nl

A GARLAND FOR GISSING

Edited by Bouwe Postmus

Amsterdam/New York, NY 2001.
(Costerus NS 138)
ISBN: 90-420-1477-6 € 60,-/US$ 60.-

The crown upon the continuing vitality and popularity of Gissing studies in the final decade of the twentieth century was the publication of *The Collected Letters of George Gissing* (1990-97). The editors of that mammoth undertaking, Paul Mattheisen, Arthur Young and Pierre Coustillas, had long been an inspiration to the younger generation of Gissing scholars, and their presence at the International George Gissing Conference at Amsterdam in September 1999 explained the success of the encounter between Gissing's older and younger critics.

Ever since the reappraisal of Gissing's works began to get under way in the early 1960s through the publication of many new editions of the works and ground-breaking critical studies by Arthur Young, Jacob Korg and Pierre Coustillas, it has become impossible to ignore the high status he now enjoys by rights, which resembles the position granted to him long ago by his contemporaries, as one of the leading English novelists of the late nineteenth century.

This collection of essays is remarkable for its emphasis on women's issues addressed in Gissing's novels, ranging from the inadequate education of women to the struggle for greater female independence, within and without marriage. Several contributors seek to define the precise nature and quality of Gissing's achievement and his place in the canon and, in the process, they open up fascinating, new opportunities for future research.

Editions Rodopi B.V.
USA/Canada: One Rockefeller Plaza, Ste. 1420, New York, NY 10020,
Tel. (212) 265-6360, *Call toll-free* (U.S.only) 1-800-225-3998,
Fax (212) 265-6402
All Other Countries: Tijnmuiden 7, 1046 AK Amsterdam, The Netherlands.
Tel. ++ 31 (0)20 6114821, Fax ++ 31 (0)20 4472979
Orders-queries@rodopi.nl www.rodopi.nl

PETER CONSENSTEIN

Literary Memory Consciousness, and the Group Oulipo

Amsterdam/New York, NY 2002. 252 pp.
(Faux Titre 220)
ISBN: 90-420-1438-5 EUR 45,-/US-$ 45.-

The question of memory intrigues us more and more as industrialized societies move further and further away from the written word. In the past the role of memory was integral to literary history, precise mnemonics served as the support systems for erudition, and Mnemosyne was mother of the Muses. The group Oulipo, born in reaction to the Surrealists, proposes, invents, and applies novel literary constraints. Using memory, and best of all conscious memory, as a theoretical starting point, the implications of writing under constraint are analyzed. First, writing under constraint is viewed as a new mnemonics; second, the spiritual component of such a practice is shown to redefine a notion of inspiration; third, constraints and their relationship with games and society is highlighted; finally the manner in which they build a literary consciousness is studied through the lenspiece of contemporary neurobiological research. For the first time the work of the group Oulipo, and the member's emphasis on the function of literature, is placed in historical, cultural, and philosophical context.

Editions Rodopi B.V.
USA/Canada: One Rockefeller Plaza, Ste. 1420, New York, NY 10020,
Tel. (212) 265-6360, *Call toll-free* (U.S.only) 1-800-225-3998,
Fax (212) 265-6402
All Other Countries: Tijnmuiden 7, 1046 AK Amsterdam, The Netherlands.
Tel. ++ 31 (0)20 6114821, Fax ++ 31 (0)20 4472979
orders-queries@rodopi.nl **www.rodopi.nl**

Literature and Musical Adaptation

Edited by Michael Meyer

Amsterdam/New York, NY 2002. VIII,191 pp.
(Rodopi Perspectives on Modern Literature 26)
ISBN : 90-420-0812-1 Bound EUR 70,-/US$ 70.-
ISBN: 90-420-0802-4 Paper EUR 30,-/US$ 30.-

It can safely be said that when literary texts are utilized or adapted by a musician to create a new work of art, it is seldom that a diminished or lessened product results. Rather, such a merging usually enlarges and enhances both text and tune, perhaps significantly changing the message of the original. Discovering exactly what the new form has to offer and how it relates to the text or melody that preceded it is often a daunting task, requiring a close examination of both the author's and the composer's intent.

The essays in this collection offer an analysis of several adaptations, some successful, some not so successful, and attempt to assess just what the musicians or writers have modified or changed from to the originals they re-form it into an altogether different media. Ranging from Pasternak's appropriation of Tchaikovsky to Britten's operatic versions of Billy Budd and the *Turn of the Screw,* from Celan's use of fugal technique in his "Todesfuge" to the way that the musicianship of several women writers found voice in their writing, a broad spectrum of collaborations is examined. As readers examine an author's respect for a long dead musician (Hopkins' admiration of Purcell) or as they discover how John Harbison worked to transform Fitzgerald's musicality in *The Great Gatsby,* it will be evident that musical adaptations often provide a richness that the originals did not possess and that the potential for greatness is heightened when the arts intersect.

Rodopi

Editions Rodopi B.V.
USA/Canada: One Rockefeller Plaza, Ste. 1420, New York, NY 10020,
Tel. (212) 265-6360, *Call toll-free* (U.S.only) 1-800-225-3998,
Fax (212) 265-6402
All Other Countries: Tijnmuiden 7, 1046 AK Amsterdam, The Netherlands.
Tel. ++ 31 (0)20 6114821, Fax ++ 31 (0)20 4472979
orders-queries@rodopi.nl **www.rodopi.nl**

FLIGHT FROM CERTAINTY
The Dilemma of Identity and Exile

Ed. by Anne Luyat and Francine Tolron

Amsterdam/New York, NY 2001. VIII,254 pp.
(Rodopi Perspectives on Modern Literature 23)
ISBN: 90-420-1595-0 Bound EUR 57,-/US-$ 57.-
ISBN: 90-420-1585-3 Paper EUR 23,-/US-$ 23.-

Editions Rodopi BV
USA/Canada: One Rockefeller Plaza, Ste. 1420, New York, NY 10020
Tel. (212) 265-6360, Call toll-free (U.S.only) 1-800-225-3998
Fax (212) 265-6402
All Other Countries: Tijnmuiden 7, 1046 AK Amsterdam, The Netherlands
Tel. ++31 (0)20 611 48 21, Fax ++31 (0) 20 447 29 79
Orders-queries@rodopi.nl **www.rodopi.nl**